THE GOOD BODY GUIDE

Dr Carole Hungerford became a general practitioner in 1975. After working for five years in London she has shared her time between her rural practice in Bathurst, New South Wales, and her inner-city practice in Sydney. She has helped educate young graduates for the Royal Australian College of General Practitioners, and she is also a fellow of the Australasian College of Nutritional and Environmental Medicine.

THE GOOD BODY GUIDE
A FAMILY DOCTOR'S UNCONVENTIONAL GUIDE TO HEALTHY LIVING

DR CAROLE HUNGERFORD

MARION BOYARS
LONDON · NEW YORK

Published in Great Britain and the United States in 2009 by
MARION BOYARS PUBLISHERS LTD
24 Lacy Road London SW15 1NL

www.marionboyars.co.uk

Printed in 2009
10 9 8 7 6 5 4 3 2 1

First published as *Good Health in the 21st Century* by Scribe Publications
Pty. Australia, 2006

A CIP catalogue record for this book is available from the British Library.
A CIP catalog record for this book is available from the Library of Congress.

ISBN 978-0-7145-3171-7

Set in Bembo 11/14pt

Printed in England by J.H. Haynes & Co. Ltd., Sparkford

CONTENTS

List of Diagrams

ACKNOWLEDGEMENTS

Many people have helped me in writing this book. The following list is not complete and I offer apologies to those who have been omitted. The opinions and mistakes are all my own.

My thanks go to: Dr Robert Buist, who started me on this path, Dr Bill Hensley, whose love of biochemistry infected many of his students, Drs Joachim Fluhrer, Chris Reading, Archie Kalokerinos, Iggy Soosay and Lindsay Wing, and Professors Ian Brighthope and Ray Kearney, who have taught me much of what I have learnt; Prof. Donald Sheldon, who always taught that 'received wisdom' should not be accepted uncritically; The Australasian College of Nutritional and Environmental Medicine, who have provided a world-class forum in which such doctors can teach other doctors; Drs David Allen, Trish Pearse, Ian Dettman, Ross Walker and John Fitzherbert, who have read and commented; Pauline Shelley, Deborah Corrigall, Pamela Dickinson, John Mattes and Mary Coupe, who have read as lay people and advised; Mike 'Pred' Carlton, who read the sections on Genetics, Immunology and Cancer, and whose stellar intellect was tragically extinguished at the age of just 33; and my patients, especially Di Boyle, Emily and Joy, who placed so much trust in me.

And finally to: Kate Grenville, who mentored this book from its inception, and so generously gave of the wisdom of her enormous writing skills to help make it readable — her friendship and moral support throughout the entire process made it possible; Dr Ron Brookes, who knows how he has helped; Janet Mackenzie, who is the best editor anyone writing this book could ever have hoped for; Scribe Publications, for giving a first-time author a hearing; Elinor McDonald, who rescued the graphics at the last moment; my family, Jocelyn, Guy, Zoe and Jude, for moral support, computer and research skills, and being the subject of their mother's dietary theories; and their dad, Keith, whose tireless enthusiasm, and technical and scientific skills made it all happen.

PREFACE

This book is written as a direct response to the questions my patients ask:

- 'Why is a good diet not enough?'
- 'Why are so many diseases — cancer, allergies, depression — on the rise?'
- 'Why do I need medication to stay healthy?'
- 'Why are there so many new diseases such as autism, SARS and AIDS?'

My patients want to know the science that underpins a medical model based on health. Naturopaths, dieticians, herbalists seem to have a good grasp of what it is to be healthy — does this natural medicine have scientific merit?

If you arrive at the doctor's surgery saying, 'I feel great and I'd like a few tips on how to stay that way,' you will probably be met with bemusement. Your doctor would be likely to have a better idea what to do with you if you turn up with a disease. Doctors find it challenging to cure disease, but they tend to forget about health. The simple restoration of health may require only that we give the 'good guys' — vitamins, minerals, essential fatty acids and others — a chance to do their health-giving work.

As a general practitioner I was often torn between received wisdom and a biochemical approach to my patients' problems. I sought professional training in 'alternative' fields, although it grates that the scientific basis of nutritional biochemistry is labelled 'alternative'. In grappling with my patients' questions, I had to challenge many of the things that I had been taught. As mainstream medicine becomes ever more dogmatic, its self-belief strengthened by the doctrine of evidence-based medicine, the voices of my patients begin to sound like the chorus in a Greek drama, sowing seeds of challenge and discontent.

Western nations are worrying about the problems of an ageing population. But current longevity predictions are based on a population born between World War I and World War II, for whom sugar, fat and motor vehicles were luxuries. By the time junk food came into being, their eating habits were well established. Pesticides did not permeate the food chain, and good husbandry prevailed in farming and horticulture. If we take into account the health trends in younger generations — the rising incidence of asthma, depression, obesity, and younger diagnoses of many cancers — we arrive at a frightening prediction: for the first time in human history, we have produced a generation which is not expected to outlive its parents.

Doctors throughout the developed world are beginning to question a health industry based on a model of 'curing disease'. The role of the pharmaceutical companies in this 'health' industry causes increased disquiet. This book is dedicated to my patients, to the doctors whom I have the privilege to teach, and other patients and doctors like them.

Chapter One
MEDICINE AND PROGRESS

*The doctors of today prescribe medicines of which they
know little, to cure disease of which they know less,
in human beings of whom they know almost nothing.*

VOLTAIRE: 1694–1778

*Progress is all very well, but it has gone on
long enough.*

OGDEN NASH: 1902–1971

THE WAITING ROOM

IT IS MONDAY MORNING in the waiting room of an imaginary general
practice on the outskirts of the inner city. The patients include
students from the nearby university, factory workers, shift workers,
business people. Many ethnic groups are represented. Let us suppose
that I work in this busy practice with four or five other doctors. We
all get on well together and often discuss difficult cases with each
other. All of us have areas of special interest in medicine, and we
have a wide range of outside interests. Mine is a hobby farm in a
bushland environment a few hours out of the city. These various
interests form the subject matter of many of our lunchtime
conversations.

In the waiting room on this busy morning are a group of typical
patients who could be in any city, any suburb. Some have cuts or

sprains from weekend sporting activities or need a routine check, but most have chronic health issues such as high blood pressure, depression, menstrual disorders, headaches.

My colleagues and I have recently been to courses on nutritional and 'alternative' medicine. We felt that it was time we learnt about the safety of the things our patients are taking. Lately they have been asking us about treatments such as St John's wort and glucosamine. One of us has a pregnant wife who is taking vitamin supplements. Does my colleague know that this is safe? She eats well, why would she need them? Is there any scientific evidence?

My first patient of the day is Mary, who is 28 years old. She has come to see me because of chronic, low-grade depression and a feeling of 'just not being well'. She has a job which she enjoys and good friends. A two-year relationship ended amicably a few months ago, and she currently does not have a partner. She says she wants her own space for a while. She eats reasonably well, although she admits to a sweet tooth and perhaps more coffee than she ought. She drinks a fair bit of tap water because she has heard that this will help to keep her bowels regular. She drinks alcohol within a safe range and is a non-smoker. She gets some exercise, although admits she hasn't had a lot of energy lately.

Her medical history includes mild asthma with seasonal exacerbations, for which she has a range of puffers. She uses at least one of these most days, but regards her asthma as fairly easy to control. Her bowels are usually okay, but if she's not careful she can become constipated. She is on the oral contraceptive pill although she has no current need for contraception. She has been on the pill on and off since she was 16 and says she is scared to come off it because she will have heavy cramping periods and her skin will break out. When she first went on the pill she was still at school and did not need contraception. The doctor she was seeing at the time said it would be the best thing for the cramps that were keeping her away from school one or two days a month, and it would also help her troublesome acne. At the time of commencement she had never had a migraine. She has had three or four migraines since, but the doctor thought that it was okay for her to take the low-dose pill.

Her blood pressure went up a bit on the pill, but as it is in the normal range she and I have agreed just to keep an eye on it. We plan to do this regularly, because I am also treating her mother for mild hypertension. Mostly the pill controls Mary's painful periods but sometimes she has to take an anti-inflammatory. She is totally dependent on these when she is giving the pill a 'rest'. At those times, she often has to take antibiotics for her skin as well. She gets mood swings around the time of her period, and thinks these are a bit better on the pill, although she suspects that her overall well-being is reduced. She has discussed with me her lack of interest in the things which used to give her pleasure. We have talked about an anti-depressant, but she is not keen to take that path yet.

There is probably a Mary in every doctor's waiting room every morning of the week, and few doctors would argue with the treatments she is on. After all, one in four Australians now has a lifetime expectancy of asthma, and although this is one of the highest rates in the world, other developed nations are not far behind; in the UK, 5.2 million people are receiving treatment for asthma and that figure is 20 million in America. And it's known that certain illnesses such as asthma, migraine, depression, dysmenorrhoea and irritable bowel cluster together—in individuals, in families and in cultural groups.

So it's *common* for these conditions to occur together, and we've also come to accept it as *normal*. But have we accepted Mary's symptoms too readily? When we see whole families of asthmatics and migraineurs we think of shared genes, but how can such conditions be shared by whole cultures?

If we look at Mary, and the thousands like her, from the perspective of a hundred years ago, or of a rural dweller from the rapidly vanishing tribal peoples of the world, her diagnoses and treatments are nothing short of astonishing. Here she is, still in her twenties, a healthy individual, and yet she has been, or is, taking:

- a beta adrenergic bronchodilator
- oral or inhaled corticosteroids
- synthetic oestrogen and progesterone
- long-term antibiotics
- a non-steroidal anti-inflammatory pain killer
- a specific anti-prostaglandins medication.

As if this is not enough, an antidepressant could soon be added if things don't look up. Most of her medications require a prescription, or at least dispensation by a trained pharmacist, in Western countries. A look at the associated list of side effects, precautions, drug interactions and warnings of use in pregnancy soon explains why. These medications are not to be taken lightly.

If we look at the various treatments Mary has had, there is no underlying pharmacological consistency. Each has targeted a specific problem. The bronchodilator she takes for her asthma is unlikely to do much for her mood swings or her tendency to constipation. If these conditions tend to cluster, it seems intuitive to expect that a treatment for one might have a favourable effect on the others — assuming that the relationship between the conditions is at least partly causal, which commonsense seems to dictate.

But Mary's medications lack logical connection with each other. Some are potentially incompatible. This incompatibility may be pharmacological — that is, the drugs themselves interact in a negative way — or it may be to do with the symptoms. The action of the steroid medication could well worsen the depression. If Mary is among the 20 per cent of asthmatics who are sensitive to aspirin, the medications she takes for her period pain may make her asthma worse. If she were a severe asthmatic this would rapidly become apparent, but as she is usually well controlled the overall deterioration over time may not be connected to her intermittent use of aspirin-like painkillers.

Even a few decades ago, patients like Mary would have had a much narrower range of medications at their disposal. There might have been something for her asthma, and some aspirin or paracetamol for her pain. Under the age of 40 or 50, only an unusually sick patient would have been taking more than a couple of prescription medications on a regular basis.

What is so bad in the human design that one in four now needs drugs in order to breathe normally? What is so maladaptive about a menstrual cycle that it regularly puts a significant number of women to bed once a month? Mary has not got asthma because she has a Ventolin deficiency, and menstrual cramps are not caused by Ponstan deficiency. Why does she — like thousands of others — have such a constellation of medical problems, and such a galaxy of pharmaceutical solutions to them?

These are the questions that we are beginning to debate in our lunchroom at work. To begin to answer them, we have to start a long way back, at the moment when some humans decided that hunting and gathering was too hard.

AGRICULTURE: THE UNFINISHED EXPERIMENT

Beginnings of Agriculture

At some time in a distant past our hunter-gatherer ancestors came to the conclusion, or had it forced upon them, that life would be easier if they were not continually on the move. Food grew from seed; animals grazed on plants. Maybe people would have more control over their lives if they planted those seeds and domesticated those animals.

It was long accepted that agriculture began around 10,000 years ago in the Middle East. Nowadays we believe that it originated in several places, and much earlier than previously thought.[1] The reasons for the adoption of agriculture varied. For example, in North America the end of the last ice age saw the extinction of many of the large game animals, forcing hunter-gatherers to turn to cultivated plants.

But the transition from a hunter-gatherer society to one based predominantly on agriculture brought with it not only profound social change but also unprecedented biological challenges.

Seeds of change

It is easy for us to conjure up a scene of a pastoral idyll, where contented farmers plough their fields with yoked animals. Compared with the stress and pollution of the cities of the modern world, those fields indeed appear as a picture of Elysian bliss. But along with the seeds of those early crops, the seeds of the diseases of civilisation were being planted. Even in those early days, the skeletal remains of Stone Age farmers showed more signs of tooth decay, infectious disease and malnutrition than their hunter-gatherer forebears.[2] The suggestion is that wheat and barley were grown as much for the production of beer and luxury items as for a staple.

Over time, however, these crops came to provide staples, in addition to whatever their original use had been. And with settlement came the motivation to construct more permanent and secure shelter. We began to lose some of our adaptation to cold and to food deprivation. Being settled in one place provided both the opportunity and the motive to construct food storage vessels. We were no longer confined to a rotational diet, no longer had to eat seasonally.

Food storage also provided protection against hunger. Chapter 8 discusses the concept of the 'thrifty gene'. This gene, or genes, enabled people to slow down their metabolism and thus reduce their energy usage in times of starvation. Some people have thrifty genes; some do not. Those who have them fare well in times of famine. Civilisation allowed those without thrifty genes to survive, which was an appropriate evolutionary step. The disadvantage for those retaining the genes was that they found themselves in a world where starvation was rarely a problem. In the face of dietary excess, they became prone to obesity and diabetes.

Over time, changes occurred in the crops that humans grew and the animals they tended. These changes reflected changing social needs, such as ease of handling animals or the timing of the harvest, but sometimes they worked against human biochemical needs.

Evolutionary science indicates that biological systems evolve in parallel. But this takes time and, in the meantime, evolution is a ruthless game of trial and error. Not all change is beneficial. Moreover, evolution never counted on our ability to thwart it. The domestication of animals provides an example of this. Like us, wild animals depend on essential fatty acids (EFAs), such as omega-3 fatty acids, for protection against cold, defence against inflammatory disorders, and many other aspects of health. By and large, omega-3s are derived from plants—animals have limited, if any, ability to manufacture them from dietary precursors. We must eat the plants which contain them, or eat animals which have eaten those plants. One of the richest sources, especially of omega-3 fatty acids, is algae. Another source is seeds that need to withstand extremes of weather, particularly cold spells.

As humans bred animals for their thick hides and wools, their docility and their tolerance of enclosure, and as they turned wild mountain sheep and buffalo into placid merinos and tranquil cows, and wild turkeys and ducks into the modern flightless equivalent, they also reduced their reliance on omega-3s. We kept these animals warm in barns and completely changed their diet. We fed them the crops we grew, which in turn reflected needs other than nutritional. Yield, ease of harvest—such factors took precedence over a chemistry which we did not yet understand.

Thus we produced animals more tolerant of a lowered level of EFAs in their tissues. Wild animals with thick coats can endure the cold, and domesticated animals are provided with shelter. As a result, there was a lower level of EFAs in our food supply — to which, we now know, we are far from adapted. Domesticated animals will incorporate EFAs into their tissues if they are in their diet. Any resistance to deprivation has not erased the need for these essential nutrients.

Free-ranging animals have access to ground plants and seeds. A free-ranging domestic hen ignores her 'layer pellets' and works hard to extract some tiny seeds from a plant we regard as a weed. Perhaps, in our ignorance, we would even prefer to poison the plant. No wonder fish remain one of the best sources of EFAs — all that algae, all that choice. Wild animals in zoos often fare badly, perhaps because they suffer the problems of EFA deficiency. The fleet of foot, the wild and unsheltered, the animal surviving on its wits, the animal which has to endure extremes of temperature — these typically have flesh which is high in omega-3 fatty acids.

When it comes to plants, the story of dietary change is even more interesting. While early humans continued to trap wild animals and fish to conserve their precious herds and flocks, the cultivation of plants created the potential to narrow the dietary intake to a relatively few species — corn, wheat, barley, rice, and some vegetables and herbs. When these were supplemented with game, milk and eggs, our forebears were well fed. But humans had opened the door to the development of monocultures. No longer did we eat whatever we could find, going further afield when that proved inadequate.

Although agriculture opened up possibilities for an increase in variety, one look at the predominance of staples such as wheat and dairy in today's world shows us that the ultimate trend was actually in the direction of narrowed choice. The medical consequences of this will be discussed throughout this book.

Some anthropologists feel that humans have always to some extent been farmers, but Stephen H. Leckson of the University of Colorado is less compromising. He writes:

> Farming is an unfinished experiment. ... Two million years
> ago our genus first appeared; we've been farming for less than
> 12,000 years. Fully modern humans have been farmers for
> less than one-third of Homo sapiens' chequered past on this
> planet. It's too soon to tell if this farming thing will work
> out: It's not natural.[3]

Agribusiness

Whether we began to live with agriculture 10,000 or 20,000 years ago, there have been two distinct, if overlapping phases. The first was gradual; the second has taken place in the last century or so. In this second phase, the rate of change has paralleled the explosion in industrial, technological, scientific and medical knowledge. If the transition to agriculture posed challenges to human biology, it is a mere hiccup in comparison to the transition from agriculture to agribusiness. Indeed, this second phase is arguably responsible for what are loosely termed 'the diseases of modern civilisation'.

We are not restricted to ancient records to understand how our forebears ate, lived and died. Anthropologists and archaeologists provide all the evidence we need. There are surviving cultures still primarily hunter-gatherer, or who practise a form of agriculture more like that of the last 10,000 years than the last 100. We look more closely at the diets of some of these people in Chapter 10.

When we look at the early hunter-gatherers, or their modern equivalents, one of the things which stands out is the variety of foods they could access. This is in part a consequence of the abundance of plant and animal species in the natural world, and in part a matter of necessity. When you are really hungry, you eat what you can get—a concept alien to the average urban dweller.

Doctors who suggest excluding wheat and dairy products from the diet commonly get the response 'But what is there left to eat?' What indeed, if breakfast is a bagel and a café latte, lunch a cheese and tomato sandwich, and dinner pasta with cheese and tomato sauce or a pizza? Between them, meat, milk, wheat, potato and tomato, provide the bulk of the nutritionally significant part of the Western diet. Young people at the supermarket checkout may ask their customers the names of certain fruits or vegetables. Unusual items such as okra, starfruit or taro we might understand, but I have been asked to name parsnip, brussels sprouts, and—twice in one week at different shops—beetroot.

In Britain consumption of leafy greens has halved during the past 50 years, and less than one in 10 children could name a cauliflower when shown one. In 1995 an Australian survey of 3000 young people aged 2–18 showed that one-quarter ate no fruit and one-fifth ate no vegetables on the day of the survey. If fruit juice was excluded, 40 per cent had eaten no fruit. Potato was the most commonly eaten vegetable, and much of that was eaten as fried chips. Less than 20 per cent of surveyed children had eaten any cruciferous vegetables (mustard, radish and the cabbage family) in the last 24 hours, and only one-third had eaten any carotenoid vegetables, such as carrot or leafy greens. In the USA, a survey spanning two decades and surveying almost 25,000 adults found that only 11% of adults reached the minimum recommendations for both fruit and vegetable intake. The researchers also noted that 65% of the people surveyed said they don't eat any fruits and 25% said they don't eat any vegetables on a typical day.

Freshness, seasonality and diversity

The hunter-gatherers' diet was not only diverse; it was composed of food that was fresh and in season. How long have our fruits and vegetables been in cold storage?

Seasonality was a feature of old-style agriculture, but not of the modern diet. It has two interesting implications. First, we were effectively on a permanent rotation diet, sometimes called the Stone Age diet. The idea is that the constant consumption of any particular food group presents a challenge to the immune system, and this can be the basis for the development of food allergies. Health practitioners sometimes treat medical conditions such as migraine and irritable bowel syndrome by limiting the frequency with which any one food is consumed (Chapter 8).

Second, there is the fascinating theory that defence mechanisms which a plant developed to adapt itself to the local climate and environment could possibly confer similar benefits on people and animals sharing that environment.

Variety is one of the areas most worthy of future research. The food family lists in Appendix 2 may come as a surprise. *The New Oxford Book of Food Plants* (see Further Reading) is also cause for wonder, not only for the abundance of natural produce but also for the amount which the modern diet omits.[4] And yet both of these sources merely scratch the surface. The bush foods of Australian Aboriginals show what else there is in the natural world.[5] Tribal Aboriginals consumed many hundreds of kinds of plants — roots, seeds, legumes, fruits, sea vegetables, fungi, crustaceans, insects and animals (Chapter 10). (In a theme central to this book, the idea of food as medicine blurs with food as nourishment in Aboriginal culture.) Add to this the fruits and vegetables of the Amazon, the African jungles, the herbs and berries of Asia and New Guinea.

Compare this bounty to the total number of plant or animal species that you have consumed in the last week, the last year. And even if you do occasionally eat the more unusual vegetables, such as beetroot or rhubarb, how often do you do so?

As we move away from the old idea of the five or seven basic food groups to a more sophisticated understanding of human biochemistry and its necessary nutritional inputs, we start to see extraordinary complexity. Terms such as 'phytochemicals', 'leucopenes', 'essential fatty acids' and 'ultra-trace elements' are coming into everyday language. Many of these substances are required in small, or even tiny, amounts. Although they may not be essential for survival, they may be essential for optimal health. The distinction between survival and optimal health is only gradually gaining acceptance in the medical world.

Folk wisdom in Japan says that one should eat 30 different food types every day. Counting herbs, spices, oils, nuts and seeds, it is estimated that the typical Italian diet contains approximately 60 different food groups. The comparable estimate for the typical Western diet is just 20 food groups. So it may not be the high olive oil content and low levels of saturated fats in the Mediterranean diet which confer the well-known benefits: it may be the variety as well. This would certainly help explain the French anomaly, where the consumption of butter, cream and cheese is legendary, but where freshness and variety of herbs and vegetables are also paramount. (There are also other reasons why the French may fare better than their British and German counterparts; see Chapters 8 and 10.)

In a delightful essay British science writer Colin Tudge elaborates this theme, suggesting that modern, agricultural human beings, are 'pharmacologically impoverished'.[6] This essay significantly altered my own thinking. Until then I had assumed that some nutrients were important for the maintenance of optimal health, and others were essential for life itself. Inevitably things would sometimes go wrong, and at that point one would look to a pharmaceutical, either a modern drug or a herbal remedy, to fix things. Tudge takes this thinking one step further. These natural 'medicines' were perhaps an *integral part* of an original diet, taken regularly to prevent disease. This theme is developed in Chapter 10.

Agribusiness takes over

We have looked at what might prevail in an ideal hunter-gatherer world or an agrarian society before industrial farming methods were introduced. Western agriculture today has undergone a shift of exponential proportions. Changes have happened so rapidly that there has barely been time to consider the biological effects on the environment, let alone the more subtle biochemical impact on humans and animals, or on the birds, insects, earthworms, plants, fungi and soil micro-organisms on which depends the entire food chain.

The social changes that have accompanied the shift from an agrarian society to an industrial one are obvious; dietary changes deserve equal attention. The new technologies made it possible to preserve or refrigerate food, thus allowing it to be kept much longer, and changes in transport allow food to be moved over vast distances in a relatively short time. It is no longer possible to tell what season it is simply by looking at the fruits and vegetables on display in the local supermarket, as was true just a few years ago.

Now people can eat their favourite food all year round; indeed, they often do. This increases the likelihood of developing a sensitivity to that food, while similarly restricting the range of foods they do eat. You don't like the brassicas—cabbage, broccoli, brussels sprouts, traditional winter vegetables? No matter, eat baby spring peas all year round. Easy to prepare, no shelling required, straight from their frozen plastic pack. Your children get the message. They've never eaten a brussels sprout, and in their Saturday job at the supermarket they will ask the customer the name of this strange vegetable. The supermarket manager gets the message: hardly anyone buys this item, so it always looks stale and unattractive, spoiling the display. The farmer gets the message and plants more peas and less cabbage. So it goes.

In an affluent society, we no longer eat what is available: what is available is what we will eat. This in itself would not necessarily be a bad thing were the choices not so frequently based on convenience. The most commonly given reason for not eating fish or cabbage is not dislike, as one might imagine, but the messiness of preparation and the persisting smells in today's enclosed kitchens

If the changes taking place in the supermarket and the kitchen are profound (and that's without weighing into the debate about freezers and microwaves), what is going on out in the paddocks? In those Elysian fields, we toiled by the sweat of our brow (no Syndrome X there). We fertilised fields with the manure of our animals (not to mention our own); we relied on the birds for pest control, the worms for soil aeration, the trees for topsoil.

Biodiversity

Australia is a country which is already 90 per cent desert. To our knowledge, this has not been largely the result of human activity, but of climatic and geographical events over very long periods of time. However, since European occupation two centuries ago, trees have been felled at such a rate that tree coverage is a mere 10 per cent of what it was at the time of Captain Cook's arrival.

In England and much of Europe the reduction in woodland in the last century or so has been of similar proportions. This has had devastating consequences for both the environment and human health. Biodiversity experts have estimated that individuals, communities and whole ecosystems are becoming extinct at a rate as great as 10,000 times the 'normal' level. (One has to acknowledge that there have been other rapid changes brought about by ice ages and asteroids, but these were out of human control.)

> As a general rule, for a plant species that becomes extinct we can expect 15 animal species to follow. The toll for Australia's plant species amounts to 76 extinctions and more than 300 currently endangered species (not including algae, moss lichens and liverworts, the status of which is unknown). This means that there are probably more than 1000 species of extinct animals, most of which are likely to be invertebrates, and more than 4000 threatened animal species. ... The flow-on effects of this are clearly devastating. Globally, half the known extinctions of the last 2000 years have occurred during this century. Whereas for the past 250 million years approximately one species became extinct per year, we are losing about fifty species every day.[7]

The implications of the loss of biodiversity are manifold. We lose plant species before we have even begun to tap their pharmaceutical potential. The world's frogs begin to disappear, and we don't know why. Who is to say that we are not next? The outlook for human survival is only as good as the quality of human sperm.

The web of life

As we continue to deforest in order to make way for the combine harvester, we might look at other health consequences.

If Dog is our best friend in the animal world, then Tree is our best friend in the plant world. It provides us with shade and shelter, timber for boats and fence posts, aesthetic and other purposes. It is a carbon sink and a vital link in the food chain. It supplies shelter for farm animals and for the birds which eat pests. In a Queensland pilot program, the use of rodent poison on sugar cane dropped steeply when reafforestation brought the owls back.

Trees hold the topsoil together, preventing its loss to wind and weather, and they renew that topsoil. Minerals which are taken up from the soil by plants and are then sold off-farm are lost to the farmer forever. If they end up in the city sewage, they are lost to the food chain as well, because their destination is often the ocean. The tree puts down roots deep through the clay, breaking up rocks and releasing minerals into the soil. These minerals nourish other plants and are also taken up by the tree itself. Here they nourish the leaves which later fall from the trees and are decomposed by the micro-organisms sustained in and around the tree roots. In this manner, depleted soils have opportunity to renew themselves. Even in climates and lands as barren as Australia, when topsoils become devoid of minerals, there often remains an untapped supply in the rocks and soils below.

If tree felling on individual farms is a worry, the clear-felling of rainforests to establish cattle and Western agriculture is a global tragedy. As global warming increases, tropical diseases spread. Malaria is now increasingly identified in northern Australia, a phenomenon rare in modern times. Worldwide, epidemics of unknown bugs are expected to emerge, as if nature were exacting a terrible revenge.

In summary, the equation does not consist of humans, a tree, a rock and a sheaf of wheat: every protozoan, fungus, nematode and pollinating insect must be taken into account in this delicate web of life. We have come to regard some of these creatures as pests, but over millennia nature struck a balance that we interfere with at our peril. Farmers realise that when you poison a slug the birds that feed on slugs die, either through starvation or poisoning; so you need to use more poison, which means more expense, and more birds die and then the bugs become resistant to that poison, and so it goes on, with the poison manufacturer earning more than the farmer.

And what of these poisons? Despite massive cover-ups, political and medical indifference, hostility and denial, the evidence continues to mount against agricultural chemicals. They are implicated in the causation of an amazing range of diseases — autism, infertility, cancer, Parkinson's disease.

In animal breeding when you select for one trait, such as beauty, you may lose another, such as vitality. The loss of nutritional value for the incorporation of poison resistance could well be a metaphor for 21st-century agriculture.

Soil health

The relationship of humans to soil can be summarised in one word: minerals. A plant cannot make minerals. For a mineral to be in the food chain, it has to have been in the soil in the first place. This is in distinct contrast to a vitamin, which is an elaborate structure, but is made of a few simple elements. Given a bit of water, a plant can make a vitamin literally out of thin air, using just the hydrogen, oxygen, carbon and nitrogen that surround it. We make use of this phenomenon when we put a few mustard or cress seeds in some water, and eat their vitamin-rich sprouts a few days later.

In the case of minerals — calcium, magnesium, iron, zinc, selenium, iodine, manganese, copper, boron — if it's not in the soil there will be none in the plant. Many factors determine the soil levels of minerals — the underlying geology, how much weathering of rocks has taken place, how many trees remain, how many generations of farming have occurred, whether that farming has been sustainable or not. Geographical location is a crucial determinant, and can vary over short distances. The concept of 'microclimates' within a few acres has recently become of interest both in agriculture and ecology. A further extension of this is the variation of soils and the micro-organisms which inhabit them, again within very short distances. Basalt soils from weathered volcanic rocks are most prized by farmers.

Soil health and human health

Dust to dust …

Slowly, we are beginning to realise that current farming practices give rise to acid soils, salination, and ultimately, desertification. Nowhere on earth is this more apparent than in Australia, where modern technology and wealth clash with ancient and fragile ecosystems. And nowhere on earth, I shall argue, can we better learn about serious health problems such as asthma, depression, and even cot death. Australia (along with New Zealand) is in the unenviable position of having the world's highest incidence of these conditions.

How does this happen?

We know that many of the nutrients needed for human health are needed also by plants. These include calcium, nitrogen, phosphorus and potassium. Nitrogen is essential for growth, yield and quality of the plant, and is an essential constituent of the plant's protein and chlorophyll. Phosphorous is needed for root development, cell division and growth, and potassium for the transport of sugars and other carbohydrates within the plant. Overworked soils lack some of these elements, and so farmers apply fertiliser. Superphosphate provides phosphate and calcium, while NPK provides nitrogen, phosphorous, and potassium. Calcium in plants has several roles, including a structural one analogous to the human skeleton.

Magnesium, too, is important. Among the roles of magnesium, the most fascinating is the formation of chlorophyll. This compound is almost identical to the 'heme' part of human haemoglobin, except that it has an atom of magnesium at its centre rather than an atom of iron. Anaemia in humans, which makes us look pale and sickly, is often due to iron deficiency. 'Plant anaemia' is caused by lack of magnesium, and like human anaemia it can go neglected, often for a long time. With inadequate magnesium, plants cannot properly form chlorophyll and suffer from 'yellow leaf', a particular problem in citrus plants.

The need for the major nutrients, with the exception of magnesium, is usually met. But elements which are present in trace amounts in the soil are required in trace amounts in both the plant and animal world. The quote above indicates that our bodies reflect the composition of the soils which sustain them. Life may still be possible despite sub-optimal quantities of those trace elements. But the metabolic, enzymatic, gene transcription (how our genes are read) and immune systems supported by those nutrients will not function at their best. And here a difference between the plant and animal world emerges, important in degree though not in kind.

We may share more than 40 per cent of our genetic material with a nematode (worm) — or worse still, a banana — but animal biology is generally more complex than that of plants, and mammalian biology is more complex than that of insects. So soil which sustains a plant may not provide all that is needed by the animal which grazes on that plant. The increased system complexity of the animal may require more nutrients.

Acid soils

If nutrient deficiency is only a matter of depleted soils, perhaps the problem will be solved by fertilisers which contain the missing trace elements. But there are other problems with synthetic fertilisers. Recurrent applications tend to increase the acidity of the soil, reducing its fertility. This problem is widespread throughout the modern agricultural world.

Many minerals, such as magnesium, molybdenum and selenium, can only be taken up by a plant when the soil is neutral — neither alkaline nor acidic. Even when soil analysis reveals adequate minerals, they may as well not be there if the soil is so acid that they are unavailable to plants.

Farmers often apply lime to counteract acidity; but this, too, is fraught. Many lime products contain calcium, which in a calcium-deplete soil may be advantageous. But the chemistry of calcium, one of the most abundant elements in the earth's crust, is similar to that of magnesium. As calcium and magnesium compete with each other at a cellular level, an over-application of calcium can worsen magnesium depletion. High calcium can also reduce selenium absorption (see below, Putting the Evidence to the Test). Magnesium and selenium depletion may play crucial roles in the modern epidemics of asthma, osteoporosis, depression and obstetric intervention (Chapters 4, 7 and 9). Even if the correct ratio of calcium to magnesium is preserved, over-liming brings with it a risk of deficiencies of boron, manganese, zinc and iron, and their associated health problems.

Selenium, too, is an important case in point. In human health this mineral has long been poorly understood and consequently neglected. Some recent American trials have prompted a medical rethink of selenium in relation to asthma, certain cancers, depression and infertility (Chapter 4). Oddly, although selenium-dependent enzymes have been described in primitive life forms such as micro-organisms and phytoplankton, selenium currently is thought to have no known role in plant physiology. Certain plants such as seaweed, garlic, onions and other members of the allium family concentrate it selectively, but the land plants survive, indeed thrive, in a selenium-deplete environment. Moreover, there appears to be no mechanism for active transport of selenium into the plant. It is concentrated by a passive mechanism which, critically, does not operate at all in acid soil conditions.

Similarly, cobalt is essential in Vitamin B12 metabolism, and a deficiency can lead to pernicious anaemia, especially in vegetarians, and yet vegetables can grow well in the absence of cobalt.

To spell out the obvious, a healthy plant from an unhealthy soil may fail to meet the nutritional needs for humans in critical ways. From the farmer's perspective, if the soil is so acid or salty that commercial crops cannot be grown, corrective action is a necessity. (Salination is not discussed here, but it is just as critical as acidity.) Under commercial pressures, applications of minerals that the plant does not need are not a priority. By contrast, if animals grazing on such pastures develop deficiency diseases, there is a strong motive for change. Now, though, they are slaughtered so young that they may not live long enough to develop some of the diseases of deficiency. Mature animals, which are the breeders, may get extra nutrition, but it is not the breeding animals which appear on your dinner table.

The matter of taste

If we are going to want to eat a varied, nutritious diet, it has to taste good. The arguments which follow regarding the taste of mature fruits apply equally to the lost culture of eating mature animals. Most people over the age of 50 remember the flavour of mutton, and of tomatoes, apples and other fruits and vegetables of their childhood. Is this just nostalgia, or did they really taste better?

Green harvesting and salicylates
It is during that last phase of ripening that most of the vitamins, minerals and natural sugars are concentrated into fruits and

vegetables. Seed dispersal depends on attractive and tasty fruits and nuts. Mother Nature does not want the seed eaten in the early stages of development, because this will not help the species survive. So she fills the fruit with salicylates, making it bitter and unappetising. As the fruit matures, these bitter compounds are replaced with the sugars and nutrients which make the fruit attractive to the creatures that will spread the seeds.

Those vitamins, minerals and natural sugars (and numerous other important compounds discussed in Chapter 10) give home-grown food its characteristic appeal. As youngsters my children showed disappointingly little interest in many of the fruits and vegetables we offered to them. It was not until a visit to their grandfather's orchard, where they encountered mature fruit, that I began to understand why. Grandfather was an old-fashioned farmer who lamented his buyers' demand for small, unripe fruit. Hard green specimens survive transport, packaging and handling over distances and time periods which would turn mature fruit into mush. High in salicylates and low in nutrients, unripe fruit lacks flavour. No wonder kids don't find fruit delicious, and 'salicylate sensitivity' is so frequently diagnosed.

Home-grown versus commercial products

Sceptics ask whether there is any hard evidence that today's commercial produce is inferior to the organic or home-grown item. Various surveys produce claim and counterclaim, but the trend favours home-grown and organically grown food. In a 2000 British study, David Thomas scanned past editions of the respected authority *The Composition of Foods*, by McCance and Widdowson, and found some alarming trends.[8] The overall decline of calcium in all fruit and vegetables was 46 per cent, of copper 75 per cent. Carrots had lost 75 per cent of their magnesium, broccoli 75 per cent of its calcium. An Australian study conducted by the Organic Retailers and Growers Association of Australia was also compelling. It examined beans, tomatoes, capsicums and silver beet for levels of calcium, potassium, magnesium, sodium, iron and zinc.[9] Nutrient ranges in the organic products were commonly ten or more times higher than in commercial specimens. Perhaps the discrepancies between the two countries reflects the fact that the ancient Australian soils were in a more parlous state to begin with and are now flogged to adapt to an agriculture to which they are not suited. In either case, the figures are deeply disturbing.

Other research confirms these findings. In Britain, rats fed organic fruit and vegetables 'were slimmer, slept better and had stronger immune systems than those given conventionally grown produce. Japanese researchers reported that organic milk had higher levels of vitamin E, omega-3 essential fatty acids and antioxidants.'[10]

GM foods

The topic of genetic engineering, like that of soil chemistry, is complex. Many nutritional scientists and doctors have deep reservations—not only about the supposed advantages and who will benefit from them, but also about what will happen to thousands of years of slow evolution in the delicate interdependent web of life.

Assurances that we have been genetically modifying food since the agricultural revolution bring little comfort. The story of gluten and casein makes this point vividly (Chapters 2, 9 and 10). A new breed of brussels sprouts has been developed to lose the characteristic taste and smell of the brassica family; this is achieved by drastically reducing the plant chemicals that are thought to protect against a wide range of common cancers. One wonders whether hungry British children during the food shortages following World War II found the smell of brussels sprouts as offensive as do their modern counterparts. But more, one is left breathless by the audacity of humans who blithely ignore the possible consequences of 'improvements' to millennia of gradual adaptive evolution.

Genetic modification takes these concerns into a new realm altogether. Selective breeding is not the same as putting fish genes into corn. An audience of farmers in Sydney heard a startling story from a visiting American, Professor Elaine Ingham of Oregon State University, in 1999.[11] It appeared that the US Food and Drug Administration had been within an ace of approving for release a genetically modified soil bacterium, developed to convert crop residues into useful products, including alcohol. At the eleventh hour, it was found that the alcohol would leach into the soil, poisoning it. Ingham's conclusion was that, had this been released into the environment, the potential for soil organisms to exchange genetic information is such that it could have resulted in a widespread agricultural disaster.

WHAT CAN DOCTORS LEARN FROM VETS?

When I was in medical school, it was a standing joke that veterinary science was much easier than medicine because you could shoot your mistakes. Later, when farming brought me into contact with some rural vets, I wondered what it would be like to deal with owners whose livelihood depended on the health of their animals. Animals have kidneys, livers, hearts, like humans. What would you do if half of your cows needed blood pressure tablets and cholesterol-lowering agents? Would you mix them in the feed or put them in the drinking water?

It is not usually apparent that the health of the soil has a direct impact on the health of the humans and pets that are sustained by plants grown in it. On the farm this relationship is inescapable.

The importance of diet

Doctors who sit in with vets will notice one big difference between human medicine and veterinary medicine. Whether it is a sick household pet or an ailing stud bull, one of the first questions is always 'What are you feeding this animal?' Although a 'good diet' was discussed in medical school, we were never taught that this line of enquiry might help us when a child came in with his fourth middle-ear infection for the winter, or recurrent abdominal pain, or chronic constipation.

Would we confess to the vet that Rover had had Coco Pops for breakfast or routinely finished lunch with an iced donut? Zoos are bedecked with signs saying: 'Do not feed the animals'. The zoo vet fears that we will give the animals the same junk food that our kids are eating on their day out.

The importance of field work

Vets have a significant advantage over doctors as a result of the requirements of the pastoral industry. Far from shooting their mistakes, vets are expected to stand between the farmer and bankruptcy. Where farming provides a significant part of the economy, there might even be government interest in keeping farm animals healthy.

The outcome of this financial interest provides further contrast between human and animal medicine. Comprehensive data exists on animals' nutritional requirements, and farmers aim to meet those requirements from the resources of the farm. Textbooks of veterinary medicine and agricultural science stand in silent admonition to the texts on human medicine.

Most telling is the issue of recommended daily allowance (RDI; Appendix 1). The farmer whose livelihood depends on the meat, milk or wool of an animal knows that this is crucial. If the pasture does not supply enough selenium for the reproductive needs of the animal, it must be supplemented. Farmers cannot afford to dismiss such needs with 'you can get all the vitamins and minerals you need from a healthy diet'. Despite the shortfalls of fertilisers, this topic is at least up for discussion and the health consequences of nutritional depletion are not trivialised.

Contrast this to the human situation. During the last part of the 20th century, Australia and Britain had no human RDI values for most minerals other than iron and calcium. The vet was taught how much selenium his patients needed to stay healthy, but the doctor was not. In 2006, in both Australia and Britain, the values applicable to humans are still not taught in medical school, and are not known by the average doctor.

Putting the evidence to the test

With a limited number of genetic and environmental variables, the vet is much better placed than the doctor to understand what is making patients sick. On the farm controlled experiments are taking place all the time, even if this is not the conscious intention.

The farmer's herds or flocks are of closely related animals; they may all have the same father, because farmers usually aim at conformity for desirable characteristics. So if a farmer decides to topdress one paddock with magnesium or add selenium and Vitamin E to the drench, and the stock yield goes up 50 per cent, this provides valuable data. If word of improved yield gets around, the neighbours might decide to topdress or drench in a similar manner. If their stock yield goes up as well, the database grows. If the neighbours have similar breeds, similar soils and similar clinical problems, before long the vet starts to see the point of all that nutritional stuff she learned for her final exams.

If the particular treatment benefits only cows but not sheep, the vet has learnt something about cows. If it benefits the sheep, the alpacas and the farm dog as well, it may demonstrate something about placental mammals.

Do humans also benefit from this knowledge? Let us compare some entries in the leading standard texts for doctors and vets respectively. The textbook *Harrison's Principles of Internal Medicine* is the most comprehensive English-language medical textbook; *Diseases of Livestock* by Thomas Hungerford (a distant relative) was a major reference in 1990 in both Britain and Australia. It was still being used in 2005.[12] The index under 'zinc deficiency' has four entries in Harrison and nineteen in Hungerford. Similarly, for 'magnesium deficiency' Harrison has no entries while Hungerford has eleven; and for 'selenium' Harrison has five references, none relating to deficiency, while Hungerford lists over fifty for selenium all up, and thirty-four for deficiency.

Selenium deficiency in the veterinary text makes interesting reading, especially in contrast to Harrison, whose entry is notable for its brevity and contains no deficiency listings at all. The author of the veterinary textbook wrote about such omissions:

> In the past thirty years, each time I have written a new edition of *Diseases of Livestock*, I am appalled at the fact that white muscle disease is a well recognised and common condition in lambs and sheep, goats, cattle and, to a lesser extent, in horses, pigs and rarely other species, but no comparative observations are available on humans.
>
> If a veterinarian has multiple cases of cardiac failure with sudden deaths in lambs, calves or kids he automatically looks for myocardial infarction and selenium deficiency, and with clinical pathology and biochemical backup may find it as the common cause. If a medical man in humans has a cardiac arrest and myocardial infarctions, on post mortem, he automatically looks for coronary occlusions, thromboembolic emergencies or atheromatous conditions, and may find them. He thinks in terms of cholesterol excess, nicotine, alcohol, etc. but never in terms of selenium deficiency as one possible cause.
>
> In the animal field we all know of the relationship between selenium and sulphates, nitrates and calcium, so that sulphates, nitrates and high dietary calcium decrease the

absorption of selenium in cattle and has been associated with muscular dystrophy, metritis, clinical mastitis and retained placenta. In this context note the human fact that post-menopausal women are encouraged to take more calcium by recommendation of dieticians. Indeed, the matter of trace mineral inter- relationships is very delicate. Think of dietary intake of molybdenum, sulphur, zinc, iron, cadmium and calcium — all decrease the availability of dietary copper to animals ... To summarise, selenium deficiency and its possible inter-relationships with heart and muscle conditions in humans needs critical investigation. *The veterinary profession has so much data at its fingertips it is a tragedy if this is not brought to the forefront of thought by the medical profession.* [my italics][13]

In 1989 vets knew that selenium deficiency could cause mastitis and retained placenta, and yet in 2005 doctors still treat the former with massive doses of antibiotics, and the latter remains a serious cause of birth trauma. Why are we still encouraging menopausal women to ingest obscene quantities of dairy products in order to 'get your calcium', with scant regard to the intake of magnesium and other minerals? Perhaps it is time for doctors to leave their comfortable offices and do some compulsory field work?

The problem is not confined to selenium. Let us imagine a young doctor, raised in the city, but keen to explore the idea of country practice. He decides to do the country thing, and buys himself a few acres and a small herd of cows. He knows nothing about animals or farming, but is confident that his medical knowledge will be transferable. When the time comes for his cows to calve, he finds that the first cow to give birth is in trouble. Rolling up his sleeves, he proceeds to do an assisted delivery, only to find that the next cow is in a similar predicament. Envisaging a long night ahead, and noticing that several other cows are 'down', he calls the vet.

Does what happens next change his thinking? The vet arrives and produces the largest horse syringe he has ever seen. He goes around the herd, injecting the afflicted animals. And, one by one, they get to their feet and deliver their calves, with no further assistance.

'*What* is in that syringe?' the young doctor asks.

'Didn't they teach you about grass tetany, eclampsia, or delayed labour in medical school?' the vet replies. 'You have one of the most magnesium-deplete soils in the world around here. Magnesium is necessary to relax the uterus. No magnesium, no calf. No mum either, if you're not careful.'

His thoughts turn to his patient in the maternity ward, now entering her second day of labour. He adds some magnesium solution to her intravenous infusion, and a grateful patient delivers soon after, with minimal assistance.

Will his colleagues applaud his actions—or will he be in trouble for treating his patients as if they are cows?

Why magnesium is so spectacularly effective in conditions such as eclampsia and obstructed labour is explained in Chapter 4. (In eclampsia a rapid and malignant rise in blood pressure threatens the life of both mother and baby. Western medicine treats it with a cocktail of antihypertensives, and if this does not work, an urgent caesarean section.) The incidence of caesareans in England reached an all-time high in 2002 of 21.5 per cent; in some hospitals it was nearly 30 per cent. In 2005, one in five of all babies born in Australian capital cities was delivered by caesarean section and in the same year the rate in the United States was 30.2%. These figures are rising. While some of these cases are driven by the fear of litigation, anyone with obstetric experience knows that it is extremely difficult to impose surgery on an ideally progressing normal labour.

The World Health Organisation recommends a caesarean rate of 10 per cent or less. In Bangladesh eclampsia is treated with magnesium sulphate before a patient is referred to hospital.[14] Perhaps they have less money for frivolous surgery, or perhaps they just have more sense.

Caesareans for 20 per cent of the herd would rapidly send a farmer bankrupt. Do we tolerate bad medicine because we can afford to do so? The bigger brains and bigger heads of humans can result in difficult labour, but are we so much different to other species?

It would be wrong, of course, to imply that all cases of eclampsia or delayed labour are simply a result of magnesium deficiency. Zinc and selenium are known also to be important in all aspects of reproductive health. Animal breeders and farmers have been using these minerals to improve fertility for decades. It is extraordinary that human IVF clinics and obstetric hospitals still do not.

Do vets ever get it wrong?

Rover, rather like his owner, usually eats a wide-ranging and omnivorous diet. Sometimes it is leftovers; vets often advise against this but in an affluent society Rover may be getting the most nutritious part of the family meal. Compared with iced donuts, the diet of Mogsy and Rover may be superior to that of their owners. They may be lucky enough to be raised on bones and natural foods. If they are fed processed food, they may need treatment for diabetes, kidney disease and arthritis as they age. Even to discuss diseases of affluence in animals is a matter of regret. But if an animal's diet and lifestyle have little evolutionary precedent, it is as much at risk as its owner. It is not an Orwellian vision but a sad reality that today's vets need electrocardiograph machines, that they do hip replacements and even prescribe Prozac. But there may be signs that the tide is turning: one dog food company is reported to be making a food which benefits animal learning and behaviour.[15]

Certain vets are taking a stand. Vested interests donate to the veterinary faculties of universities and furnish the waiting rooms of many surgeries. The dog and cat foods advertised in this way supply the vet with a steady stream of chronic ill-health. In protest against these insidious inroads, some vets have resigned from their professional organisations. Books such as *Grow your Pups with Bones* tell it all.[16]

Do animals ever get it wrong?

If doctors and vets might learn from each other, what might we learn from the animals themselves? Does Mogsy eat slush out of a can because she prefers it, or because it is what's on offer? Experimental animals, given access to 'cafeteria' feeding, will choose a perfectly balanced diet.[17] If this is true, why do humans with seemingly unlimited choice get it so wrong? Are animals really smarter than us?

Recently I watched one of my free-range hens. After getting her 'fix' of essential fatty acids from tiny seeds in the weeds, she strutted over to a window and demolished two red-back spiders in rapid succession. Next on the menu was a small frog, rescued from the pond. After that, it was a beeline for a half-eaten corn husk. This particular hen has even been seen eating a small snake. (It's a fair bet that *her* eggs will be full of omega-3 fatty acids.) Of course, the hen does not get imprinted by television advertising telling her that sugar and salt are 'rewards' for some undesignated achievement. She obviously 'knows' that she needs a broad diet. How does she achieve this? Why do commercial pellets (which look alarmingly like many breakfast cereals) hold such little appeal?

A dog is by nature easy-going. It is a scavenger in the wild, eating whatever is edible, and will gobble canned food or leftovers with the same cheerful ease. But it seems happiest when gnawing on a bone. This keeps the teeth in good shape, and the cartilage on the ends of the bone supplies the necessary ingredients for the dog's own cartilages. The owners meanwhile, who prefer instant soup to the messy process of simmering bones for stock, carefully take their glucosamine tablets and are on the waiting list for hip replacement surgery.

Mogsy is more difficult. A hungry stray will eat anything that looks like meat and even things that don't. A pampered cat often has a hierarchy of food preferences, with canned fish at the top and dried food accepted with reluctance. Some cats prefer one brand of food over another, and often the chosen brand has a much higher salt content. The cat's owners notice that it is drinking a lot of water and using the litter tray several times during the night. The vet wonders about diabetes and kidney disease. Blood tests show that Mogsy has signs of early renal failure.

Why does the cat's instinct not warn of salt overload? Probably for the same reason that ours does not. It is only with the advent of modern technology and affluence that the possibility has arisen of consuming sugar and salt in excess of that found in nature or of eating 'non-foods'. These are the topics of the following chapters.

Chapter Two
THE POLITICS OF HEALTH

Modern medicine has become a major threat to health and its potential for social, even physical, disruption is rivalled only by the perils inherent in the industrialised production of food.

IVAN ILLICH, 1974

A single death is a tragedy; a million deaths is a statistic.

JOSEPH STALIN

ALTHOUGH A FEW STUDENTS may enter medicine because of the perceived status or income, the desire to heal lurks in the breast of most young medicos. It is what happens along the way that may lead to blind spots, bias, conservatism or cynicism.

Once they enter medical school, students have to work hard. Often there is no spare time for extra-curricular activity, and the focus can become very narrow. From an early stage a sense of responsibility is impressed upon them. This is right and proper, as there are few professions where such trust is placed in a total stranger.

The young interns watch with great respect as their teachers save lives and execute difficult procedures. This is not an environment in which creative thinking flourishes. No-one is interested in a novel idea for removing an appendix, least of all the patient.

Once on the wards, newly graduated doctors face life-threatening emergencies in obstetrics, cardiology, psychiatry. They are often short on sleep; there are multiple new skills to acquire; they are grateful for any tips given by seniors; they are constantly aware that errors cost lives and result in lawsuits. This is hardly an environment in which to challenge the status quo. As they become increasingly confident of their ability, they teach other anxious interns what they have been taught. If they decide to enter a speciality they will be involved in research and clinical trials. The trial, the medications, the salaries, possibly even the furnishings in the ward itself, are funded by some organisation, very often the pharmaceutical industry.

And so the pressures mount. There are punishing exams to pass, inhuman hours to work, younger doctors to supervise, medical students to teach, training obligations to fulfil — and soon, perhaps, a family and a mortgage to support. A certain confidence — one might almost call it arrogance — can come from the social status of being a doctor. Scientists may know a lot more, but doctors preside over the dramas of birth, life and death. It is much easier to make a television series about the doctor in the Emergency Room than about the scientist in the lab peering into a microscope or a test tube.

If some painstaking research in molecular biology or biochemistry demonstrates a role for zinc or folic acid in the transcription of genes, this will be published in a journal of molecular biology or clinical nutrition; it may fail to filter through to the medical journals. The research done by a pharmaceutical company on its latest drug or vaccine has more exposure, more advertising funds, and finally more respect from doctors, than the results of some under-funded university laboratory on a non-patentable natural substance.

In short, the medical profession is, by and large, conservative, and it is in the business of disease rather than the business of health.

EVIDENCE-BASED MEDICINE

For Brutus is an honourable man;
So are they all, all honourable men.
Julius Caesar, Act III

A new scientific truth does not triumph by convincing its
opponents and making them see the light, but rather because
its opponents eventually die, and a new generation grows up

that is familiar with it.
Max Planck, *A Scientific Autobiography*, 1949

Evidence-based medicine relies heavily on the clinical trial. The 'gold standard' is the random controlled trial, or RCT, and evidence provided by meeting *all* the criteria of the ideal RCT is referred to as level-1 evidence. In an RCT the people studied are randomly selected to represent the population under surveillance. So, if we are looking at the effect of a drug to prevent stroke in high-risk males over the age of 60, the patients selected are chosen in such a manner that their risk is representative of *all* high-risk males over 60. For a controlled trial, there must be a similarly sized control group, fulfilling all the same requirements. One group is given the active drug; the other receives a placebo or 'dummy' drug. Neither the persons administering the medication, nor the recipients, know which group is receiving the active medication. Such a trial is referred to as 'double-blind'. The trial is interrupted only if it becomes grossly apparent that one group is being so significantly benefited or harmed that continuation would be unethical.

For various reasons, many trials do not conform to the RCT standard. In certain circumstances the nature of the active treatment cannot be disguised, or is so risky that only terminally ill patients are invited to take part. Sometimes the trials cannot be conducted for long enough to give the highest level of evidence because of either lack of funds or unpleasant side effects of the medication.

Not all evidence is gained from clinical trials. Some comes from animal experiments, and some studies are carried out on human cell cultures in test tubes. Sometimes a large group of people is followed over a long period in an epidemiological study. The long-running Nurses' Health Study and Physicians' Health Study in the United States, and a similar one in Australia, are of this nature. An emerging science, known as bioinformatics, analyses the masses of biological data already to hand in fields such as genetics, biochemistry and molecular biology, calling on skills from disciplines as wide-ranging as physics, computer modelling and medicinal chemistry.

Many established treatments will probably never undergo a clinical trial. The removal of an appendix for acute appendicitis is one example.

Problems of clinical trials

If the benefits of clinical trials are obvious, the problems are somewhat less so. They may include: the design of the trial; the conduct of the trial; the nature of the questions asked; the question of who is paying for the trial; and the biases of the pharmaceutical companies.

The design of the trial

In designing a trial, medical scientists have two aims: to gain approval to conduct the trial and to use the product at the end of the trial.

The tension between these aims often shapes the trial design. The emphasis on safety and the control of extraneous influences may determine who can enter the trial. As a result, the drug may be tested on a population very different to the one which will use it. If a drug is tested on a very sick population, for example, it may not demonstrate increased morbidity or mortality because other ills mask the damaging effects.

The trial may exclude, for instance, people of a certain age, or those suffering from renal or liver disease, or smokers. When we add simple refusal to take part in a trial, the population tested in drug trials is very much narrower than the population that will eventually take the drug.

Other aspects of trial design may be suspect. Many trials have been criticised because they have trialled a high dose of a new drug against a lower dose of an old one. When the public is told that a new drug is more effective than an older one, they are not told that this higher dose can have side effects such as demands on the detoxifying enzymes in the liver.

The conduct of the trial

The conduct of the RCT often has problems which go unremarked. Research at Johns Hopkins University and the University of California LA indicated that a large proportion of volunteers failed to take the treatment as instructed. The researchers concluded that the unexpectedly large number of people failing to comply raised serious doubts about the validity of clinical trials.[1]

As doctors we remember the Hippocratic oath: 'First do no harm.' We expect, as does the public, that the treatment will not harm the patient. We expect a trial to analyse risks and benefits.

Safety is clearly a priority, but safety is a relative concept.

The substances being tested may not result in acute toxicity, but there are other effects that are more subtle or harder to establish. Because of the economic imperative, drug manufacturers are keen to market drugs as soon as trials have been completed. But many effects do not show up in the time-span of the trials, which are sometimes measured in just months. For example, the drugs known as ACE inhibitors (because they work against the angiotensin-converting enzyme) produce an asthma-like cough in a significant percentage of users. These observations only emerged after the drug had gained approval and was well established.

Cancer has a long latency period. Concern has been expressed that cholesterol-lowering drugs, some hormonal treatments and various other medications may have an effect on later cancer development because they affect critical biochemical pathways. Some research has suggested that statin may interfere with the metabolism of selenium.[2] Patients are rarely told of these risks because they are deemed to be small and hypothetical.

Long-term effects on the foetus are even more worrying. Cervical and breast cancer developed in women whose mothers took diethyl stilboestrol (DES) during pregnancy. The harm was done years, or even decades, before the effects became apparent in the offspring.

Some aspects of safety can only be established as disasters unfurl. The ability to cause foetal malformation (teratogenesis) is tested in laboratory animals and cannot always be extrapolated to humans. The thalidomide tragedy is the best known, although not the only, example of this.

Let us look a case of dubious safety in a clinical trial. Celebrex is a selective prostaglandins-2 inhibitor within the family of non-steroidal anti-inflammatory drugs, known as NSAIDs. (It is also a prototype of the drugs known as COX-2 inhibitors. COX stands for *cyclo-oxygenase*. See Chart 5.3 for the place of this enzyme in the synthesis of certain prostaglandins.) Celebrex was developed to treat arthritis without the problems such as gastrointestinal bleeding which limited the use of the older agents derived from aspirin. Its safety was a key selling point. As the drug was most useful to patients with chronic arthritis, the elderly constituted both the trial population and the target market.

After a few months some users were beginning to develop heart failure. Was this because it had been trialled in elderly, but otherwise healthy, arthritics? Did the design of the trial exclude people with heart conditions? Were the trials long enough, and in large enough numbers, and high enough doses, to unmask the patients with incipient heart failure? Soon doctors were advised that a drug found to be very safe in clinical trials should not be given to patients with suspected heart failure, predominantly the elderly.

Problems also began to emerge in young people. Celebrex had become an effective and popular treatment for the pain and inflammation of sporting injuries. If this medication was 'safe' for older, frailer people, surely it would be safe in the young? But the drug appeared to seriously impede bone healing in an age group normally associated with the *rapid* mending of broken bones.[3] Delayed healing may not have been noticed in elderly, arthritic people, where fractures and soft tissue injuries are notoriously slow to heal. Applied inappropriately to a different population, the drug seemed to be doing more harm than good.

If you are old and in pain, impaired healing may be worth the relief. For a young person, tolerating the pain may be the better option. Despite all this, the drug was still in wide use in 2004 for sporting injuries in the young. The manufacturer left it to the discretion of the doctor, and the doctor is shielded by the fact that the drug company has not banned its use in the young. The young person, keen to get back on the sporting field as soon as possible, gives no thought to the possibility of increased risk of arthritis in the future by an altered healing response now.

When a drug gains approval, look-alikes follow as soon as the patent laws allow. Although the look-alikes also have to undergo trial, the general acceptance and apparent safety of the parent drug usually results in rapid acceptance for the second generation. The next COX-2 on the market was Vioxx, released in June 1999, which became as popular as Celebrex.

If a drug is well received, the manufacturer starts to look for new applications for it. The COX-2s, as already mentioned, are intended as a refinement on aspirin. Since aspirin has proven benefit in preventing bowel cancer, maybe Vioxx could do the same thing, with fewer side effects. Another trial was begun.

Three years into the trial, on 1 October 2004, every practising doctor in Australia was phoned and faxed: all patients on Vioxx were to be urgently recalled. After 18 months on the medication, taken for whatever reason, the risk of an adverse cardiovascular event such as heart attack or stroke was increased significantly. This represented approximately 4740 Australian patients at risk. By early 2005, warnings came out for Celebrex. When the data was specifically analysed to uncover harmful effects, they were not hard to find. Celebrex has not actually been withdrawn, but the limitations now placed on its use make the original fanfare around its 'safety' read like a parody.

The questions asked

Traditionally medical trials, especially RCTs, are designed to test hypotheses—for example, that drug X will have beneficial effect Y on patients with heart disease. These trials are very suitable for single-factor testing.

This approach suits the 'disease' model. It cannot be applied to nutritional medicine because nutrients work interactively. Yet this is precisely the tool that has been used to evaluate various nutrients in the management of illness. Trials have had to squeeze themselves into the RCT mould to gain acceptance and publication. Not surprisingly, many of them have 'failed to show benefit'.

Take for example the trial set up to determine whether beta carotene was better than a placebo in preventing lung cancer, in which the vitamin actually seemed to *increase* the risk of lung cancer. The trial used one or two companion nutrients but no selenium, which alone should have invalidated the findings. But the real problem lies with the unnatural use of a single carotenoid. In real life, and in better-quality supplements, mixed carotenoids are always present.

As fat-soluble vitamins, the carotenoids compete for absorption from the gut.[4] The large dose of a single agent may well have reduced the uptake of other equally important forms of Vitamin A. In short, it may well have been the *absence* of essential carotenoids, rather than the presence of beta carotene, which gave rise to the excess cancers.

There was a second problem: *synthetic* beta carotene was used. Synthetic beta carotene is only one of 272 stereo-isomers (molecular forms) of the vitamin. Notably, the most important isomer, 9-*cis* beta carotene, was missing from the supplement; this is the isomer most strongly associated with anti-cancer activity. As one letter to the *New England Journal of Medicine* said: 'how a particular beta carotene came to be selected for world-wide testing is neither hard to understand nor easy to forgive'.[5] It is no surprise that the placebo fared better.

This study highlights the difference between the pharmaceutical and the biological approach to healthcare. When a drug is introduced to the treatment regime, it is brought in as an outsider, a trouble-shooter, something which does not belong in the system but which may have a beneficial effect. It *always* has side effects, but it is hoped that these will be minor compared to the benefits. It is appropriately tested as a single agent.

By contrast, nutrients work as essential cogs in a very complex mechanism. To dump in large doses of one nutrient is rarely appropriate. Perhaps the designer of this trial was unaware of the importance of a mixture of carotenoids, but the whole exercise highlights how the RCT has been designed to test single rather than multiple factors. Yet still, in 2005, this trial is regularly quoted to 'prove' that beta-carotene—and often, by implication, other supplements—does more harm than good.

Who funds the trial?

By their nature, trials are expensive to run; the rigid criteria of ethics committees and safety rules add further costs. Trials most likely to be conducted in the approved manner are usually funded by drug companies. Other, smaller trials may be more relevant and just as well run, but they cannot afford to meet criteria such as duration or numbers.

Many small trials never get off the ground at all. Good therapies are rejected because there is 'no evidence'. Detractors of these small and therefore 'inconclusive' trials fail to accept that 'absence of evidence is not evidence of absence'.

Britain, at least in regard to cancer research, is an exception because much funding comes from charitable organisations. Often these bodies have some input into trial design and conduct, opening up the possibility for greater independence of thought.

Bias from the pharmaceutical industry

Drug companies are, first and foremost, business enterprises. Unless they also sell natural products, they are unlikely to examine the role of vitamins, minerals and essential fatty acids in the prevention and treatment of disease, simply because these things are not subject to patent laws.

If a drug company spends a large amount of money in trialling a product, it needs to have a monopoly on that product to regain its investment costs and to make a profit. So long as governments are happy to leave the bulk of medical research in the hands of the pharmaceutical industry, it stands to reason that the cures found will be drugs. 'If the only tool you have is a hammer, everything looks like a nail.'

Drug companies engage in selective reporting. An analysis undertaken at the University of California showed some worrying characteristics.[6] Results of 359 drug trials published in five major international journals between 1989 and 1999 *all* expressed the risk reduction resulting from the use of their medication in terms of relative risk. Relative risk is by far the most favourable-*looking* statistic. By contrast, only eight trials reported the number of patients a doctor would have to treat (number needed to treat, NNT) before one received a benefit. The NNT could have been calculated on the data available at the conclusion of the other trials, but it was not.

Moreover, it is long-standing practice that only *favourable* trials are reported. Suppose a company does 20 trials on its latest drug and 19 fail to show any benefit for those taking the medication, or possibly even show deleterious effects. The company keeps quiet about the 19 trials and publishes the one indicating a favourable outcome.

In 2004, some prestigious journals rejected the role of mouthpiece for the pharmaceutical industry. They have collaborated in refusing to publish trials unless the evidence of *all* relevant trials is made available. The International Committee of Medical Journal Editors has declared that its members will not publish trials which are not announced publicly at the outset. Included in this collaboration are such prestigious journals as *The Lancet, The New England Journal of Medicine* and *The Journal of the American Medical Association*. This step is expected to go a long way towards redressing the problem of silence on negative studies.

SUSPECT ALLIANCES

The pharmaceutical industry has found many ways to influence the medical profession. It is well known that sales representatives from pharmaceutical companies visit doctors with handouts of drug samples and small gifts such as notepads, appropriately branded. Drug companies also host lunches, seminars and conferences, some of which qualify as part of the continuing education doctors must undertake to retain their vocational registration. This is all done with the approval of accreditation bodies such as the Royal Australian College of General Practitioners, Royal Australasian College of Physicians, Royal Australian and New Zealand College of Psychiatrists and many other similar bodies across the world.

'Unbiased advice': assessing drug trials

The promotional activities of drug companies influence doctors' clinical decisions. This is to be expected. But doctors often fail to recognise the influence.[7] A spokesperson for the Royal Australian College of General Practitioners has claimed that the new generation of GPs is well equipped to critically assess claims made by drug companies. But drug companies, well provided with marketing experts, would not bother to spend millions courting doctors if they felt these activities had no impact.

Even if doctors can resist the blandishments of the drug companies, they still need a degree of sophistication in both the language and mathematical reasoning of statistical analysis. 'Statistical significance' does not always equate to 'clinical significance', although it is natural to assume this would be so. Numbers that look impressive in one form lose their impact when put another way.

Suppose I tell a woman with breast cancer that the drug Tamoxifen will reduce her risk of recurrence by 20 per cent. We discuss the fact that it increases her risk of uterine cancer, but it is breast cancer she has now; she's more scared of breast than uterine cancer and she opts for the treatment. But if I say to her that her overall risk of *recurrence* of breast cancer is only 20 per cent, and Tamoxifen, by reducing that 20 per cent by 20 per cent in fact reduces her *real* risk by a mere 4 per cent, she may think twice. It seems that this is the more honest figure to give, and yet, as with the discussion on numbers needed to treat, the real risk reduction is rarely quoted.

NNT is the most appropriate expression of benefit. In my personal experience it is certainly the one that patients can relate to. If I tell that woman I will have to treat 30 women in her situation before just one will gain a benefit, she is fairly positioned to make her decision.

Let us look at the results of a study reported in the *British Medical Journal*.[8] Assume that you have a serious medical condition and four new drugs have been trialled. For simplicity we'll say that none of the treatments will have any impact on the quality of your life; they will only affect your chance of survival. Which one would you prefer to have? Do the quiz yourself and see if you fare better than the health authority executives did.

- Drug A reduced the rate of deaths by 20 per cent.
- Drug B produced an absolute reduction in deaths of 3 per cent.
- Drug C increased patient survival rate from 85 per cent to 88 per cent.
- Drug D meant that 33 people needed to be treated to prevent one death.

Doctors are not statisticians. The question was a trick one: all four sets of figures have almost identical outcomes. Of 140 respondents who answered the quiz, exactly three picked that there was essentially no difference between the four drugs.

And how would these drugs be reported in the media? Headlines sell newspapers. The Tamoxifen results, in almost every case around the world, were represented like Drug A. But these comments are not confined to Tamoxifen. New 'wonder drugs' always make their debut in the most favourable light.

Even where NNT is provided, it may be presented misleadingly. On my desk is a brochure for a cholesterol-lowering drug; the cover says in huge type, 'WRITE 17 SCRIPTS. RE-WRITE SOMEONE'S LIFE.' In other words, you have to treat 17 people to benefit just one. And what of the other 16? Well, in tiny type much later in the brochure we find that 2.5 per cent of users will suffer abdominal pain, 2.5 per cent will experience constipation, 2 per cent will have flatulence, 0.8 per cent will develop diarrhoea, 1 per cent will get headaches, 0.5 per cent will suffer insomnia. A smaller proportion will get the very dangerous myopathy/rhabdomyolysis. And not yet proven but suspected to be associated are: depression, leucopenia (low white cell count), impotence, loss of protein in the urine, and bruising. Also suspected is a linkage to the often fatal Stevens–Johnson syndrome.

Disease creation

Another tactic, and one which is creating ripples within the most conservative of medical establishments, is the process of 'disease creation'.

One example is Syndrome X, discussed in Chapter 8. There is no mystery about the way in which diet and lifestyle can lead to obesity and diabetes, but the labelling creates the perception that there is some mystery factor involved. The X factor provides an opportunity for new medication, and in fact a whole industry of Syndrome X drugs has mushroomed. Syndrome X education is heavily funded by the manufacturers of the relevant medications.

Another 'new disease' is ADD (attention deficit disorder and its many variants). This is a collection of several conditions, most of which can be approached without medication. But here, too, a large range of drugs has emerged to treat what is portrayed as a mystery disorder. These drugs are far from benign; they include amphetamines and anti-depressants. Perhaps ADD stands for 'anti-depressant drug deficiency'.

Minor problems with sexual performance (Chapter 7) and with sleep have been similarly medicalised. The *British Medical Journal* has expressed concern that the pharmaceutical industry is exaggerating both the size and severity of medical problems to create markets for its drugs.[9] It is heartening to see such mainstream journals acknowledging the enormous influence that vested interest can wield.

More tactics

However, vested interest has many cards to play. Not content to create new ills, the drug companies have set about publishing magazines. 'Awareness' journals, presented as educational, are a thin disguise for advertising. Often they contain articles written by eminent doctors, whose remuneration for such participation is not disclosed. Worse still, journal articles are sometimes ghost-written, occasioning in 2005 a crack-down by the World Association of Medical Editors.

Widening the goal posts is another strategy. For instance, SSRIs have been prescribed for children, even though children were not included in the original trials of the drugs.

Confidentiality in the consulting room can be compromised

when voices can be heard in the waiting room. An ideal solution is a television set. What a coincidence, one of the drug companies has been doing the rounds installing them. Are we surprised that the television shows infomercials on conditions treated by products made by this obliging company?

Another opportunity comes with software. The best software for medical information is expensive, but drug companies are willing to install it for you. More surprises as ads for targeted products pop up on the screen when you seek information on a condition or write a script.

It has become the practice in recent years for the sufferers of various chronic illnesses to form self-help groups. Only the most naïve can see pharmaceutical companies' involvement with these organisations as altruistic when the group provides an ideal forum for drug trials and good press.

Another well-known tactic is the televised infomercial. They are often shown on late-night slots, when not much has happened since prime-time news. It is not technically a lie to present research not yet scrutinised by peer review. 'Promising new research has given doctors hope that the cure for cancer/asthma/schizophrenia might just be around the corner.'

Sometimes the tactic is frank bribery. How generous that cognitive behaviour therapy was offered free to the patients whose doctors prescribed the sponsors' drug (Aropax, made by GlaxoSmithKline) for anxiety disorders.

A question of ethics

Drug companies undertake trials in developing countries where they can ignore ethical guidelines. Sometimes the 'volunteers' do not understand the nature of the trial, are not told of the risks, and are not offered medical treatment in return for their co-operation. *All* of these factors breach the rules for conducting trials in Western countries.

In the late 1990s AZT was trialled in Africa to determine its effect in preventing transmission of the HIV virus from mothers to babies. In the trial a placebo was used, something that would breach all ethical constraints in Western countries because the drug had already be demonstrated to be effective at certain doses. By the middle of 2002, only 30,000 of an estimated 30 million AIDS sufferers in sub-Saharan Africa were receiving the benefits of the drugs which had been tested on them in this way. Yet the drug companies have held firm against reducing the cost of the drugs for these impoverished nations. The companies are utilising desperate populations to conduct trials in a manner which would be prohibited at home, but they are unwilling to pay back that debt to the nations concerned. Developing countries are becoming medical sweatshops.[10]

CANCER

It is almost 30 years since President Nixon famously declared war on cancer. Since then, billions of dollars, much of it wasted, have been spent around the world in almost every arena of the cancer drama. 'Research', 'screening' and 'treatment' all receive funding and media attention. The exception is 'prevention', the one area most likely to make a difference. Blame for the rising incidence of many cancers can be sheeted home to environmental and lifestyle factors. Few politicians are prepared to confront such influential forces.

War bulletins or propaganda?

It is hard to tell whether the cancer war is being won or lost. British epidemiologist Sir Richard Doll represents the optimists, claiming that cancer rates are steady and will fall as lifestyles become healthier. By contrast, the American epidemiologist Samuel Epstein claims that the cancer rate has escalated in recent decades to the extent that Americans now face close to a 50 per cent lifetime risk of developing cancer.[11]

There are several reasons for such disparate views. One is the long delay between the events that initiate a cancer and the cancer developing to a diagnosable stage. Any prediction made on previous trends fails, by definition, to take into account new factors. Also, the parameters by which victory is judged vary. They can include:

- reduction in the diagnosed rate of a common cancer
- rise or fall in the rate of a previously uncommon cancer

- an increase in the survival rate of people diagnosed with any given cancer.

When the war is going badly, should we add a positive spin to maintain morale? Or should we tell it like it is, and run the risk of losing public confidence?

Here are some of the factors shaping cancer bulletins:

- An increase in the survival rate is often presented as a win, but it may just reflect earlier diagnosis.
- Cure rates may rise, but if the rate of that particular cancer is also rising that 'win' is a dubious advance. Cures for lymphomas and childhood leukaemias have improved spectacularly in recent decades, but the rates of these cancers are also increasing.
- Causes may be found, such as cigarettes and lung cancer. However, city living is now regarded as the equivalent to smoking 10 cigarettes a day.[12] It is hard to see such findings as a win.
- Terms such as 'five-year survival' are often regarded as indicating a cure, but they may only signify a delay in time of death. If much of the extra time has been spent sick and debilitated from the treatment, the value of such a 'win' is questionable.
- By using the tactics discussed in the section on clinical trials, *real* increases in survivor time are often represented by the more favourable *relative* values. The media, too, prefers relative values. Everyone gets the cosy feeling that a cure is just around the corner.

The reports of the 'success' of Tamoxifen in breast cancer are a case in point. Although as we have seen the real risk reduction for most women stood at around 4 per cent, the press reported the relative risk reduction of 20 per cent. These trials were conducted on women who had seen no spread of their cancer at the time of diagnosis, who had a good prognosis anyway. Furthermore, the important side effects of Tamoxifen were hardly mentioned. Reports of collateral damage were not allowed to spoil the success story.

And this was not the time to focus on another uncomfortable fact: the lifetime risk of breast cancer has risen steadily over the last few decades.

We are seeing increases in the incidence or the death rate, or both, in certain cancers. Testicular cancer, oral cancer in men, myeloma, bone marrow cancer and breast cancer have all risen in the last few decades. More cervical cancers in young women, and melanomas in young men and women, are being diagnosed, and the death *rate* from prostatic cancer in men and pancreatic cancer in women has risen.

Identifying the enemy

If we continue the warfare metaphor, we need to define the enemy. Is it the cancer cell itself? Or are our genes to blame? A closer look at the biology might help to answer these questions.

The cancer cell

Cancer, by and large, occurs when the normal controls on cell division break down. Cells which previously duplicated themselves for tissue repair start to make mistakes. They don't know when to switch off. They become autonomous.

Every time cells replicate, this risk of error occurs. However, the body exercises several defence mechanisms against this eventuality, including repairing the mistake in the DNA or destroying the cell in question.

Cancer can be seen as a communication breakdown. Cells normally proliferate in order to repair a wound, to replace old cells, or to defend the organism through an inflammatory response. When cells are informed that the threat has been contained, they switch off. If communication is not established, they may continue to proliferate inappropriately. The transformation to malignancy is the last step in a long line of failed communication.

Oncogenes

Oncogenes supposedly are genes that mark one out for cancer. They were first identified as a result of the observation that cancer often ran in families. The BRCA1 and 2 genes, and their association with the risk of breast, and possibly prostate, cancer, have gained near-mythic status. Some women who have these genes take the drastic step of having prophylactic (preventive) mastectomies.

Oncogenes are DNA or RNA sequences within cells which

allow uncontrolled cell proliferation. *But only under certain circumstances.* Not all people with these genes go on to develop cancer. We are not simply the sum of our genetic material (Chapter 3). The expression of the genetic code is a dialogue between the gene and what is going on around it.

The so-called oncogene is a gene which says, 'I am one of the weaker links in your genetic makeup. Please look after me.' It signals difficulty in protecting us from cancer, rather than giving us cancer. How we might look after our weaker genes is a major theme in this book.

Other suspects

In this war the enemy may be defined as anything that might affect genetic material. Some damage is the result of oxidation with the production of free radicals. Some comes as a result of chemical alteration of the structure of the DNA. There is no shortage of suspects:

- toxic exposure: radiation, air pollution, smoking, chemicals
- hormones (outsiders and home-grown)
- nutrient depletion (lack of vitamins, minerals and essential fatty acids)
- obesity and/or a junk food diet
- lifestyle (stress, lack of exercise, fresh air, sunshine or healthy recreational pursuits)
- genetics.

Some of these are actively harmful influences. Some are defined by their *lack*. Some are internal to the system itself, such as the genes or hormones. Hormones such as insulin, cortisol and oestrogen are essential to life, but in certain circumstances they can increase the risk of cancer.

Nature supplies a lot of buffer systems for the effects of these 'bad guys'. Repair enzymes are discussed in Chapters 3 and 4. Many buffer molecules come from the diet, but not from the typical Western diet. We neglect these defences at our peril.

Government

Leaving aside for the moment the complex area of genetics,

everything in the list above has political implications. Attempts by lobby groups to have nuclear reactors either closed down or moved to safer sites have brought political opposition. Smoking was banned in public places only after incontrovertible evidence dictated that no other course was conscionable.

Approximately 1000 toxic chemicals are released around the world every year. When long-term effects are shown to be deleterious, few governments are prepared to risk their standing with powerful industry groups. Instead of a ban, we see 'phased withdrawal', 'limited use' or 'self-regulation by the industry'.

The particular association between chemicals and cancer deserves attention here. Many years ago, Rachel Carson sounded a timely warning in her seminal work, *Silent Spring*. Samuel Epstein, Professor of Occupational and Environmental Medicine at the University of Illinois, has carried on where Carson left off. He was the key expert in the inquiry which led to the banning of DDT, aldrin and chlordane in the United States. He warns of the hazards of using synthetic bovine growth hormone, not to mention sex hormones, in the beef and dairy industries. His book *The Politics of Cancer Revisited* describes political obfuscation, denial by industry and government, and breathtaking indifference on the part of the medical profession in regard to known carcinogens.

Epstein comments that, despite the $20 billion spent since Nixon launched his war in 1971, there has been little, if any, improvement in the treatment or survival rate for most common cancers: 'The cancer establishment remains myopically fixated on damage control—diagnosis and treatment—and basic genetic research, with, not always benign, indifference to cancer prevention.'

According to Epstein, the US National Cancer Institute spends less than 1 per cent of its budget on researching occupational cancer, although these cancers account for at least 10 per cent of all adult cancers. Of the 1976 cancer research budget of $51.4 million, just $1 million was spent on research into carcinogens. This proportion has been roughly maintained into the 21st century.[13]

Epstein gives chlorine in water supplies as an example of environmental chemicals. Chlorine reacts with organic compounds and carcinogenic pollutants to produce trihalomethanes (THMs). This can occur at the reservoir or, worryingly, in the human gut. Neither the chlorine nor the THMs are fully removed by filtration plants. According to Epstein, more than 10,700 people in the United

States die every year due to THM-induced rectal and bladder cancer.14 The pecuniary cost of screening, diagnosing and treating these cancers alone would justify improved filtration systems. The idea that chlorine is needed to prevent cholera, typhoid, cryptosporidia or giardiasis is not in question. Adequate filtration is.

It is easy to see the political dilemma here. If the government admits that the water supply is causing cancer, then it becomes obliged to make expensive changes to the system. Much easier to abrogate responsibility. Fund the medical profession to find the 'magic bullet'.

Industry

In the case of science and medicine, government must rely on its advisers. Without the collusion of doctors and researchers, would government be able to ignore the fact that cancer is caused by carcinogens?

Chapters 4 and 5 discuss the roles of nutrients such as selenium, zinc and Vitamins A, C, E and D in the cancer equation. We might argue that it is hard to justify the expense of some of the current research when application of *what we already know* is neglected.

Most cancer clinics are subsidised by the makers of anti-cancer drugs. Many drug companies are concerned about, if not openly hostile to, the addition of any treatment which would confound the results of the trial regime. Doctors in these clinics defer to the wishes of those who are funding them, without seeing in it anything sinister. They assume that someone else will be researching selenium or factor X.

War cynicism

There comes a time in many wars when the public becomes cynical about the costs and begins to suspect the motives of those supporting the war. The term 'cancer industry' has entered common parlance. The cynics argue that the drug companies, the researchers, the oncologists, the manufacturers of screening devices do not want the cure for cancer to be found. Their livelihoods are at stake.

Let us look at screening, for example. There are certain rules associated with screening of any kind:

- It should be cost-effective.
- Early diagnosis should make a difference to the natural course of the disease.
- An effective treatment must exist.
- Results must be reliable and easily confirmed, creating no anxiety.
- Most importantly, the test itself should do no harm. If it *does* cause harm, this has to be seriously weighed against the benefits of making the diagnosis in this way, and at this time.

All babies are screened for phenylketonuria (PKU), and this is regarded as an ideal model. Although rare, PKU is a devastating cause of mental retardation, brought about by congenital deficiency of an enzyme. The test is cost-effective, requiring only a drop of blood obtained from a heel prick at birth. The treatment is both highly effective and affordable.

How does cancer screening compare? According to *Scientific American*, 'Cancer screening is notoriously unreliable: a positive test often does not indicate disease, and a negative result does not mean that the patient can walk away with a handshake and a smile.'[15]

Screening is not without value, and there are success stories. But as a battle tactic, issues around breast cancer are worth a look.

Breast cancer: a case in point

It is not hard to understand why breast cancer screening receives so much publicity and funding. The current figure for a Western woman's lifetime risk is rising radically. The trend indicates that the risk now approaches one in *seven* for girls yet to reach puberty. What is worse is the number of *young* women developing a disease once associated with their grandmothers. Breast cancer in post-menopausal women is often a slow-growing disease, but in young women it can be aggressive. Often these women have young families.

Early surgical treatment when the disease is still confined to the breast has a reasonably good outcome. If it has spread to the axillary lymph nodes, results are less promising; if it has spread to distant organs, the prognosis is very poor. Therefore, early detection gives the best chance of survival.

But this is the right answer to the wrong question. The best chance of survival comes from not getting cancer in the first place.

The mammogram is the main tool of detection. It is promoted in ever-increasing frequency to ever-younger age groups. Sometimes a mammogram, along with a rather perfunctory breast check, makes up all of the woman's breast health consultation.

When mammograms were introduced, women were advised to undergo testing every two years from the age of 50. The debate is now current as to whether the screening age should be dropped to 40. In many places, an *annual* mammogram has become the norm.

Breast tissue is radiosensitive, and repeated examinations may be dangerous. I have heard a specialist say, 'The irradiation dose is such that maybe the only women we should be screening are the ones at high risk. And yet, they are the very ones we *shouldn't* be irradiating.'

At a seminar, a molecular biologist described the way in which gene breakage is induced when studying DNA damage in cultured cells. The cells are irradiated while being subjected to shearing forces. Instinctively I remarked that it sounded like having a mammogram. Few women who have undergone the procedure would argue with the words 'shearing forces'. He explained that to induce maximal damage, you need to compress the cell and irradiate it, both *at the same time*. The damage induced by mammography may not be simply measured in rads. The fact that the cells are under compression stress at the time of irradiation affects their vulnerability.

Such concepts are accepted in both biology and physics. The lost hiker's fate depends not on absolute temperature but on the wind chill factor. After Hiroshima, the original calculations of radiation levels necessary to cause disease were found to be wrong because they failed to take into account the *angle* at which the radiation had been received. The implications from re-examination of the figures in the late 1980s are that radiation safety margins are much narrower than had previously been thought.

A 2002 study from the University of Newcastle (UK) indicated a link between the nuclear industry at Sellafield in Britain and an excess of childhood cancers.[16] The jury is still out on the tolerance levels of ionising radiation in human health and the operation of the many variables which affect it.

Mammograms: the balance sheet

The arguments are that the benefits of mammograms outweigh the possible risks. But do they? Remember that we are discussing *screening*— healthy women having a check-up. This is quite different from a woman with a detectable lump about which decisions must be made.

In screening for breast cancer we have at our disposal several possible tools:

- self-examination by the patient
- manual examination by a doctor
- breast ultrasound
- mammogram
- other, including techniques based on thermography, which may be considerably safer than mammograms but are not yet widely available.

Various studies of each of these methods have not had clear results. Women were encouraged to regularly examine their own breasts, until some studies seemed to indicate that this had no effect on the cancer death rate. Doctors fared pretty well when the results of screening by manual examination were analysed. In fact, it has been surmised that they might be as reliable as a mammogram at detecting a cancer.[17]

Ultrasounds are an under-used resource in screening for breast cancer; they emit no ionising radiation and are unlikely to have any harmful effects. They are the diagnostic tool of choice in young women, in whom breast tissue tends to be too dense to give accurate mammogram information. Mammograms tend to find the lump when it is smaller, but the ultrasound often gives better definition, showing whether it is solid or cystic.

What is the value of using a mammogram to detect lesions at a very early stage? If the mammogram finds the cancer when it is the size of a lentil, whereas the ultrasound does not find it until it is the size of a pea, does this translate into increased survivor time?

According to a study in *The Lancet*, finding the cancer earlier did not translate into improved survivor time.[18] (There is no doubt that finding a lump before it reaches the size of a cherry is worthwhile, but by this stage the patient has almost certainly found it herself and it will probably show up on most diagnostic techniques.) The report said that of the seven world-wide trials which had supposedly shown the value of mammogram screening, five had been seriously flawed. The all-important process did not meet agreed standards. The remaining two trials showed screening had no effect on overall death rates. Even more uncomfortably, there was an *excess* of cancers in the screened group. The idea that the screening itself had contributed to these was hard to avoid.

The publication of this study caused a furore. Early detection was the policy, and now the facts seemed to be opposed to it. The editorial board of the Nordic Cochrane Centre rejected the original report of the study. Normally esteemed for its work in compiling objective assessments, the Cochrane Centre clearly had trouble in confronting the politics. They insisted the review be rewritten to present screening in a more favourable light. Instead, one of the authors, Peter Gotzsche, sent the unedited version to *The Lancet*.

In 2005 it would seem that he has been vindicated, with new findings that mammography does little to alter death rates.[19]

The *Lancet* study suggested that lentil or pea size made little difference to the ultimate outcome. And in the meantime, much angst had been caused. When the mammogram suggested a small nest of malignant cells, the next procedure was biopsy. The difficulties in locating such small lesions are well known, and the procedure can be traumatic. Detection is still subject to the risks of both false positives and false negatives. Patients go through an anxious few months waiting to see if the lesion grows. There is a case to be made for waiting until the lesion has reached a size big enough both to see on ultrasound, and to access for biopsy. There is no safety limit on the frequency with which the ultrasound can be performed. It can be repeated as often as thought necessary.

It would be wrong to imply that mammography never has a place in screening, but it should be the job of the patient and her doctor to discuss the way in which she reduces her risk of breast cancer.

Conflict of interest
General Electric is a major producer of mammogram machines. It is also a major user of polychlorinated biphenyls (PCBs). There are 210 organochlorines making up the PCB family, and collectively the PCBs have been classified by the US Environmental Protection Agency as 'probable human carcinogens'. Several studies have linked

PCBs to breast cancer.

The primary sponsor of National Breast Cancer Awareness Month in the United States is AstraZeneca, a British-based multinational which manufactures Tamoxifen. It also manufactures fungicides and herbicides, including the carcinogen acetchlor. Its chemical plant in Ohio is the third-largest source of potential carcinogens in the United States. As Sharon Batt and Lisa Cross note, 'Any mention of the role such chemicals may be playing in rising breast cancer rates is missing from the Breast Cancer Awareness Month Promos.'[20]

In 1992 the Breast Cancer Prevention Trial in the United States and Canada involved 16,000 *healthy* women, deemed to be at high risk of breast cancer. It was terminated 14 months prematurely in 1998, seemingly on the grounds that the drug was so beneficial that it would be wrong not to make it available as early as possible. But were there other motivations for this early termination? By 1998 Tamoxifen was already known to have unpleasant side effects like uterine cancer, deep vein thrombosis and pulmonary embolism.

The Lancet commented on trials involving thousands of high-risk women in Milan and London:

> The failure of these trials to confirm the results of the US study … casts doubt on the wisdom of the rush, at least in some places, to prescribe Tamoxifen widely for prevention. Longer-term follow-up of completed and current trials is clearly required, to clarify the relative preventative benefits and risks. … Most importantly, none of these trials provides reliable data on mortality, which should be the ultimate endpoint.'[21]

Samuel Epstein agreed: 'At the very best, chemoprevention with Tamoxifen is an *exercise in disease substitution rather than disease prevention,* and the rationale for its use in healthy women is thus highly questionable.' Epstein's criticism is not confined to the drugs and their trials. He continues:

> This is a conflict of interest unparalleled in the history of American medicine. You've got a company that's a spin-off of one of the world's biggest manufacturers of carcinogenic chemicals, they've got control of breast cancer treatment,

they've got control of the chemoprevention [studies], and now
they've got control of cancer treatment in eleven centres
which are clearly going to be prescribing the drugs they
manufacture.[22]

Conflict of interest over breast cancer is not confined to the
pharmaceutical industry. The cosmetic firm Revlon sponsors events
to raise funds in the 'battle against breast and ovarian cancers'. Hair
dyes have been associated with mammary and liver cancer in rodents.
One ingredient in modern fast-drying nail polishes is a significant
hormone-disrupting chemical. It is absorbed into the bloodstream
and acts to aromatise hydrocarbon, effectively raising the potency of
the female hormones. There may also be a link between deodorants
and breast cancer, because the preservative parabens, added to many
deodorants, has been found inside the cancerous cells removed from
breast tissue. Would it be excessive to expect that Revlon, and other
cosmetic manufacturers, remove such products from the market
until the question is settled?

The solution to breast cancer lies neither in better diagnosis nor
in better treatments. As one doctor I know recently commented,
'Once you have diagnosed a cancer, the war has already been lost'.

HORMONE REPLACEMENT THERAPY

First, do no harm.— Hippocrates

Hormone replacement therapy, or HRT, is based on the principle
that women produce oestrogen and progesterone throughout their
lives, and that this production, which is maximal in the period
between puberty and menopause, needs replacement in the post-
menopausal years. Women also produce testosterone, although in
much smaller amounts than men. HRT therefore may contain a
mixture of oestrogen, progesterone and, less commonly,
testosterone. In different formulations, HRT is sometimes also
prescribed for men.

It is now approximately 40 years since doctors decided that this
was another area in which Mother Nature could be improved upon.

Every imaginable combination and permutation of oestrogen, with or without progesterone, was on offer to post-menopausal and peri-menopausal women. There is a dizzying array of treatments that a woman could have, and that her doctor is expected to keep up to date with. There was also much talk about 'natural' products to appease the women who felt uncomfortable about putting synthetic hormones into their bodies. Unfortunately 'natural' usually meant natural to horses. The inhumane way in which these animals were kept so that not a drop of their precious urine would be lost is another story.

Benefits

Short-term use

The symptoms of menopause are well known: mood swings, hot flushes and irregular and heavy periods. Also common are weight gain, skin and vaginal dryness, insomnia and loss of libido.

For many women, HRT brought relief. Less commonly discussed were the *new* symptoms some women acquired when they commenced HRT. Some were relatively harmless, such as modest weight gain, but some women experienced worsening headaches and migraines or even developed migraines for the first time.

Long-term use

Throughout the 1990s the list of benefits of HRT grew. First there was protection from gynaecological cancers. It was observed that women who developed breast cancer while on HRT seemed to fare better as a group than those who did not. One explanation may be that the breast cancer had actually been caused by HRT and was more easily controlled once the offending drug was withdrawn. In the meantime, the statistic was interpreted as if the therapy was actually *protective* against the more virulent forms. As for cervical, uterine and ovarian cancer, the studies were inconclusive.

Osteoporosis was another disease thought to benefit from HRT. Obese women suffer fewer osteoporotic fractures than their thinner sisters, probably because fat functions as an endocrine gland and can produce oestrogens. The promotion of oestrogen as an anti-ageing medication was the next step. Soon, cardiovascular disease, Alzheimer's and senile dementia became indications for HRT treatment. Then it was depression. And if oestrogen did so much for women, maybe the chaps should have some, too.

And then the final bold leap: we were now suffering from 'hormone-deficiency disorders'. Once you accept that you had a disorder which responded to hormones, 'deficiency' of the hormone was not implausible. Therapy was clearly the solution.

Problems in hormone heaven

Then other evidence began to appear. Environmental scientists noted that in sites contaminated with the degradation products of plastics and pesticides, male animals were turning into females or having difficulty reproducing due to underdeveloped genitalia.[23] The epidemiologists realised that in populations in which breast cancer was uncommon, women did not experience menopausal symptoms when their periods stopped. The Japanese famously did not have a term for the event. Soy products suddenly became popular in the West.

Early research had indicated that HRT was protective against heart disease, but now it looked as though HRT might be useful for people who already had heart disease but might increase the risk of those who did not. Further studies seemed to indicate that actually nobody benefited.[24]

And then in July 2002 came the headlines about a halt in a major US study of HRT, because it appeared to cause a significant increase in the risk of breast cancer, stroke and heart disease.[25]

The trial, involving 16,608 women aged between 50 and 79, was described as one of the biggest and best yet conducted. Interestingly, it was carried out not by a drug company but by a group called the Women's Health Initiative. The trial showed that for every 10,000 women taking HRT, eight more would develop invasive breast cancer, seven more would have a heart attack, eight more would have a stroke and 18 more would suffer from blood clots, than the women not receiving such treatment. This represented a figure of one woman in 250 having a life-threatening event in a five-year period as a result of treatment. These were ailments that HRT was supposed to be *benefiting*.

The trial was halted as soon as the risk for breast cancer was established. In fairness to HRT, it should be noted that there was a reduction in the number of cases of osteoporotic fractures and bowel cancer in the treatment group. The latter may be due to the mildly laxative effect of high levels of the hormone, as constipation is often linked with bowel cancer.

The advocates swung into damage control and reassurances came thick and fast. Ageing celebrities were dragged from their Botox appointments to endorse HRT. But the news was not good. With one-third of all of the women on HRT in Britain taking this particular preparation, 1200 deaths or life-threatening events were assumed already to have occurred as a result of this 'safe' elixir of youth.

Not all of this was a surprise. For some time there had been suggestions that there might be a link between HRT and breast cancer and that the cardiovascular effects were complex. But doctors had begun to believe their own spin. The more enthusiasm there was for the health benefits of HRT, the harder it became to think critically.

VACCINATION

Vaccination is one of the miracles of modern medicine. It arose in the 1790s when Edward Jenner observed that people who had suffered cowpox seemed to be immune to smallpox. He proved that an infection with a weaker strain of a virus or bacterium provoked an immune response which offered protection against more virulent forms.

Politicians love vaccination programs because saving babies has feel-good value. But what if the parents don't want their child vaccinated? Questions of civil liberties arise. Things can get quite heated.

It is human nature to gamble. If the vaccine itself carries risks, some people would prefer to take their chances on catching the wild strain.

The fear nowadays within the medical profession is that a population of young parents, never exposed to the realities of diseases such as diphtheria, polio and tetanus, are likely to be complacent about their babies' vaccination. Part of the anxiety relates to the 'critical mass' required to produce an epidemic. Until a certain proportion of the population is affected, any disease outbreak remains contained; but at a critical percentage, the infection spills into the wider community.

Thus vaccination rates have to reach a certain level to hold epidemics at bay. The onus to be vaccinated therefore is seen both as a protection against personal risk and a community obligation. It is argued that healthy people who refuse vaccination selfishly risk infecting others.

The issue is not whether vaccination confers benefit: it clearly does. It is the politics of the vaccine debate which concern us here. The issues include freedom of choice, ethics, safety, and the balance of costs and benefits.

Freedom of choice

Voices of discontent have been heard from the outset and have reached a crescendo in recent times. Several years ago there was an outcry when it was realised that the whooping cough component of triple antigen sometimes gave rise to fits and even brain damage. Children who had had a feverish reaction to their first shot were subsequently given a vaccine omitting this component. Some parents elected to have the scaled-down version from the start, and others opted for no vaccination at all.

Early polio vaccines were crude by modern standards and had an unacceptable rate of complications. Having seen problems with the whooping cough vaccine, the public was becoming wary. Then concerns were raised about the measles-mumps-rubella (MMR) vaccine. Thousands of parents refused the vaccination; about half a dozen children died of measles, which was presumed to have been due to their not receiving vaccination.

Governments began to pressure doctors to conform to official guidelines, and they in turn pressured parents. In both Britain and Australia, doctors were offered significant financial incentives to increase vaccination rates. Naturally, some parents disliked the feeling of coercion. Beginning in the early 1990s, state primary schools refused to admit children without a certificate stating that they were fully vaccinated. Receipt of child benefits also carried this caveat. In both cases, were the parents to object, certification from a doctor was required. Parents who normally avoided doctors for religious or any other reasons were brought into contact with mainstream medicine. Sometimes this was handled sensitively; sometimes it was not.

Vaccine-preventable death is regrettable, but how does it stack up against other preventable deaths? Think of the number of children who die unrestrained in cars. Smoking households have a greater incidence of child illness and death from asthma, meningitis, ear, nose and throat infections, and the bacterial illness HiB. Yet there are no sanctions against smoking parents, and driving the kids unbelted gets only a fine.

Most fears can be assuaged by statistics. If one in a thousand children in a given community will die or be left permanently brain-damaged by catching the wild measles virus, and one in a million will be similarly injured by the vaccine, the choice is obvious. But the parents' reasons for refusing vaccination should at least be heard impartially.

Ethics

World-wide eradication of any disease benefits everyone, so surely the extension of vaccination programs to the developing world is a humanitarian act. The development of the polio vaccine illustrates why ethical considerations must never be dressed up in philanthropic disguise.

The early testing of polio vaccines raises two issues. First, the trials were conducted in Africa on impoverished and malnourished orphans. On just about every selection criterion they would have been deemed unsuitable candidates in a developed country, even under the relatively liberal ethics of the day. Second, and much more controversially, it has been claimed that the use of monkey kidney to incubate the polio virus was the beginning of the AIDS epidemic. In fact, it probably wasn't—but maybe this was due to good luck.

The possible link is explained thus. The virus for the polio trial was incubated in monkey tissue which may have carried the simian AIDS virus. When this was injected into the children their immune systems were challenged by the polio virus, making them more susceptible to any other virus which might be around. This is one of the conditions which increase the risk of pathogens jumping species. By introducing a simian virus into a group of children who were *already malnourished and immune-compromised*, the researchers created ideal conditions to allow the virus to jump species.

It was argued that Africans had a history of eating monkey brains, so the exposure to the simian AIDS virus was not new. But when we eat a pathogen, it has to pass through membrane barriers designed by nature to protect us (Chapter 3). No such barrier exists when material is injected. The failure to take this into account reflects poorly on the understanding of the scientists involved.

Safety

In the vaccination equation are the reputations of individual scientists, of pharmaceutical companies, and of various governments. Also there are the countless millions which might be made as future profits, or lost in compensation. In short, it is hard to see how any of the evidence in these controversial issues can truly be called objective.

If objectivity and, worse still, integrity cannot be assumed, the public has a right to know the track record of the medical profession. After all, parents who refuse vaccination of their children may suffer sanctions. Remember that government scientists less than 20 years ago were reassuring the public that they had nothing to fear from eating BSE-infected meat. BSE, mad-cow disease, raises the same immunological dilemmas as vaccination.

BSE is caused by a rogue prion. The significant point is that the infected meat containing the prion was ingested by *vegetarian* animals. Their gut-related immune system was never designed to handle meat or its pathogens (Chapter 6). With breathtaking recklessness, the scientists of the day allowed these hapless animals to consume not only meat products but, it was rumoured, meat from sheep declared *not fit for human consumption because they were infected with scrapie*, the ovine form of prion disease. Idle rumour or cover-up, the feeding of meat to herbivores breaks every rule of common sense. Once the infective agent gained entry into the cow's biological system, which had no natural defences against it, the disease jumped from sheep to cows. In such circumstances, the virulence may be unprecedented. Because political and economic considerations took precedence over health, a disease was enabled to jump from one species to another.

There are serious proposals to use animals that are genetically engineered to provide xenografts as 'spare parts' for humans. People who are on dialysis or have transplanted organs are often on steroids or other immune-suppressive agents. The comparison to the malnourished African children on whom the polio virus was trialled is uncomfortably close. As one scientist has commented, 'What if we were trying to design the ideal experiment in which a new virus that would infect humans would be cross transmitted from pigs to humans? We would be hard pressed to come up with a better experiment than what is planned to be done with xenografts.'[26]

Costs and benefits

The undoubted benefits of an intervention have to be weighed against the various costs.

Value for money

Meningitis is one of the most feared of all diseases. The word means 'inflammation of the meninges', which are the coverings of the brain. The commonest clinical presentations are usually either viral or bacterial. Effective — though sometimes controversial — vaccines have been developed against disease caused by the tubercule bacillus, pneumococcus and, of course, the measles virus. But let us focus on one kind of bacterial meningitis which has deservedly given meningitis its bad reputation. It can kill rapidly and, because it most commonly strikes children and adolescents, the loss is particularly poignant. This is just the kind of health issue that has a feel-good effect for both the community and the politicians. To this end the Australian government recently undertook an expensive campaign to vaccinate the vulnerable population against the particularly nasty meningococcal form of meningitis.

In Australia annually, meningococcal meningitis causes approximately 24 deaths and a significant number of severe disabilities (loss of limbs etc.). The vaccination protects only against the C form of the disease, which causes about 40 per cent of all cases. In 2002 the scheme to vaccinate against meningococcus C was costed at around $200 million.[27]

Up to 90 per cent of all cases of meningococcal meningitis occur in smokers, or children from smoking households. It is thought that damage to the mucosal barrier, brought about by smoke inhalation, enables the germ to defeat the immune system's first line of defence. Therefore, we are spending large sums to prevent less than a dozen deaths from what is effectively a smoking-related disease. The benefits to those who lose limbs also have to be considered, but we still have to ask if this is the best value for the health dollar.

Natural resistance

If dollars count when we are costing an intervention, they pale into insignificance when the interventions cause harm. We have already discussed direct harm in the case of whooping cough vaccine.

When we wander through a 19th-century churchyard and see the graves of whole families of children lost in infancy, we might conclude that safety benefits outweigh cost. But this is an emotional rather than an epidemiological response. On balance, the protective effects of vaccination will probably win the day, but there remain some indirect effects which warrant discussion.

To understand these we need first to look at how Mother Nature does it.

Babies over the millennia encountered infection. Every day they had another small dose of bacteria, dirt and foreign antigens. Before birth they were protected by the antibodies received from the mother, which crossed the placenta and remained active in the body for some months. These antibodies reflected the immune status of the mother, and provided the baby with a passive defence against the infections the mother had had in her lifetime.

At the same time the infant was receiving a top-up of its immunity through breast milk, including defence against any illness the mother might currently be exposed to. As the infant and the mother were rarely far from each other, the infections which could threaten the baby were also encountered by the mother. Antibodies which she made to those illnesses appeared in the breast milk, affording the baby significant protection. Meanwhile, protected from many ills in this way, the babies' own immune systems developed. Through exposure to new germs, they gradually gained primary immunity.

The contrast to the modern baby could not be greater. It is guarded jealously against common or garden germs; everything is sterilised; pets and sick siblings are kept at bay. But then the baby is vaccinated. An immune system which has had little practice is suddenly put into overdrive.

Educating the immune system

Chapters 6 and 7 discuss the hygiene theory; the essence of this debate is how the immune system learns its job. Relevant here is the thought that when we inject germs directly into muscle tissue, we diverge from the way in which nature normally exposes a baby to germs. Moreover, we present not one but *several* germ antigens, along with foreign proteins and viral particles from the growth medium, and preservatives and adjuvants including aluminium and thiomersol. We have to question what exactly we are teaching the baby's developing immune system.

As such, vaccination becomes part of the later discussion about the hygiene theory.

The effect of vaccination on disease profiles

Originally we hoped that when enough of the population was vaccinated worldwide, certain diseases would simply die out. Although smallpox was declared to be eradicated, samples were retained in selected laboratories. With the emergence of bioterrorism, states preserve material from which to make vaccines in case known germs are used for germ warfare.

But there is another consideration. Animal studies indicate that the concept of a disease 'dying out' might be simplistic. Evidence is emerging that vaccinating chickens against avian flu virus may be accelerating the evolution of more virulent strains. The vaccine protects the vaccinated bird, but the germ itself becomes more lethal.[28] Such concerns attract surprisingly little debate. Let us consider some of them.

One issue is multiplicity of vaccines. Giving more than one vaccine at a time may lessen the effect of the individual components. And yet children receive so many vaccines that separate administration has become practically impossible.

Although such questions cannot be tested with the gold standard RCT, natural outbreaks can give clues. In South Africa in 1992 a single vaccine showed an efficacy rate close to 100 per cent, compared with triple vaccine at 74 per cent.[29]

Worryingly, rules for testing animal vaccines are more rigorous as regards both safety and efficacy than those relating to humans. When a combined bovine measles–pneumonia jab was given to cows, the measles component suppressed the immune system, and the pneumonia element did not work properly. Measles is a well-known immune suppressant so it is a poor candidate for a combination vaccine.[30]

For human infants, studies in Israel and Finland on the effects of multiple vaccination raised concerns that vaccines which shared a common protein component reduced the immune response when given simultaneously. The vaccines under investigation in this case were diphtheria-tetanus-pertussis (whooping cough), oral polio, tetanus, HiB, influenza type B, and a pneumococcal vaccine.[31]

A second issue is the attenuated immunity conferred by the vaccine. Vaccines do not provoke as strong an immune reaction as does acquiring the disease naturally. Before vaccination, a woman who got a wild virus developed an immune response that was strong enough to last her whole life; it also gave adequate protection to any future foetuses until they were old enough for their own immune systems to do the job. Nowadays, her entire immunity comes from her own vaccination and it is much weaker — more on that presently.

Newborn babies still suffer significant illness from whooping cough, even in communities where vaccination is widespread, because they are too young to be vaccinated. It has been suggested that couples contemplating pregnancy should receive booster vaccines, and that 15- to 17-year-olds should have routine booster shots. But welcome to the real world! Many pregnancies are unplanned, especially in the most vulnerable demographics. How many adolescents are up to date with vaccines as basic as tetanus or hepatitis B? Does the average teenager plan for the children they may have in 10 years' time? Is there any ceiling on the number of vaccines which will have to be topped up, and how will this be regulated?

Chickenpox is a viral illness, normally contracted in childhood; after the acute initial infection the virus remains in the central nervous system for life. With age, or under conditions of significant stress, immune suppression of this dormant virus may weaken. The patient gets shingles, an extremely painful and unpleasant condition which can lead to severe debility, loss of sight and even death.

Adults who live in close contact with children are less likely to get shingles, apparently because exposure to infected children acts as a booster. The estimate is that to vaccinate a population the size of the United States' over 50 years would prevent 5000 child chickenpox deaths. However, there would be 5000 extra deaths in the over-60 population, and an extra 21 *million* cases of shingles.[32] How do we do a cost–benefit analysis on that?

In terms of people who are alive today, vaccination is comparatively recent. Several generations grew up with nothing more than a tetanus shot. But what of young parents now? If the mother's vaccination provokes a weaker response than she would have had with the naturally acquired disease, can she give adequate coverage to the child in the uterus or in those early months after birth? She may have enough antibodies to protect herself, but can she protect her infant in the way her mother protected her?

Perhaps the advantages she gained in infancy will be lost in later life if her only exposure to common germs has been from vaccination. And what happens when there is insufficient wild virus to boost the adult, as once would have happened?

By 'improving' on Mother Nature we may be producing a generation of infants whose immunity *in utero*, and in the early months of life, is *lower* than at any other time in human history. We may have created a generation whose survival, as a result of vaccination programs, is now *dependent* on those programs. Our concerns for the future, and how we might assess them, can be summarised as follows:

- *The strength of the immune response:* From studies done with animal vaccines, it is known that measurement of antibody level is in fact a poor measure of immune status. For many diseases, particularly viral, it is what is happening *in the immune cells* that will determine the response to the infecting agent. So even if we ask the questions posed above, there is no reliable way of answering them. Would this situation be countenanced in other clinical trials?
- *The loss of herd immunity:* 'Herd immunity' refers to the situation where most people in the population have been exposed to an infectious agent. In this case, the disease does not easily spread to the non-immune for the simple reason that it does not make most people sick. Their immune systems halt any disease proliferation. If we develop a population with no exposure to wild strains, in times of warfare or natural disaster when supplies of vaccine might be interrupted, the whole population can be wiped out. The lack of herd immunity destroyed many tribal peoples when first exposed to European explorers.
- *Risk of new diseases:* As fast as we deal with old diseases, new ones emerge. One reason for this is the relentless

march of civilisation. As we clear forests we drive out animals. These wild creatures have increased contact with humans and spread contagion. The destruction of forests has been linked to outbreaks of the dreaded Ebola virus and *Yersinia pestis* (bubonic plague). Some animals learn to adapt and begin to share their lives with humans. The sight of foxes trotting through the city demonstrates this. We cannot know how many new diseases we are releasing through this increased contact. How many vaccines will we need to protect our babies from them?

- *Risk of old diseases:* Is our confidence in vaccination falsely placed? In Slovakia, where 97 per cent of the population is vaccinated against polio, the last known case was in 1960. But in 2005 the public health authority reported that 72 different strains had been found in sewage systems—'some almost identical to wild polio virus'. The thinking is that weakened strains used in vaccination may have reverted to the pathogenic form.[33]

Do we have our paradigm wrong? Perhaps the childhood illnesses have served their purpose over time to prime the immune system in such a way that outbreaks of Ebola and new diseases had a less devastating impact than they do today. Bacteria produce microbicides (natural antibiotics). That is how they protect themselves from attack by other pathogens. These infections, in short, may be protective.

To take a viral example, people infected with a common virus known as GBV-C appear to be less likely to die of HIV infection than those not so infected. Are we 'conquering' ancient viral illnesses which protected us against even more dangerous diseases?

Over time, an ecological balance, an uneasy harmony, has developed between germs that occupy the same territory, the same host. The elimination of one germ has the potential to disrupt the entire ecosystem. (See Chapter 6: Immune System Disorders.)

MMR: a case in point

The MMR controversy brings together many of the arguments already considered Early combination vaccines were released in the late 1980s with many safety reassurances. One produced by SmithKlineBeecham around 1988 contained the Urabe strain of the mumps virus. At the time of its first release there were concerns about the safety of this strain, but the company continued to market it for another 10 years until an outbreak of meningitis in Brazil led to its withdrawal.

After the introduction of the measles–mumps–rubella vaccine, Dr Andrew Wakefield, a British paediatric gastroenterologist, and Scott Montgomery, an epidemiologist from the Karolinska Institute in Sweden, published a paper called 'Through a Glass Darkly'.[34] They suggested that MMR had been introduced without adequate safety trials; that the measles virus has long been known to cause a persisting central nervous system disorder; and that it has a predilection for the gut. They pointed out that few trials done either before or after the introduction of the vaccine had followed the children for more than four weeks. Dr Wakefield had begun to notice an unusual phenomenon. He was seeing children who had severe inflammatory bowel disease combined with autism. Autistic spectrum disorders are widely accepted as being on the increase, but this was a regressive autism. It is rare for children who have reached normal milestones to regress into autism. Similar handicaps are sometimes seen after severe infection, particularly meningitis, but in such a case the cause is clear.

At the same time reports were emerging of an increase in some inflammatory bowel conditions, including, notably, conditions resembling Crohn's disease. Not only was the frequency of this condition increasing, but it was appearing in countries such as Japan, and in populations such as children, where it had been rare. Wakefield claimed to have identified measles protein in the lymphoid tissue of the gut in 24 patients with inflammatory bowel disorders. A Japanese researcher was finding much the same thing in Crohn's patients. In Sweden, Dr Anders Ekbom found that the younger a baby was when first exposed to measles virus (including *in utero*), the greater the subsequent risk of developing Crohn's.

In 2008 the international consensus appears to be that Wakefield had it wrong. But the whole saga is a sorry tale of bias, arrogance, and a refusal to give a fair hearing to someone who dared to challenge the status quo.[35] Every possible criticism that could be levelled at bad medical science is well represented here, including corruption within the pharmaceutical industry, misrepresentation of statistics by drug companies and government departments, and indifference by the British Committee of Safety of Medicine (CSM).

The detractors of the Wakefield theories kept stating that there was 'not a shred of evidence to support them', although his data conformed far more to best practice than any put forward to dismiss him. For example, when challenged to look at case reports on affected children, the CSM sent questionnaires to their GPs instead. Half of these doctors failed even to reply.

In Britain the system used to record adverse reactions is known as the 'yellow card'. It had earlier failed to detect the meningitis outbreaks associated with the Urabe strain of mumps. As an epidemiological tool, it is almost worthless. A 1995 study published in *The Lancet* demonstrated that when hospital records were matched to GP records, *five times* more vaccination reactions were picked up.[36] Although this evidence was common knowledge, the yellow card method of reporting was used to refute one of the most serious health concerns of recent times.

The important thing to emerge from this story is not whether Wakefield was right or wrong: far more important is the question of how challenges to the status quo are handled.

MILK AND BREAD

Milk and wheat are staples of the Western diet, yet there is good evidence that they are responsible for many common health problems. Gluten allergy and lactose and dairy intolerance are discussed in Chapters 6, 9 and 10, but more general questions are discussed here. The milk and wheat we eat today are not the same as the products consumed in the early days of agriculture. Often they are not even the same as those consumed by our grandparents.

Milk and wheat both contain opioid substances. These are peptides, breakdown products of the proteins we eat. Casein from milk, for example, has eight distinct amino acid sequences that display opioid function, which are known collectively as 'caseomorphins'. The source in wheat is exorphin.[37]

Has Mother Nature somehow drugged our food with opium-like substances? That question derives from a simplistic view of food. A lot of food is a compromise. We co-evolved with the plants around us. Some effects were beneficial; many were more complex than we have yet realised. We go back to Colin Tudge's argument (Chapter 1). Food is a rich pharmacological mixture. Some of it builds bodies or provides energy. Some of it acts as a preventive medicine. Some, in small doses, heals us when we are ill. In large doses, like any medicine, it can harm us.

An opioid has various possibilities. It can calm us. It can encourage us to eat more of it. After all, why would we bother eating at all if it did not give us pleasure? Pleasure may come from a good taste, relief of hunger, or other more subtle means. Nature has many cards to play when ensuring the survival of a species.

The opioid chemicals are widespread. Grains other than wheat, such as corn rye and oats, also contain psychoactive peptides. Those derived from the gluten-containing cereals are sometimes referred to as 'gluteomorphins'. Soy and peanuts (legumes) also can exhibit similar but less active properties, but rice is thought to contain few if any of these substances. Also found in some of these 'addictive' foods are chemicals which can mimic dopamine, which is a feel-good neurotransmitter in the brain. They are referred to as 'dopaminergic' compounds and, like opioids, they act on the reward centres.

This line of thinking leads us to a theory which is truly astounding: that the 'drugging' effect of the opioids and dopaminergic compounds actually made possible the agricultural revolution.

Before the dawn of agriculture, people lived in small tribal bands of perhaps 20 or more related individuals. Agriculture provided the benefit of co-operative farming, but it had the disadvantage of having to trust people you didn't really know well. Wheat and milk cultivation preceded vegetables and fruit by several thousand years. Perhaps the effects of these food chemicals took the edge off aggression against strangers and made cohabitation possible.[38]

If we argue that psychoactive compounds have an adaptive benefit, many dilemmas arise. We have to ask about the cultures which for thousands of years did not adopt agriculture. And we have to ask why the foods in question appear to have so many harmful effects. After all, dental decay and degenerative diseases were noticeably apparent in agricultural societies from the earliest days (Chapter 1).

The answers take us to the heart of the complexity of the human race. Non-agricultural societies have been slow to 'civilise'. If we argue that civilisation is beneficial, addictive foods may be simply the price we have to pay. If there are disadvantages in consuming milk and wheat, what has happened in the last century has magnified that problem out of all previous experience. Food processing, plant and animal breeding programs, affluence leading to the exclusion of other important food groups, unnatural chemicals—all these things have created a toxic load which is unprecedented in the history of our species.

Some argue that the results include mental illness, autistic spectrum disorders (Chapter 9), cancer and autoimmune disorders.

Milk

The idea that milk is good for our health is entrenched in Western medical thought. Medical advice about the consumption of milk and cheese often sounds like an advertisement for the dairy industry. The thought that the lack of dairy products will cause us to succumb to osteoporosis as we age, or stunt our children's growth, remains one of the commonest food fallacies. Many women in pregnancy override frank dislike for the 'sake of the baby's bones'. Why?

For thousands of years of human history, milk has played a role as a nutritious food source. But this does not apply in all societies. Australian Aboriginals, for example, managed to stay osteoporosis-free and produce healthy children without animal milk for more than 40,000 years before white invasion. The most we can say is that dairy products may be a useful adjunct to the human diet; they are not, and never have been, essential after weaning.

The cultural concept of dairy as an essential food is highlighted not only by its place in the food pyramid, but by the response of parents when it is suggested that their child's emotional problems, asthma, eczema, reflux or recurrent abdominal pain may be due to milk sensitivity. The spectre of milk deprivation looms larger than all of these debilitating problems put together.

A fuller discussion of the possible health problems associated with dairy consumption is in Chapters 7 and 9. It is the political aspect of this debate which concerns us here.

Cultural and political aspects of the dairy industry

A staple food becomes a serious economic determinant. The

increased availability of a narrow range of foods produces an economic benefit. This cycle is perpetuated as government subsidies, agricultural and educational programs increase availability of the product. Agricultural degrees focus on beef and dairy production. Veterinary science reinforces the trend. Suddenly, food which is good for us has become food which is essential for us.

In this climate people come to think of dairy as the *only* good source of calcium. That their doctors and dieticians can share this view, and neglect alternative sources such as fish, nuts and vegetables, reflects ignorance rather than conscious collusion.

Milk is promoted as a natural food. But once an industry becomes as big as dairy is in the Western world, any semblance of 'natural' departs. Long before genetic engineering became technically possible, farmers were breeding cows for increased milk production. Nowadays, the typical dairy cow can no longer be drained of her milk supply by her own calf. She is dependent on the farmer to give her relief. This has a direct health consequence for the consumer. She is prone to mastitis, and is frequently dosed with antibiotics that pass into the milk.

A1 and A2 milk
About 80 per cent of the protein in milk is casein. There are several variants of casein, of which beta casein predominates. Beta casein comes in two forms, A1 and A2. Cows carry two genes for beta casein, one from each parent. If both genes code for A1, then the milk is designated A1 milk, and similarly with A2. If a cow has both genes, the milk has a mixed genetic profile.

Older lineages such as African and Asian cows, as well as yaks, buffalo, sheep and goats, all produce A2 milk, suggesting that A1 is either a rare variant or a recent mutation. Since wide-scale domestication of cows, selective breeding has favoured the A1 animals, which happen to have a higher milk output. The result is that only an estimated 20–40 per cent of animals in the national herd produce pure A2 milk. Jersey cows often carry A2 genes, but have had A1 genes introduced as other characteristics were selected for in the breeding programs.

In recent times, A1 milk has been linked to an increased risk of autoimmune disorders such as Type 1 diabetes. It has also been linked to premature coronary artery disease. The health issues are far from resolved. Milk sensitivity seems to have increased in the

Western world, as have the illnesses which *may* be linked to A1 milk. But whether A1 milk is in any way responsible will be hard to test.

From the dairy industry's point of view, such findings would be a disaster. Years of selective breeding would be rendered useless, and the cost would be enormous. In Australia and New Zealand, preliminary research in the early 2000s funded by a philanthropist met hostility from the dairy boards.

This is not to say that either doctors or farmers would resist change if health damage were proved. But as is so often the case, resistance and inertia are likely to slow investigation for the foreseeable future.[39]

The dairy industry employs many unnatural processes, some of which are dressed up as health improvements. Some, such as pasteurisation, probably confer real health benefits in an era of mass production. But closer scrutiny of many practices reveals that economic factors dominate.

Suspect production methods

Like all farmers, dairy farmers are under pressure to make a return on their investment. We will look at the results in breeding, housing and disease, feeding, and the use of supplements, chemicals and legal additives.

Animal breeding
One of the consequences of breeding animals for maximal milk output is the increased tendency to mastitis. Mastitis begins initially as an inflammation of the milk ducts, and rapidly spreads to include infection. Indeed, for some women the experience of mastitis is as painful a memory as the experience of childbirth itself. It is hard to imagine Mother Nature designing an animal as prone to this distress as the cow created by today's breeders. In humans or in cows, mastitis can drag on for months and can lead to long-term problems and, in extreme cases, death.

To reduce losses, the farmer often treats animals with antibiotics, possibly even administering them preventively. Inevitably the antibiotics enter the human food chain, creating bacteria that are resistant to antibiotics and, in some cases, sensitising the human recipients. An antibiotic received through milk products may alter the gut flora in babies fed cow's milk, and this can contribute to

altered immune defences. Babies who are not breastfed have a higher
rate of asthma and autoimmune problems, both in infancy and later
life. Several mechanisms operate in this regard, but neonatal exposure
to antibiotics can be one of them.

Animal housing and disease

To produce maximal returns, animals are often crowded into intense
living conditions which increase the potential for diseases such as
tuberculosis. Milk is an ideal culture in which to grow all manner of
bacteria. Friendly bugs such as the lacto and bifido bacilli thrive; but
so, too, do many pathogens.

Pasteurisation was originally developed to combat the organism
responsible for Q-fever (*Coxiella burnetii*). *Mycobacterium tuberculosis*
is well known for its ability to produce TB. Less well known is *M.
paratuberculosis*, the organism responsible for Johne's disease, which
causes debility and even death in cows, sheep, goats and alpacas
through chronic diarrhoea and wastage. The organisms that cause
Johne's disease may survive pasteurisation. They have an interesting
and at this stage unresolved relationship with human Crohn's disease
and irritable bowel syndrome. The incidence of Crohn's disease has
increased dramatically throughout the developed world, and has
begun to appear in cultures such as Japan and Asia, wherever the
Western diet is adopted. Association does not prove causality, but the
possibility must be considered.

Listeria monocytogenes is a disease which came to public notice in
the mid-1980s. At that time some well-publicised cases caused a
British government warning that soft cheeses should not be
consumed by pregnant women, babies, the elderly and the immune-
compromised. Listeria causes meningitis, septicaemia and, in 30 per
cent of all cases, death.

All of these conditions are more common where farming is
overcrowded and intensive. They are a considerable economic loss
to the farmer. Animals may die, and the infected products cannot be
sold. Pasteurisation reduces, but does not eliminate the problems.

Animal feeding

The perils of abnormal feeding practices, exemplified by BSE or
mad-cow disease, have already been discussed (see Vaccination).
Other examples include diets which differ from the wild diet,
weakening the immune system and resulting in more disease. Less

variety, fewer mineral resources from food grown with artificial fertilisers, the feeding of grain to ruminants, are all included in this catalogue. Humans are affected directly by reduction of nutrients, or indirectly by the increased medical interventions. The lack of omega-3 fatty acids in most human meat sources is an example discussed in Chapter 5.

Antibiotics and agricultural chemicals

Many animal diseases respond to antibiotics. Instead of improving the environment in which the animals live, antibiotics are frequently used — and often misused, as discussed above. Not all illnesses are responsive to antibiotics, of course, and susceptibility to viral and other infective diseases also increases with less-than-ideal living conditions. These animal illnesses may not seem to pose a threat to humans, but the BSE crisis shows our incomplete understanding of how infectious agents operate, and how they learn to jump species.

Perhaps the most worrying of all practices is the widespread use of agricultural chemicals. Obviously the long-term health effects of even individual chemicals cannot be known until they have been in use for a long time. For those which *have* been around for a few decades, the data are hardly reassuring. Many, such as the organochlorines, have been withdrawn from use as the story of their toxicity unfolds. Unfortunately, withdrawal is not always total; depending on the country concerned, usage may be left to the discretion of the farmer.

Furthermore, it has always been the practice to study the effects of a chemical as an independent variable. 'Synergism' is the phenomenon whereby the combined toxicity of any two (or more) chemicals may be far greater than the sum of their individual effects (Chapter 6). Farmers are not chemists, and yet they have at their disposal a wide range of toxic chemicals, many of which end up in the meat and milk of the cow or sheep.

Sometimes warnings come early. In the case of BSE, dangerous farming practices produced sick animals within a few years and scientists were alerted to the link when humans showed a similar affliction. By contrast, poisons may have a less visible link to the diseases they cause, especially if the animals are slaughtered before they have time to develop illness.

Sometimes, the contaminating chemicals do not produce overt disease in the intermediary animal. Dairy cows are not particularly prone to breast (udder) cancer. In Israel in 1978, a public outcry caused the government to ban certain organochlorines—benzene hexachloride, DDT and lindane. By 1986, breast cancer mortality rates had dropped by 8 per cent for all age groups, and by about 33 per cent for women in the age range 25–34. Such a reversal at a time when rates are rising elsewhere does give food for thought.[40]

Many of these organochlorine pesticides have been banned in other countries. They are still available for 'limited' agricultural use in Australia, often at the discretion of the farmer. The half-life of some of these poisons in the environment can be measured in hundreds of years. They are only slowly eliminated from the body.

The subject of breast, bowel and prostate cancer is dealt with in Chapters 4 and 7, but there is sufficient epidemiological evidence to link these cancers to the consumption of dairy products. The colloquial term in China for breast cancer translates as 'rich woman's disease'. We cannot say whether the link between cancer and the dairy products in the rich woman's diet is causal; that can only be established by the appropriate research.

A plant-based diet exposes the consumer to the chemicals in those plants, no more and no less. In eating meat, there is exposure to all the chemicals accumulated by the animal. Milk potentially poses an even greater problem. Nature has designed the breast tissues to concentrate many hormone-like molecules into milk. Unfortunately, many pesticides are now known to degrade to molecules very similar to hormones, earning them the epithet 'gender-benders'.

Legal 'additives'
Besides the pesticides and herbicides to which the cow is exposed, there are the chemicals which can be legally injected into the animal. Depending on the country concerned, these include not only antibiotics and anti-parasitic drugs, but hormones and related biological molecules.

This group includes prostaglandins and such pituitary hormones as growth hormone, oxytocin, follicle-stimulating hormone and luteinising hormone. The relationship of these hormones to cancer is no different to the relationship of any other hormone to cancer. That is to say, it is contentious: there are many studies showing strongly positive relationships, or purporting to deny them. Where the relationship between a hormone and a particular cancer is undeniable, there are arguments as to whether the hormone causes the cancer in the first place, or simply promotes it once it is there.

The consumption of cow products introduces into the human biological system many potent agents, some of them with strong links to malignant disease.

In those animals injected with hormones, the effect does not stop with the hormone itself. Bovine somatotrophin (BST), for example, causes a cascade of effects. The cow releases a chemical known as insulin-like growth factor (IGF-1). This chemical is biologically identical in all mammals, whether humans, cows, sheep or goats. It is a potent hormone involved in many bodily functions, including the activation of breast tissue in girls at puberty. Some research suggests that IGF-1 acts to promote breast cancer cells, and the same researchers believe that high IGF-1 levels are a predictor of prostate cancer.[41]

The levels of IGF-1 in cow's milk are much higher than in human milk. Selective breeding for milk yield, already discussed, has raised it further over recent decades. As many cows are kept pregnant while lactating, the level of growth-promoting hormones is likely to be at a maximum. IGF-1 is not destroyed by pasteurisation and, despite arguments to the contrary, there is a growing body of evidence that IGF-1 sufficiently survives the digestive process to have local effects on the gut, and also, by absorption, throughout the body. Local effects might include intestinal cancers, as some work has suggested that IGF-1 prevents programmed cell death (apoptosis; Chapters 7 and 10).[42]

The addition of BST or oestradiol implants has exaggerated the differences in levels of IGF-1. In the United States, BST has been authorised for widespread use since the early 1990s. In Europe, although BST is banned, it is legal to import affected dairy and beef products. Also in Australia, thankfully, BST remains banned, although a review in 2003 which covered other growth hormones with related effects concluded that use of these hormones could continue, despite their recognised potential for, and in some cases evidence of, carcinogenic, developmental and other effects.

Bread

Give us this day our daily bread.
Many of the issues surrounding the penetration of wheat into the

Western diet have already been discussed in the section on milk. In both cases, perhaps because of the opioid properties, these foods become a major constituent in the diets of the cultures which adopt them.

Before the advent of mass food production, any tendency to over-use these foods was held in check by seasonal and economic concerns. Industrialisation changed all that.

The heading 'bread', of course, includes all the gluten-containing cereals — wheat, rye, oats and barley — and products made from them such as pasta and biscuits. Like milk, these grains have been submitted to breeding programs to attain certain desirable characteristics, especially gluten content. But gluten differs from milk. We know that a very small number of people have a life-threatening allergy to milk and a much larger number feel that they have an adverse reaction to it. But within the current range of our testing skills, we cannot give a clear pathological diagnosis to this reaction.

Coeliac disease

With gluten, we have coeliac disease. We know the pathology: a component of the gluten peptide triggers a T-cell response in the mucosal lining of the gut. We have good (but not yet ideal) blood tests which show with accuracy close to 99 per cent whether a person has the disease. We can examine the gut with an endoscope, and under a microscope confirm the diagnosis to an even greater accuracy. We know that other illnesses are often associated; the list grows longer every day (Chapters 6, 7, 9 and 10).

The genetic predisposition to this illness depends on a white blood cell type (known as an HLA class II haplotype); it occurs in about 25 per cent of people of Northern European heritage, and to a greater or lesser extent in other groups. Historically, it was estimated that about one person in 2000 had coeliac disease. The current estimate is closer to one in 100.

From any perspective it is extraordinary that one person in 100 should have a life-threatening response to the staple food of their culture. And this number represents only the people with visible damage to the gut mucosa. As 25 per cent of northern Europeans have the genetic potential for gluten sensitivity, it is possible that one in four have some adverse health effect from the 'staff of life'. What has happened to bring about this situation? Clinicians agree that the rise in diagnoses reflects not only a greater awareness of the condition, but also a true increase in incidence.

The explanations are probably complex, and include a fascinating ramification of the hygiene theory (Chapter 6). But one aspect is simple; gluten in quantity is toxic to everyone. A 60-gram dose will produce nausea, even vomiting and diarrhoea, in most people. It is a plant poison. As with alkaloids and other plant poisons, humans have adapted to tolerate small doses of it.

But gluten has properties which we have found useful in cooking. It is the sticky substance which binds dough together and gives it elasticity. It is also known in agriculture as a 'heat shock protein'. As the name implies, this means that the grain produces gluten to increase its tolerance to drought and high temperatures.

It is easy to conceive how humans, rather than natural selection, cultivated grains for these characteristics. The morphine-like properties might have been another attraction. In recent times, however, with increasingly sophisticated selective breeding techniques (and the ever-present spectre of genetic modification), coupled with a growing cuisine of fast foods like pasta and pizza, the amount of gluten in wheat has reached an unprecedented level. In short, our ingenuity may have outstripped our genetic potential to adapt.

We have research tools; we have no shortage of patients. We have a fearsome list of associated serious and even lethal diseases. We do not even have to worry about expensive drugs because we have a cure as simple as diet. Yet this disease is under-researched and under-diagnosed. Even the unequivocal gut-coeliac is estimated to be missed in nine out of 10 sufferers. The possibility that illnesses more *tenuously* associated, such as schizophrenia and autism, might be treated by diet is usually met with ridicule.

Are the reasons political? Are the economic consequences of disrupting one of our main staples too great to contemplate? Or is society now addicted to these drug-foods?

SUPPLEMENTS

This last entry in the politics of health is probably the most emotionally charged of all. On the one hand is the camp which says that you can get everything you need from a good diet. I agree with that but, short of those few societies still living a traditional aboriginal lifestyle, few of us are eating a good diet. Some of us are eating good food grown in bad soils, or good food that is not fresh. More of us are eating bad food that is neither fresh nor grown in good soils.

In the second camp there is a growing number of doctors, nutritional scientists and members of the public who would prefer to err on the side of taking more vitamins and minerals than they need. Compared with the profile of misadventures with prescription-medication (Chapter 6), hospital admissions for supplement overdose are very rare, despite the millions of people worldwide who take them. I belong in this camp, and feel that most, if not all, of us should be taking regular supplements.

The reasons for this are not listed here because they are an underlying theme of the entire book. The politics are interesting, however. There is a turf war between the two camps. For example, when a pharmaceutical company in Australia called PAN was found guilty of poor quality control in April–May 2003, this became an attack on nutritional supplements in general. PAN also manufactures painkillers and motion sickness pharmaceuticals, and the problem was identified through dangerous mistakes in the dosage of this latter group. Thus dangers that appeared in the company's drug products, where quality control had failed, unleashed a tirade against a different product, nutritional supplements.

I feel that this war will eventually be won by the second camp, but it will not be a clean victory. It will come about by degrees. First we decided that salt needed iodine. Then it was the B-group vitamins added to bread—a tacit admission of guilt over food processing. Next came folic acid if we wanted to prevent babies being born with spina bifida. This was soon followed by the 'discovery'—30 years after Kilmer McCully first did the work (Chapter 8)—that using several B vitamins together was important for certain cardiovascular conditions.

Do we wait until we get these problems, or do we admit the deficits in the modern diet, and do some pre-emptive striking? One authoritative publication, the *Journal of the American Medical Association*, has joined the second camp, and was reported in various other journals under the heading 'All adults should take vitamin supplements':

Some groups of patients are at higher risk for vitamin
deficiency and suboptimal vitamin status. Many physicians
may be unaware of common food sources of vitamins or
unsure which vitamins they should recommend for their
patients. Vitamin excess is possible with supplementation,
particularly for fat-soluble vitamins. Inadequate intake of
several vitamins has been linked to chronic diseases, including
heart disease, cancer, and osteoporosis.[43]

A similar injunction about minerals has not been issued. Give
it time.

Chapter Three
HEALTH PROCESSES

Chemistry gives us the solution of all the problems of physiology, pathology and therapeutics. Without chemistry, you venture into darkness.

PARACELSUS, 1493–1541

PARACELSUS MAY HAVE LIVED over five hundred years ago, but he clearly had a grasp of the value of basic sciences. Even in the 16th century he was able to separate the various disciplines of pathology, physiology and therapeutics. Physiology represented normal function; pathology was what happened to bodily systems when they became sick; therapeutics was the treatment of the abnormal. Chemistry was the key to understanding all of these.

What he called physiology remains as a discipline. But now, because technology has helped us to understand at a microscopic level what happens in the cell, we have the new disciplines of biochemistry, immunology and genetics. All of these disciplines overlap. They represent at the microscopic level what happens in physiology. They give us a basis on which to build the model of health.

CHEMISTRY

For those who have not studied chemistry, the idea that you might have to come to grips with atomic structures, or the periodic table—just to understand why broccoli is good for you—can be daunting. But I hope that some readers find the diagrams helpful. For the rest, I suggest that you just follow the story line.

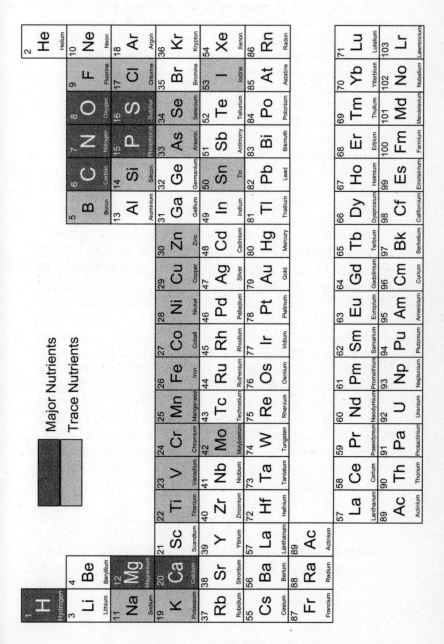

Chart 3.1: Periodic Table of the Elements

Elements

An element is the basic substance of all matter and cannot be broken down by chemical means. The naturally occurring elements range from the simplest, hydrogen, to the heaviest, uranium. Each element is made up of only one type of atom, and for general purposes, the term 'atom' can be used interchangeably with 'element'.

An atom has a nucleus which is circled by electrons arranged in orbits. The electrons, each with a negative charge, balance the positive charge of protons in the nucleus. When the number of electrons does not exactly equal the protons, there is a nett charge that can be positive or negative. Such an atom is referred to as being in the 'ionised' state.

Only the electrons in the outer orbit (or 'shell') are involved in chemical reactions. The outer shell has a maximum of eight electrons and a minimum of one.

The elements have been arranged in a chart called the Periodic Table (Chart 3.1),[1] in increasing size, such that vertical columns contain elements with the same number of electrons in the outer shell. Elements with the same configuration of the outer shell tend to have similar chemical properties. Sometimes in biology this can result in one element being substituted for another, with effects that can be good or bad. The Periodic Table indicates the roles of some key elements — major nutrients, trace elements and toxic elements. More details will be given on these in the relevant chapters of this book.

Calcium and magnesium are in the same column and look alike from the body's point of view. The importance of this is discussed in Chapter 4. Zinc, cadmium and mercury all occur in the same column. Mercury poisoning is all the more dangerous when there is a zinc deficiency. Conversely, there can be a flushing effect on mercury when the diet is rich in zinc.

Minerals

Minerals are a subset of the elements. Strictly speaking, 'mineral' is not a chemical term: it refers to those elements that can be mined. In addition to the mining done by humans, we can think of mining as one of the functions of plants in their extraction of nutrients from the soil.

It is common to refer to soil-derived nutrient elements, such as calcium and magnesium, as minerals, and to those required in lesser amounts, such as selenium and zinc, as trace elements or trace minerals.

'Metal' is another commonly used term. More than half of the elements on the periodic table can be classified as metals, based predominantly on their ability to conduct electricity. In biology, 'metal' is most often heard in the context of the toxicity of the heavy metals such as lead and mercury. However, many of the most important nutrients are metals, and so we read of 'metallo-enzymes' and so on.

The elements shown in the middle of the Periodic Table (starting at the fourth row) are often referred to as 'transition elements' because in their chemical behaviour they constitute a transition between the two left-hand columns and the six columns on the right. This chemistry makes them important in a number of biochemical reactions, particularly for their role in enzymes. Of particular note are copper, manganese, molybdenum, chromium, iron and zinc.

Molecules

When atoms combine together, the grouping is referred to as a 'molecule'. The smallest molecules have two atoms, while the largest have thousands. Many of the molecules in living organisms are very large — that is, they have thousands of atoms.

The atoms of a molecule are joined together by chemical bonds. Practically all the bonds holding together the molecules of living matter are the sort known as covalent bonds. This means that they are the result of electrons being 'shared' between adjoining atoms. Covalent bonds can be single (sharing a single electron), double (sharing two electrons), or triple (sharing three electrons).

A common type of molecule consists of a chain of carbon atoms. Fats are variations on a carbon chain. Carbon has four binding sites, and so a carbon atom can be joined by a single bond to two neighbouring carbon atoms, with two hydrogen atoms taking up the other two bonds. One of the bonds in this chain can be made a double bond by removing one hydrogen atom from each of two neighbouring carbon atoms (Chart 5.1).

If the remaining two hydrogens are on the same side of the chain it is called a *cis* bond. When they are on opposite sides of the chain it is a *trans* bond.

Free radicals and redox

A free radical is an atom or group of atoms that has an odd number of electrons — that is, it has an 'unpaired' electron. Electrons 'like' to be in pairs, so a free radical is 'restless': it will seek out and attach to any potential electron donor that it can find. Molecules that donate these electrons to free radicals are referred to as anti-oxidants.

Oxygen has a special role in chemistry. When it combines with another element, there is a change to the sharing of electrons. It obtains a share of the other element's electrons. This type of reaction is called redox, a combination of the terms oxidation and reduction. Although the name 'oxidation' implies that oxygen should be involved, it is used for any reaction which gives this same outcome. The term reducing agent is used for the element which gets a lesser share.

Both 'free radical' and 'redox chemistry' are concepts important to the understanding of biochemistry. They are discussed below under Biochemistry in Action.

BIOCHEMISTRY

Biochemistry is chemistry as it applies to living organisms. It deals with the same atoms as chemistry does, but they appear in the living micro-organisms, viruses, bacteria, algae, fungi, plants and animals which make up life on this earth.

All biological systems are made up of organic molecules, which by and large belong to one of four major classes:

- lipids (fats)
- proteins (made up of amino acids)
- carbohydrates
- nucleic acids.[2]

In turn, these molecules combine with each other to form more complex molecules. For example, a carbohydrate can combine with a protein, and we might call the product a 'glycoprotein'. Or a lipid might combine with a protein to produce a 'lipoprotein'. We look at these molecules in more detail in Chapter 4.

Mammal cells

A cell's job is twofold: to take care of its own housekeeping; and to contribute to the organism of which it is a part (Chart 3.2). The job description of a typical mammalian cell might include:

- take in an adequate supply of nutrients such as water, oxygen, glucose, amino acids, lipids, vitamins and minerals such that it can stay alive
- burn some nutrients, and store others, for energy
- dispose of its waste products, including carbon dioxide
- divide to replace older cells when they are damaged or die
- repair itself
- carry out the specific function it is designed for: a thyroid cell will make the hormone thyroxin, a muscle cell will contract, and so on
- respond appropriately to the messages sent to it from other parts of the body
- communicate with the cells around it and, in some cases, with cells in distant parts of the body.

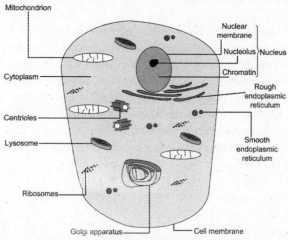

Chart 3.2: Schematic diagram of a mammalian cell

Some biochemical functions take place in almost every cell of the body, but some take place either exclusively, or predominantly, in dedicated organs such as an endocrine gland or the liver.

Enzymes

Many cellular reactions take place very slowly, because the reacting ingredients occur in low concentrations (making them unlikely to get together) or because there is a high 'activation energy'. Activation energy is like a barrier or threshold that has to be overcome before a reaction can proceed.

Enzymes speed up or catalyse many biological reactions. Enzymes are proteins, coded for by genes (more later) which help to bring the reacting ingredients together. Enzymes also help to meet or reduce the activation energy requirement. Once a set of molecules has completed a reaction, the enzyme, unchanged, goes on to facilitate further reactions.

Enzymes exist mostly in cells, although a few function in the blood, digestive tract and so on. A typical animal cell contains between 1000 and 3000 different types of enzyme. Some enzymes, such as those to do with cellular respiration or the production of energy, are almost universal; some are specific to particular cells or organs. If all the enzyme systems within a cell came to a halt, that cell would rapidly die.

Enzymes are classified into one of six groups, according to their basic chemical activity, and their names always end in -ase:

- *hydrolases and lyases:* split compounds by adding water
- *transferases:* add or subtract whole chemical 'groups' such as methyl or acetyl groups
- *oxido-reductases:* transfer electrons, thus achieving redox reactions.
- *isomerases:* produce molecules with an identical formula to the original, but a different layout
- *ligases:* form bonds between carbon and other carbons, or carbon to oxygen, nitrogen or sulphur.

Co-enzymes and co-factors

Many enzymes cannot function without the presence of co-enzymes, which are typically vitamins and minerals. In fact, one of the main functions of vitamins and (trace) minerals is to act as co-enzymes.

A co-enzyme is a small organic molecule that an enzyme utilises in the catalytic process. Not all enzymes require a co-enzyme, but many work slowly, if at all, in the absence of their particular co-enzyme. Most of the co-enzymes work by shuttling back and forth between two or more different forms—an active form and an inactive form that requires regeneration back to the active form.

A co-factor is any chemical required by an enzyme in order to function, such as a metal ion, a lipid, an accessory protein or a co-enzyme. It can include simple structures such as methyl groups. These consist basically of a single carbon atom with three hydrogens attached. Some vitamins such as folic acid are good co-enzymes because they act as a ready source of methyl groups. The addition of a methyl group to a molecule is the basis of the reaction known as 'methylation'. The importance of methylation will soon become apparent.

A metallo-enzyme is an enzyme which requires a metal as part of its *structure*. In this case, the metal is not a co-factor; it is structural. The metal is usually zinc, copper or manganese, which are all 'transitional' elements (Chart 3.1) and as such have a strong capacity to form complexes in which the metal is the central atom. The most common element to be found in metallo-enzymes is zinc.

Biochemistry in action

Biochemistry can help us to understand health and disease.

Chart 3.3 illustrates some of the biochemical pathways in the production of two neurotransmitters, serotonin and dopamine. When a brain cell is trying to communicate with other cells in the brain, it may make serotonin. It takes the amino acid tryptophan from the bloodstream, converts it to 5-OH tryptophan (5HT) and finally makes serotonin. Along the way, this reaction is catalysed by the enzymes *tryptophan oxygenase* and *5HT decarboxylase*, which in turn use Vitamins B3 and B6, and the mineral iron, as co-enzymes.

This reaction could in theory take days or months. Fortunately

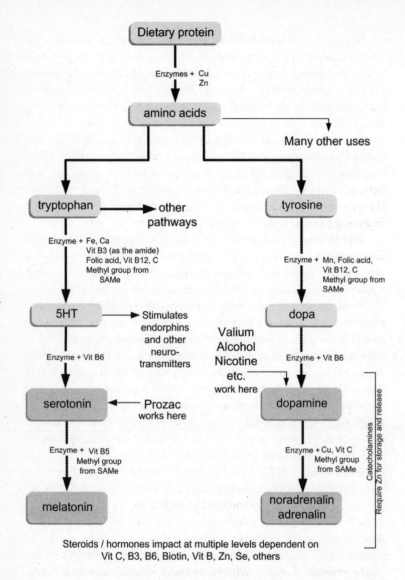

Chart 3.3: Hormones relating to mood and sleep

it is further catalysed by the biochemical reaction 'methylation', mentioned above. This occurs when another amino acid, methionine, is converted to s-adenosyl methionine (SAMe), which can act as a source of the methyl group.

However, the production of a methyl group from SAMe requires magnesium, Vitamin C, folic acid, and Vitamin B12. Some people take a commercial preparation of SAMe for depression and get good results because it raises their levels of serotonin and dopamine. Others have no response. It is not hard to see why. Low levels of nutrients such as B12 will still hold things up. SAMe represents only one cog in the machine.

Many amino acids are required as the raw material for the enzyme production line, which operates within the brain cells under the direction of genes. The genes are switched on when the cell detects a need for serotonin. When we understand that serotonin is the precursor to melatonin, the 'sleep hormone', we can see why depressed patients might have difficulty sleeping.

The diet must provide the amino acids, vitamins and minerals for this whole operation to proceed smoothly. It is no surprise that anxiety and depression are among the clinical manifestations of deficiency of magnesium, iron, B-group vitamins or protein.

SAMe is a universal methyl donor, required by almost every methylation reaction in the body. Methylation is one of the critical and most fundamental of all biochemical reactions. In health, it has roles ranging from genetic transcription to the maintenance of the health of the cardiovascular system, the joints of the skeleton and, of course, the brain (Chart 3.4).

When methylation is slow or substandard, we really begin to appreciate its role in *normal* circumstances. As such, it is a recurrent theme in our story.[3]

Homocysteine
Some truly staggering associations between raised levels of homocysteine in the blood and disease risk have been shown (Chapter 8). These include cardiovascular disease, epilepsy, Alzheimer's disease, cancer, arthritis, depression, and even the increased risk of giving birth to a child with Down syndrome.

I can think of several hypotheses about what is happening here:

- An accumulation of homocysteine is toxic in its own right.
- An elevation of homocysteine marks a deficiency of B-group vitamins, magnesium etc., and all that this implies.
- Such deficiencies slow the methylation processes so vital to life.

• An accumulation of homocysteine results in a lowered production of glutathione (derived from SAMe).

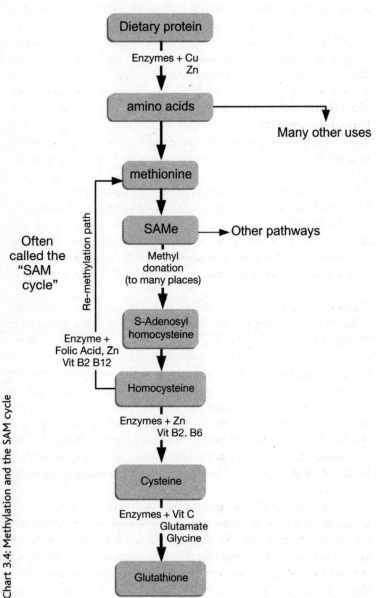

Chart 3.4: Methylation and the SAM cycle

About 50 per cent of the population have a less efficient genetic variant of one of the enzymes involved in processing homocysteine through the methionine cycle (*methylenetetrahydrofolate reductase*), and between 5 and 25 per cent of the population are homozygous for this less efficient form.[4] In such individuals, the enzyme is present but less active, thereby increasing the risk of raised blood levels of homocysteine. This could be seen as one of Mother Nature's stuff-ups, a *widespread* genetic aberration with serious health consequences. Why has this gene not bred itself out of the population?

The answer takes us to one of the major topics in this book: the 'deleterious' genes which are only unmasked by our current diets. Hunter-gatherers did not usually lack folic acid (folate); nor even does the subsistence farmer of today. Indeed, half of the population might still get away with a substandard, processed diet, but some will not.

Homocysteine is easily measured, using a fasting blood sample. High levels of homocysteine are almost certainly a greater risk to your health than high cholesterol. Unlike cholesterol, there is no drug which can lower them. To correct the level you need only magnesium, zinc and some B-group vitamins—which is probably why you have never heard of it.

Cholesterol

Cholesterol has some structural roles in the body, discussed in later chapters, and it is also the raw material for the steroid messenger molecules (Chart 3.5). These include all the sex steroids, such as oestrogen, progesterone and testosterone, and also cortisol, cortisone and aldosterone.

So important to us is cholesterol that the liver can manufacture it to compensate for any dietary lack. High dietary intake should not be assumed to be unhealthy. There are various genetic defects for the handling of cholesterol, but in most of these a moderate intake of cholesterol is not harmful. For a rare few, the situation is more serious.

Raised 'bad' cholesterol generally arises in one of two ways. First, it may be caused by the consumption of cholesterol in the processed or oxidised form, especially in processed food. In the second, the raised cholesterol could resemble homocysteine: an accumulation of the end-product is bad, but it is what it says about our biochemistry that is important. To treat raised cholesterol as the problem may

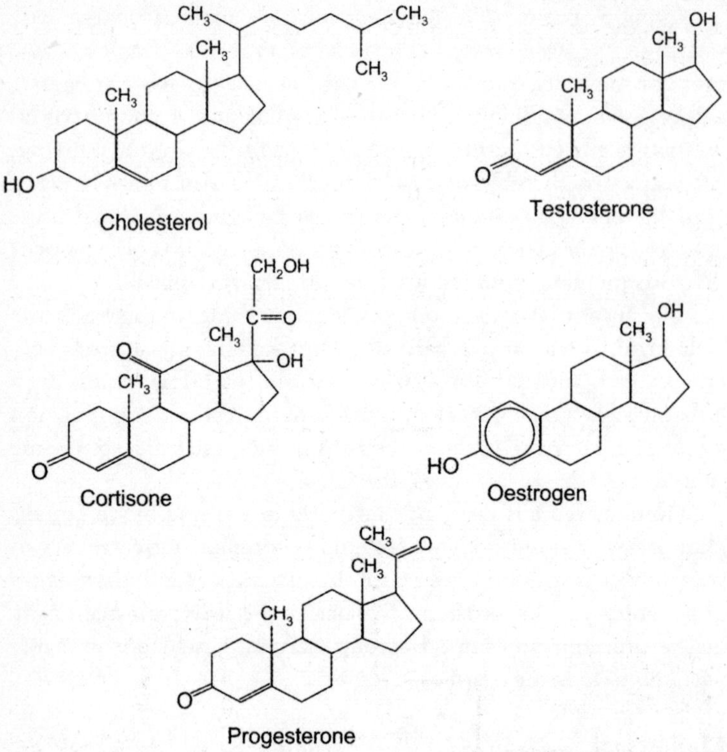

Cholesterol

Testosterone

Cortisone

Oestrogen

Progesterone

Chart 3.5: Some important steroids

amount to shooting the messenger. Perhaps the problem is that we are unable to convert cholesterol into its desired metabolites. After all, this is why Mother Nature set about ensuring that we got enough of the stuff.

Many enzymes are involved in converting cholesterol, and co-enzymes are required for many of these reactions. These co-enzymes include the B-group vitamins, Vitamin C, magnesium, zinc, selenium, boron and others. Thus many 'hormonal' disorders, not to mention stress-related illness and raised serum cholesterol, may demonstrate that a lack of these co-enzymes is interrupting the normal function of the cholesterol pathway, rather than demonstrating the 'need' for HRT, fertility treatment or cholesterol-lowering drugs.

The pathways to the production of steroids from cholesterol are set out in Chart 3.6. There is plenty of evidence to show that supplying some of the vital co-factors both reduces raised cholesterol and restores normal hormonal function. The circuit blockage has been alleviated.

Sterols

Chart 3.5 introduces the structures known as sterols. Sterols are defined by a four-ring structure as represented. These will become important shortly when we discuss gut bacteria, phyto-oestrogens and phyto-sterols, and later when we discuss gender-bending chemicals and hormone look-alikes (Chapters 6, 7 and 10).

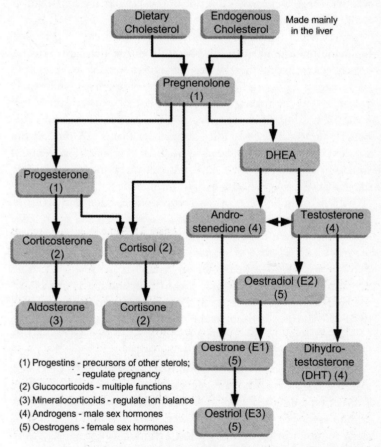

(1) Progestins - precursors of other sterols;
        - regulate pregnancy
(2) Glucocorticoids - multiple functions
(3) Mineralocorticoids - regulate ion balance
(4) Androgens - male sex hormones
(5) Oestrogens - female sex hormones

Most of these reactions are catalysed by enzymes, eg 16-hydroxylase and many require essential cofactors such as Zinc and Vitamin C. Some intermediate steps are not shown

Chart 3.6: Steroid pathways

Anti-oxidants and free radicals

Oxygen is necessary to almost all living forms. Indeed, no discussion of biochemistry would be adequate without reference to oxygen and redox chemistry. (Redox reactions were discussed earlier in this chapter.) In the simplest terms, if we think of oxygen as not only life-giving but as the source of many of the free radicals that cause so much harm in the body, anything acting as an anti-oxidant protects us from that free-radical damage. It does this by donating electrons to free radicals, thereby pairing up its unpaired or highly reactive 'free' electrons. As a result of this process the anti-oxidant itself becomes pro-oxidant.

A misunderstanding of the biochemistry involved here accounts for many myths and scare campaigns. It is true that anti-oxidants donate electrons and thereby may become pro-oxidants. Vitamin C (ascorbate) is a powerful electron donor, very non toxic, and readily available — which makes it the most important anti-oxidant. When Vitamin C donates its first electron to 'quench' a vigorous free radical, an ascorbyl free radical is initially formed. Although the ascorbyl free radical is potentially pro-oxidant because of its chemical structure, the ascorbyl free radical, relatively speaking, is much more stable than the free radical it has just quenched.

In this manner, Vitamin C (ascorbate) and other anti-oxidants 'quench' the potent free radicals that cause so much damage to cells. The ascorbyl-free radical, in turn, can self-quench with another ascorbyl radical or can donate another electron to produce dehydroascorbate (the oxidised form of Vitamin C). The dehydroascorbate is also weakly pro-oxidant and fairly unstable. In the cell, dehydroascorbate is rapidly reduced again by glutathione, thereby recycling it back to the reduced Vitamin C (ascorbate). Non–reduced dehydroascorbate breaks down quite quickly into a number of useful biochemical intermediates.

In this way, very large amounts of Vitamin C delivered intravenously or orally can quench very large numbers of free radicals. Nor does the story stop there. Some enzymatic reactions require electrons to catalyse their reactions. Vitamin C acts as an electron donor in at least eight known mammalian enzyme systems, all vital, which will be discussed presently. (See also Chapter 5.)

Two of the body's main defences against the accumulation of free radicals are anti-oxidant enzyme systems, and molecules which can act as anti-oxidants in their own right. The seleno-enzymes are a good example of the former. Vitamin C also acts as an anti-oxidant in its own right. Because a lot of Vitamin C is passed out in urine, cynics often observe that people who take supplements of Vitamin C pass 'expensive urine'. They fail to understand how metabolically active that Vitamin C has been in transit.

Ratios

In nature, vitamins, minerals and essential fatty acids tend to occur in ratios which parallel the needs of the animals and plants within their ecosystem. Not only is there a minimum absolute requirement of nutrients, but for the health of the organism the *ratio* in which these nutrients occur is very important.

A move away from a natural diet produces not only deficiency disorders, but imbalance of nutrients. Table 3.1 gives some examples of nutrient ratios which have been identified as causing problems to biochemical systems. Other examples are suspected, but have yet to be identified or quantified.

Table 3.1: Some important ratios in biochemical systems

Ratio	Ideal estimated (approx.)	Level in current Western diet (approx.)
omega-3 EFAs to omega-6 EFAs	1:1	1:16
magnesium to calcium	2:3	1:8
potassium to sodium	5:1	1:2

THE IMMUNE SYSTEM

Immunology shows that is impossible to separate 'biochemistry' from 'immunology' from 'genetics' from 'molecular biology'. The same nutrients, the same stressors, the same defence mechanisms, all crop up. Still, the distinctions help to corral a vast amount of medical knowledge into digestible pieces.

The immune system evolved to protect complex organisms from invasion by pathogens (germs, viruses, etc.). These pathogens can enter the body in two ways:

- They may gain access across barriers such as skin and mucous membranes, which, of course, have been designed to resist such invasion. Other barriers are hair (especially in the nostrils, the ear canals and the pubic region), stomach acid, wax, oil from oil glands, and genital secretions.
- They may gain direct access, as in the case of a flesh wound. The 'wounds' may be large, as happens in trauma, or small, as with an insect bite or vaccination.

Over time, the immune system has come to counter threats other than pathogens. Thus pollens, foreign bodies, food allergens and even animal dander have become targets of the immune response. The immune system is made up of both cells and organs, and these can be divided into further categories.

Cellular components

The immune system has three main kinds of cells: leukocytes, auxiliary cells and tissue cells.

Leukocytes

These cells, also known as 'white cells', may be subdivided into three groups. In varying degrees they reflect the evolution of the immune system from simple to complex.

- *Phagocytes* are named from the Greek *phagos*, 'devouring'. Phagocytes do just that; they engulf the invader or swallow it whole. Phagocytes are non-specific. If they recognise anything as foreign, they will try to swallow it. They are therefore regarded as a primitive (but effective) part of the immune system.
- *Lymphocytes* are the predominant cell of the 'lymphatic system' and are also common in the bloodstream. They include B-cells and T-cells (B-lymphocytes and T-lymphocytes), and their actions are much more sophisticated than simply swallowing the enemy. B-cells produce antibodies after they 'recognise' a *specific*

threat. T-cells produce chemical messengers known as *cytokines*, designed to kill cells which are virally infected. T-cells have entered common parlance through the understanding of HIV-AIDS. We will learn more about T-cell function, in terms of Th1 and Th2 responses, in later chapters. Another kind of lymphocyte is known as a large granular lymphocyte (LGL); it can produce cytokines, and is also good at recognising cells which are somehow wrong. It can 'nuke' such cells, which gives it the name 'natural killer' or NK cell.

- *Basophils* produce inflammatory mediators, such as histamine and serotonin. These mediators are helpful in protection against parasites, but their actions are wide-ranging.

Auxiliary cells

This term includes mast cells and platelets. (Basophils can also be classified as auxiliary cells, just to show that classification was not meant to be easy.) Auxiliary cells have various functions, but in the context of this chapter, their role is to produce inflammatory mediators. (See Inflammation on page 96.)

Tissue cells

Ordinary body cells often act as part of the immune system. These cells produce *cytokines,* including various *interferons*. Cytokines are small proteins which are responsible for speeding up and slowing down immune reactions. They usually act on the cells which produced them, or on the cells in their immediate vicinity. More than 100 human cytokines have been identified, and more are being discovered all the time. They rarely act in isolation but are part of the complex network of immune response. Some of the better-known cytokines include interleukins, interferons, tumour necrosis factors and growth factors.

Organs

Any individual cell may have immune function, but when we think of the immune system in structural terms, it is usually the lymphatic system which we have in mind.

The organs include the spleen, the bone marrow, the thymus gland, lymph glands or 'nodes', and patches of lymph tissue in the lining of the gut, the respiratory tree and the genito-urinary tract. We know some of these without thinking of them as part of our immune system. For example, the tonsils and adenoids in humans are an aggregate of lymphoid tissue in the respiratory tract. When they are surgically removed, we lose part of our immune system. As often as not, this surgery represents shooting the messenger.

By contrast with the tonsils, the gut-associated lymphoid tissue (GALT) does not have a high profile. You probably have not heard of it. It is so important to health that I shall discuss it separately below, (see also Chapter 6).

Connecting all of the lymph tissues are low-pressure channels called lymph vessels, through which lymphatic fluid flows. The lymphocytes can travel between both blood and lymph systems.

Inflammation

We all recognise inflammation, with its redness, swelling, and usually a degree of tenderness. Although this can represent the painful side of a wound or infection, and is certainly the means by which allergic reactions promote discomfort, it clearly has a purpose.

As blood flow increases and capillaries become more permeable, there is an influx of enzymes, antibodies and other immune molecules into the trouble site. The swelling and hardness act as a physical barrier to contain the infection or immune challenge to that part of the body under threat. This limits further spread of associated germs, antigens or toxins. Such a response occurs when the cells of the immune system release chemicals known as 'inflammatory mediators'. Some inflammatory mediators are histamine, serotonin, platelet-activating factor (PAF), bradykinen, certain prostaglandins and leukotrienes. Cytokines are also part of this process.

Inflammation is about waging war on 'bad guys', and there are a few rules. You don't go to war to keep the soldiers occupied; you do it to keep a real threat at bay. You keep your soldiers well equipped and feed them properly. You watch out for trigger-happy soldiers and discipline them. And, most importantly, you make sure that no one dies from friendly fire.

The inflammatory mediators are the foot soldiers. It is this aspect of the protective process which is jeopardised by the Western diet

(Chapters 5 and 6).

There are also factors which can provoke an inappropriate or ineffective inflammatory response. Chronic exposure to toxic chemicals is one such situation. This is tantamount to increasing the ranks of the enemy while poisoning the troops you expect you fight it. The various ways in which the immune response can become pathological are discussed in Chapter 6.

The gut's contribution to immunity

Gut bacteria are found in most species, including the invertebrates. These bacteria are also known as bowel or intestinal flora, friendly bacteria or normal commensals. The generic term is 'probiotic'.

Such friendly bacteria are found throughout the entire length of the intestinal tract, from mouth to anus. Concentrations are lower in the stomach, increase markedly in the small bowel, and are maximal in the large bowel. Several hundred species are known, and others await identification. Their distribution varies according to the location in the gut, and the stage of life of the host organism.

Most of the species of these bacteria cultured for humans belong to the lactic acid genera. Patients often assume that this means they come from milk, but it just signifies that they can be grown on milk. The predominant species include:

- *Lactobacilli:* There are many of these, the best-known being *Lactobacillus acidophilus*, and thus one often hears the term 'acidophilus' as if it were a generic.
- *Bifidobacteria:* The bifidobacteria are phylogenetically different to lactic acid bacteria, but have many similarities in their ecology and function.
- *Another group of non-lactic acid bacilli:* Sometimes used therapeutically, this group includes such species as non-pathogenic *E. coli* and saccharomyces.
- *Other bacteria:* These await identification, but they may play a vital role in immunology in the future. In this regard we should remember that 95 per cent of all gut bacteria are anaerobes — which means that they can only thrive where there is no oxygen. This has severely limited our study of them, but other researchers are working to overcome the technical problems with

promising outcomes.[5] See also Chapter 6, Postscript 2008: Where are we now?

The bacteria to date that are most commonly isolated from the gut, and whose various contributions to the overall picture are therefore best known, are *L. acidophilus, L. rhamnosus, L. casei, Bifidobacterium bifidum* and *B. longnum*. Human babies have a predominance of bifidobacteria, and probiotic treatment in infants is best done with *B. bifidum*.

Other micro-organisms in the gut include yeasts, moulds and fungi. It is the task of the friendly bacteria to keep these, and pathogenic(disease-causing) bacteria, in line. When the normal flora is out of balance, or unfriendly micro-organisms are present, the resulting ill-health is known as 'gut dysbiosis'.

It may be damaging for the human ego to regard ourselves as a colony, but there are about 90 trillion bacteria living on or in us, and a mere 10 trillion cells making up the rest of our body. Some of the 90 trillion are resident on our skin and in our noses, throats and genital tracts. The majority, however, occupy our gut, somewhere between the mouth and the anus.

These little single-cell organisms are much smaller than the other cells in our body, but altogether the gut bacteria weigh a couple of kilograms. Mother Nature is unlikely to put kilograms of anything in the body without a reason. These bugs have more functions than one would have dreamed of:[6]

- *Immune activity:* The gut bacteria do not simply support the immune system, *they are physically part of it.* As this is possibly the most important of all their functions, I shall return to it shortly.
- *Vitamin manufacture:* Although the full extent of their contribution has yet to be identified, we know that the bifidobacteria produce Vitamins B1, B2, B5, B6, and Vitamin K. One subspecies produces biotin. Other bacteria are thought to produce folic acid , and there is even the possibility that Vitamin B12 can be produced in the gut.
- *Bacteriocide production:* The gut bacteria produce chemicals which can destroy unfriendly bacteria. There is no quicker way of curing 'Bali belly' than to swallow some

of these little bugs regularly until things settle down. The vitality of the locals' gut flora has been proposed as one of the mechanisms by which they can often resist the diarrhoea which afflicts the traveller in an endemic area. (This is thought to include protection against such feared diseases as cholera and typhoid.)

- *Anti-virals:* The rotavirus responsible for much viral gastroenteritis has proved vulnerable to the friendly bacteria, as have moulds and yeasts.
- *Detoxification of poisons:* Many otherwise toxic substances appear to be broken down by the activity of the gut flora.
- *Gut repair:* The leaky gut is of growing interest in health (Chapter 6). Gut bacteria have a significant role in the repair of the leaky gut.
- *Digestion:* By assisting in acid balance and other environmental controls, the gut bacteria aid in the digestion of foodstuffs. They help digest the soluble fibre in food such as beans, lentils and other legumes, which then become the source of the short-chain fatty acids (SCFAs; see below and Chapter 7). Full digestion, of course, is the first step in the reduction of the food reactions that contribute to irritable bowel, migraine, asthma, chronic sinusitis and other related conditions. Gut bacteria play an important role in the prevention of these common health problems.

But there is more. These bugs not only to talk to each other (by means of chemical signalling and even the exchange of genetic material), but to the cells of the body. This is proving to be the most intriguing facet of their behaviour, with significant implications for our immune system.

Gut-associated lymphoid tissue (GALT)

Along the 7.5 metres of gut, and in the massive curtain-like structure (omentum) from which the gut is suspended, lie numerous lymph glands. These glands are in direct communication with the extensive lymph tissue situated in the gut wall. This includes dedicated islands of lymphatic cells (Peyer's patches), and widely disseminated lymphocytes such as T-cells.

Even the appendix, long thought to be a vestigial remnant from an ancestral predecessor, is now considered to be a significant part of the GALT. It is interesting to note that Crohn's disease sometimes first shows up in the appendix. As Crohn's is an immune disorder, its presence in the appendix may signal an immune system under siege.

The immune system of the gut is separate from the immune system of the circulation, and it functions differently. The lymphocytes of the gut 'home' back to the gastrointestinal tract, and do not remain in the mainstream circulation. This is in direct contrast to the rest of the body, where lymphocytes readily transit from the lymphatic circulation to liver, from liver to bloodstream, and back again.

This does not imply that these two arms of the immune system do not talk to each other. They most certainly can and do, through the cytokines and other immune messengers. The real point here is to understand just how specialised and important the gut and GALT are.

Foreign matter can enter our bodies through the air we breathe, through the skin, through sexual contact, and through the gut. Under normal circumstances, the amount of germs, pollution, pollen or dust-mites we inhale would be measured in micrograms to grams. The skin is such an effective barrier that it takes a significant wound to bring more than a tiny amount of anything in contact with the body's tissues. (The subject of deliberately injecting foreign matter was dealt with in Chapter 2: Vaccination; but this, too, is usually in very small amounts.) Seminal fluid is measured in grams.

By startling contrast, the amount of foreign matter, including highly reactive foreign proteins, which goes daily through the gut in the form of food and fluids is measured in kilograms. Most of this is not just in transit. It requires active absorption and assimilation, and may be 'contaminated' with immeasurable numbers of micro-organisms. It is hardly surprising therefore that the gut should have a sophisticated immune system of its own.

This is perhaps best imagined if you think of drinking a glass of milk. Assuming you are one of those who still produce the gut enzyme lactase into adulthood, and that you have no antibodies to milk proteins, then within an hour or so you will have digested the milk. Proteins, fats and sugars in the milk will have entered your bloodstream, providing you with amino acids for tissue regeneration, and fats and sugars for energy.

If by contrast, we draw that same glass of milk into a large syringe and inject it slowly into your vein, within an hour or so you will be dead, or in the intensive care ward fighting for your life.

What has gone on in the gut that renders this glass of milk safe for most of us to drink? Why is an injection of milk lethal? Certainly one reason for the danger is the physical properties of the milk. But equally important are the chemical and immunological responses that injecting it would provoke. One factor determining uneventful passage through the gut barrier is the immunological phenomenon known as 'the development of oral tolerance'.

The medical profession has more questions than answers about oral tolerance. We have learned that it begins at weaning, and that as a result of it, food antigens, recognised as foreign by the immune system of the small intestine, do not cause a reaction because the immune response is suppressed.

We know that breast milk possesses a chemical called *transforming growth factor beta*, a natural immunosuppressive agent. Breast milk may assist, but cannot be essential to, the development of oral tolerance. We know that oral tolerance is essential to survival, and that only minor abnormalities are compatible with life. We know that one of these abnormalities is coeliac disease (Chapters 2 and 6).

Perhaps the study of the gut bacteria is beginning to unlock some of the secrets of oral tolerance. By looking at the bacterial environment in the developing infant gut, maybe we will gain insight into the rising incidence of food allergies and autoimmune disease. For suggestions on maintaining gut health, see Appendix 3.

Getting it right
If we are to employ our knowledge of gut bacteria to better support our immune system, we need to understand what happens immediately during and after birth.

The general consensus is that *in utero* the foetal gut is completely sterile. During the birth process and the early hours of life the infant acquires and swallows micro-organisms from the birth canal, the hands of those assisting the birth, the skin of its mother, and the nipple it sucks.

Evidence is accumulating that these micro-organisms take their cues from chemical signals along the length of the gut, and, 'as part of an intensively interactive community that has been honed by millions of years of co-evolution … guides early colonisation'.[7] It seems that the bacteria might actually determine which part of the genome (the collection of human genes in its entirety) in any one intestinal cell might be turned on or off.

It is amazing to think that the actions of the bacteria might have localised effects on cell differentiation. Even more amazingly, the bacteria might also influence the subsequent *behaviour* of those cells. When we pause to consider that this includes immune cells, we realise the immensity of the possibility. The presence of normal healthy gut bacteria in the early weeks of life may exert lifelong immune benefit. Even when the *mother* supplements with good bacteria in pregnancy, the baby's risk of later asthma and eczema is reduced (Chapter 6).

The laboratory evidence indicates that these little bugs are the unsung heroes of the immune system. Unlike most micro-organisms, many gut bugs can pass through the protective lining of the gut wall and stimulate macrophages (one of the two main kinds of phagocyte). There are studies under way in human babies to determine what effect the bacterial count in early life has on later immune function.

At a clinical level, there is already a wealth of circumstantial evidence. Let us look at some of it.

Hygiene

Hygiene as a factor in immune disorders is discussed in Chapters 2, 6 and 7. Theories surrounding gut bacteria deserve at least as much attention. The intestine of a three-day-old baby from the slums of Lahore in Pakistan is likely to be teeming with intestinal bacteria, but a Swedish baby may have none, even when it is a week old.[8] This cannot be written off as racial difference, any more than could the differences across the Berlin wall or between urban Aboriginal children in Australia and their desert cousins (Chapter 6).

Birth-order also has a significant impact on the later development of allergic illness. Firstborns have more allergic problems than their siblings. And the benefits seem to accrue as the number of children in the family increases. There are a couple of possible explanations for this. One is that older children bring home more respiratory germs. Equally important, however, those big brothers and sisters impart gut flora through kissing, sucking the baby's fingers, giving the baby their fingers to suck, sharing food, and so on. 'Wash your hands before you play with the baby' runs counter to thousands of years of natural human behaviour.

Coeliac disease may represent yet another side of this story. In Chapter 2 we saw that its *prevalence* is on the increase, and this increase seems to be more common in developed nations. Asians living in a Western culture move from a low rate of coeliac to a higher one. Research indicates that better diagnostic facilities do not explain these differences. Like most medical problems, the causes of coeliac disease will prove to be multiple. If one in four Westerners have the genes for gluten sensitivity but only one in 25 of those go on to develop full coeliac disease of the gut, what else is happening? We know that breastfeeding is protective, but only partially. Gut bacteria may be the missing link.

A done deal

What do these little gut bugs ask in return for these multiple services? Their requirements are much the same as our own — congenial housing, shelter, companionship, interesting and productive employment, and a square meal.

For a square meal they like resistant starches and soluble fibre, such as are found in asparagus, sweet potato, onions and garlic, baked beans, red kidney beans, lentils, and the whole range of foods known as 'phyto-oestrogens'. They also consume some of the sugars, lipids and proteins in the gut, and although this could be seen as competition with our own needs, the losses are small and the benefits considerable. Included in their mixed diet are dead cells from the gut wall, bacterial debris, bile acid wastes, and some surplus cholesterol. In return for a small energy supply, they not only contribute to immune function, they modify blood lipid and cholesterol levels, and act as all-purpose waste disposal units as well.

Matters might end there, with food in exchange for services. But with an efficiency typical of Mother Nature, even the waste products of their digestion prove to be invaluable.

To make beer or wine, we take a sugary liquid and add yeasts. The yeast consumes the sugars, and as a by-product of its digestion gives us alcohol and some vitamins. Similarly, when the friendly bacteria in the gut consume their mixed diet, the by-products are vitamins and some *short-chain fatty acids* (SCFAs). The latter include lactic, acetic, propionic, citric, hippuric, orotic and butyric acid. The SCFAs have various functions that we know about, and others that we have yet to fully understand.

Three SCFAs; acetic, propionic and butyric (acetate, propionate and butyrate), have been shown to affect the manner in which tissues normally regenerate themselves, avoid inflammation, and destroy cancer cells.[9] SCFAs are fundamental to these processes. They readily enter the bloodstream. They are one of the main reasons why gut bacteria can modify, or even prevent, conditions as diverse as irritable and inflammatory bowel disease, various cancers, autoimmune disorders, psoriasis, asthma, eczema and arthritis.

Let us take butyric acid (or butyrate), for example. It supplies up to 70 per cent of the energy required by epithelial cells in the colon. The epithelium is the single layer of cells which lines the entire length of the gut. Butyric acid is also believed to induce enzymes such as *transglutaminase*, which is involved in mucosal repair, and *glutathione transferase*, an important redox enzyme. Research has suggested that a disturbance of butyrate metabolism is the underlying problem in ulcerative colitis. Colonic irrigation with butyric acid has been shown to induce remission in patients with active ulcerative colitis.[10] There is little doubt that butyrate is a key player in the prevention of colonic cancer, and possibly breast, prostate and liver cancers as well. Its role in gene transcription is discussed shortly under Genetics.

SCFAs are thought to be one of the means by which gut bacteria help to reduce the population of undesirable organisms in the gut, including some of the most dangerous pathogens. Acetic acid, produced predominantly by *B. bifidum* and *B. longum* in combination with lactic acid (see below), has been found to inhibit the growth of the organisms that cause typhoid and bacillic dysentery, and the infections caused by salmonella, golden staph and pathogenic *E. coli*.

SCFAs also affect micro-organisms that exist as normal gut dwellers, or 'commensals', but which can cause problems if they increase in numbers or develop into a virulent strain. *Helicobacter pylori*, the much vilified 'causative agent' in peptic ulcer disease, is found in the stomachs of up to 80 per cent of healthy individuals. It is suspected that this organism is problematic only when abnormal conditions allow its numbers to proliferate. In fact, helicobacter is now being researched as 'one of humanity's oldest and closest companions', a possible protective agent against oesophageal cancer and other diseases of the digestive tract.[11] Indeed, there is even research suggesting that infection with helicobacter may protect against obesity (Chapter 8), allergy and asthma (Chapter 7). We know that *L. acidophilus* and *L. casei* control the growth of helicobacter by the production of acetic acid, hydrochloric acid and, particularly, lactic acid. So is the development of peptic ulcers just another example of bacterial imbalance?

Acetic acid, the principal SCFA found in the gut lumen, has been found effective against a wide range of yeasts, moulds and bacteria.

In low numbers, the candida organism is probably a normal gut commensal. Patients who are suffering from a candidal infection complain of feeling 'groggy' all the time. The overgrowth of yeast in the gut can produce alcohol by the process described above. In the presence of sufficient dietary sugar, even the staunchest teetotaller can produce low levels of blood alcohol. No wonder people can find sugary diets addictive, and children living on junk food can behave irrationally. Only in the case of severe immune compromise, such as HIV-related illness or chemotherapy, are the means truly lacking to bring commensals such as candida under control.

Propionic acid has important roles beyond the gut: it helps balance hormone levels through its ability to stimulate the liver to produce sex hormone binding globulin (SHBG) (Chapters 6 and 7).

SCFAs are not the only means by which gut microflora can reduce numbers of unfriendly colonisers. Other by-products of the fermentation process include hydrogen peroxide and carbon dioxide. As already noted, they can produce specific bacteriocins, chemicals which are most accurately designated 'nature's antibiotics.'

Although not part of the gut, the vagina in females and urethra in both sexes are similarly colonised by friendly bacteria. They are both vulnerable to infection, and are normally colonised by specific strains of lactobacilli. Culture of vaginal lactobacilli has found them to act against a wide range of urogenital organisms, including chlamydia, gardnerella, and ureaplasma urealyticum. Any comments in later chapters about the mistreatment of gut flora are pertinent to these organisms as well.

GENETICS

And the end of all our exploring
Will be to arrive where we started
And know the place for the first time.
— T. S. Eliot, *Four Quartets*

Chromosomes

It is possible to understand the really exciting stuff about genetics without discussing the terminology or the structure of the famous double helix. This would be a pity, however, as the reality is quite poetic.

The double helix is often likened to a ladder, two longitudinal strands joined by rungs. Because this ladder is twisted, it is best to think of it as a rope ladder. Another image is a double-stranded string of pearls.

One half of this double helix or rope ladder or string of pearls is the basic unit. In chemical terms, the pearls are called *bases*. The pearls are attached to every second link of a chain. There are two kinds of links and they alternate. In chemical terms, one kind of link is called a *phosphate*, and the other is a sugar molecule called a *ribose*. The pearls are attached to the ribose links.

The two strands lie side by side, with the pearls opposite each other. Each pearl has an invisible bond *across* to the pearl opposite it in the complementary strand. Although we cannot see this bond, the chemistry is sufficiently real that the bond can be represented as a thread (or a rung on the ladder). The pearls come in four different varieties — cytosine, thymine, guanine and adenine — each known by their first letter. C and T are slightly smaller than G and A.

Along the strands the pearls are held together by the chain, and the pearls can occur in any order at all. This is called the 'sequence' and it may read like this: CGGATTGAGCCTAGCTTTACCTAG AAC. However, the invisible bonds *across* the two strands are much more specialised. Not only does a large pearl link only with a small one, but C will only link with G, and A with T.

Despite the apparent randomness of the long sequences, knowing the pearl sequence of either strand makes the sequence of the other

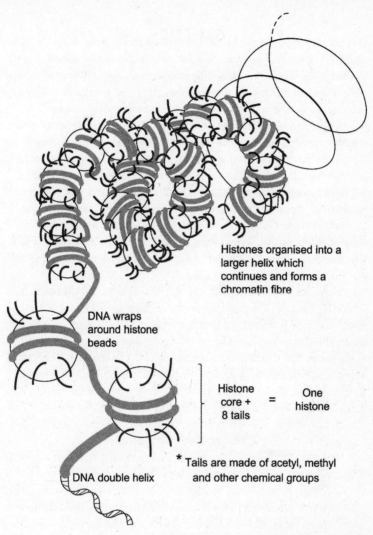

Histones organised into a
larger helix which
continues and forms a
chromatin fibre

DNA wraps
around histone
beads

Histone
core +
8 tails

=

One
histone

* Tails are made of acetyl, methyl
and other chemical groups

DNA double helix

Chart 3.7: Histone beads

strand entirely predictable. This is because every pearl must link
with the one opposite it, and will only link with its special partner.

In chemical terms, the smaller pearls are *pyrimidines* and the
larger ones *purines*. T and C are pyrimidines; A and G are purines.
The pyrimidines automatically seek out the purines, and vice versa.

The necklace is very, very long. In fact, in each chromosome
there are between 100 million and 300 million pearl-pairs. Each of
the two strands is known as a *nucleotide polymer* or a *nucleic acid*.

Linked together, the two strands have the name *deoxyribonucleic acid* or DNA. End to end, the double strand can be regarded as one molecule of DNA. And this one single molecule, with a few extra decorations, represents one *chromosome*. In some primitive life forms the ends would join because their chromosomes are circular.

In the genetic make-up of humans, there are 23 types of these double-stranded necklaces. In a fortunate vote for simplicity, they have been numbered from 1 to 23. Every person has two versions of each strand—one from mum and one from dad—giving a total of 46.

The necklaces have a natural tendency to twist, like streamers. More than that, these extremely long necklaces also have a tendency to 'pack', as if the streamers were trying to condense themselves into shorter, thicker ropes. Theoretically, there are different ways in which the necklaces could pack, but one way seems to be the preferred option. It might be imagined thus.

In the nucleus, along with the 46 double-stranded necklaces, are some large 'beads'. They are all much the same, and they are complex. Each of them is actually made up of eight smaller protein pieces, wedged tightly together. This is called the histone core. Each of the eight pieces has a little 'tail' protruding. This makes the 'bead' look hairy, as eight little fronds protrude from every bead. These hairy beads, with their tails, are called histones; they are not part of the necklace as such, but the necklace seems to wrap naturally around them.

DNA makes proteins

The whole purpose of DNA is to make proteins.

On the chromosome, bases or 'pearls' are strung along the necklace in a sequence that constitutes a highly specific code. Every set of three pairs codes for one *amino acid*. The next set of three codes for another, and so on. By reading the code, one triplet at a time, the mechanism exists for assembling amino acids, one by one, in the order dictated by the code. Amino acids, put together one by one in this manner, build up a *peptide*. Peptides put together build up a *polypeptide*, which is the basic unit of a *protein*. So if we 'read' along the necklace, we have the recipe for the different proteins, one by one.

A *gene* then, is a strip of the DNA with the code for a particular protein written on it. A slightly more formal definition is 'a nucleic acid sequence which codes for a functional polypeptide'. How many base pairs there are in any one gene depends on the complexity of the protein in question.

DNA is often referred to as a library, because of the information it contains. Under normal circumstances, the cell makes good use of this library, and is in no doubt about how, when and why its genetic material is read. It has good mechanisms for recognising where one gene ends and another starts, when one gene needs to be turned on, another off.

DNA is a library with a lot of activity. Books are being pulled off the shelf, consulted, photocopied and replaced all the time. However, there is one special feature about this library. Almost every cell in the organism contains the *whole* library, but depending on which cell it is, it only ever uses a small section of it. Thus a liver cell has not only all the instruction books it needs to operate as a liver cell, it also has the books on how to be a nerve cell, a heart cell, a kidney cell, and so on. It just never consults them. At least, that is what we think at this stage of understanding of genetics. (A stem cell, incidentally, is one which still is able to consult the whole library. It retains the ability to become any kind of cell. It has not yet become typecast.)

Notwithstanding this apparent wastage, the books that any one cell *does* need are in constant usage. When the cell needs to make a protein, either for its own use or to put into general circulation, it sends a messenger molecule into the nucleus. This molecule finds the right gene, and that bit of DNA unwinds. An enzyme in the nucleus (one of the librarians, let us say), unzips the gene for that protein, right down the middle, breaking the bond between the bases.

Floating around in the nucleus are other bases, sugars and phosphates, 'on call' as it were. These molecules attach themselves to the exposed edges of the zip, following the rules about base-to-base. The rules have altered just a bit. G still bonds to C, but A bonds not to T, but to another base called Uracil (or U), which is chemically very similar. Another difference is that the sugar that will be used this time is a *ribose*, not a *deoxyribose*. The 'photocopy' therefore is a slightly edited version of the original, and is called RNA rather than DNA.

At this stage the photocopy is just that: a blueprint of the instructions for making the protein. The enzyme, or librarian, then clips the photocopy off the original, and the newly made RNA (known as mRNA, 'm' for 'messenger'), travels back out of the nucleus and into the cytoplasm of the cell, where it 'docks' at a structure called a *ribosome*. The ribosome is a small and efficient factory, well equipped with the raw materials (amino acids) and personnel (transfer RNA, or tRNA) for reading the code and manufacturing the desired protein. Simple!

The cell is a constant production line, making the proteins that it needs to. Because the data are constantly accessed, the chromosomes are often in a state of undress in those places where they are unzipped.

Cell division

Two types of cell division are possible: mitosis and meiosis.

- *Mitosis:* When cells in an organ have undergone some kind of damage, or have simply worn out, a younger cell divides to replace the loss. The aim here is to ensure that new cells are as near as possible the same as the cells being replaced. All the chromosomes are unzipped from end to end, and attach to the available sugars, phosphates and bases in the nucleus. This is like the photocopy described above, but instead of just a part of the necklace (a gene), becoming unzipped, it is the whole necklace. Inevitably some mistakes are made during duplication. There is also a change in the length of the *telomeres*, the point at which the chromosomes pair up in cell division. These changes and mistakes are the basis of the ageing process.
- *Meiosis:* The other kind of cell division is by the formation of *gametes*, the reproductive cells (sperm and eggs). The genetic material is divided into halves during this process so the sperm and egg each carry only 23 chromosomes instead of the full set of 46. The chromosomes seek out their 'twin' (*non*-identical), known as the 'homologous chromosome'. The result of this process (and of some gene swapping as well), is that the maximum genetic mix is achieved, and the gamete gets a good mix of the characteristics of two grandparents. As the same thing happens in the formation of both sperm and egg, the chances are that the genes of all four grandparents are well represented in the resultant offspring.

Genetic variation

If human chromosomes are so predictable, how come we all look different? The fact is that variations in the code, or gene, for a particular characteristic are not only possible, but essential. Otherwise, we would all be clones.

The differing versions of a particular gene result in a protein that is not quite the same as someone else's protein. But it will still do the job. This is most evident when you compare not individuals but species. The insulin molecule, for example, starts out as a polypeptide (protein) chain of about 108 amino acids. From species to species there are some minor variations in these amino acids, and thus, we can assume, some slight variations in the base pairs which coded for them. But human diabetics have used insulin from cows and pigs, with only minor problems.

When there are minor functional variations of a particular gene *within* a species, we say that there are different *alleles* of that gene. Or we say that the gene exhibits *polymorphism*.

If the variations do not matter, the different alleles will persist in the species. Some variations may even confer benefit. Skin colour is a good example. Prior to the mass migrations of the past few centuries, people who lived around the equator all had dark skin. This protected them from the harshness of the sun's rays. As people moved north, those who had lighter-coloured skin tended to survive better. Fair skin admitted adequate light for the manufacture of Vitamin D, giving these migrants an advantage (Chapter 5).

Some variations matter enormously. The alteration of a single amino acid can so distort the structure of the resultant protein that it can no longer do the job. The shape of the protein may be so critical that no variations are allowable. Such mutations either result in disease, or are altogether incompatible with life.

Variations in genes give us the vigour that enables a species to thrive. When an organism makes a 'mistake' during the process of gamete formation as a result of background radiation, chemical input or some other factor, then a new gene is created. If the new gene is deleterious to health, it may kill the person who carries it, and it will not be passed on. If it has some advantage, it may survive and flourish. Eventually it may become the most common allele.

Sometimes, although the new gene causes ill-health, it also confers some benefit and thus survives. The best example of this is the genes for thalassaemia and sickle-cell anaemia. Both of these genes are most prevalent in the areas where malaria is endemic. Malaria has killed up to half of all the people who have ever lived, so any gene which gives a defence against malaria has something going for it. The mutations which cause thalassaemia and sickle-cell anaemia distort the red blood cells in such a way that they can cause health problems for the person carrying those genes. However, the malaria organism finds it harder to parasitise these oddly shaped cells because they are less suitable for incubating its larval phase, which therefore does not thrive. Because the people carrying the genes gain partial protection from the scourges of malaria, those genes survive. Unfortunately, the people who get a double dose of the gene (one from each parent) have such distorted red cells that they often have shortened lives and much ill-health.

Cystic fibrosis provides another example. With increased understanding of genetics we came to realise that this disease was in fact many diseases, only one or two of which caused serious illness. Others caused minor problems, and some were not much different to the healthy alleles. Here again there is the suggestion of benefit for the 5 per cent of Caucasians who carry just one copy of a defective allele. The resulting alteration in sodium and chloride metabolism not only produces salty sweat (a marker for cystic fibrosis), but also offers protection against diarrhoea, and therefore cholera.

Then there is the case of lipoprotein (a), which is discussed later as a possible contributor to heart disease. However, it appears that it may have protected us from scurvy (see Chapter 8: Cardiovascular disease).

There are about 30,000 genes in the human genome, but only a relative few are known for the trouble they cause. This is because some structures are inherently stable no matter what you do to them, and some are not. If you remove a brick from the top of a pile of bricks, the change will go unnoticed. Remove the keystone from an arch, and the whole arch will fall in. Depending on both the location of the amino acid and the *design of the original molecule*, a change in one or more of the amino acids will cause anything from 'no effect' through to catastrophe. Some proteins coded for by our genes are structurally robust, so slight alterations are of no consequence. Others are fragile; they can tolerate little alteration, or no alteration at all.

The effects of 'bad' genes

A person who has only one copy of a particular allele (good or bad) is said to be *heterozygous* for that allele. A person who has two copies is *homozygous*. Often differing alleles have a blending effect; for instance, black skin and white usually results in an in-between skin colour. Genes that consistently over-ride the effects of other alleles are called dominant genes.

There is no doubt that we all have 'bad' genes. If the bad gene is dominant, it may be enough to make us sick. Mostly, we will have a 'good' gene from our other parent which will compensate for it. This is why many people with 'bad' recessive genes never know they carry such genes unless their spouse has the same recessive gene. Even then, the couple will need to have four children (statistically speaking) in order to give birth to an afflicted child who is unlucky enough to have a double dose of the bad gene.

But the terminology of 'good' and 'bad' reduces a complex situation to the level of a B-grade movie. It is true that some genes, both recessive and dominant, are inherently lethal, but in most cases the story is not black and white.

Enzymes are proteins, and the genes that code for enzymes often exhibit polymorphism. In fact, multiple variants, or alleles, exist for up to 30 per cent of all of the thousands of enzyme systems in the human body. Health problems can arise if any one of these enzymes has a malfunctioning variant. Problems can also arise when the enzyme exists in a slightly less efficient variant, or when production of the normal variant is slow. Slow production can be due to environmental factors, but it can also be built into the genetic code.

For instance, asthma may be due to a sluggish *delta-6 desaturation enzyme*. Delta-6 helps convert dietary precursors into anti-inflammatory prostaglandins (Chart 5.3).

But reduced efficiency only matters when demand outstrips supply. In a past era, most such challenges could be met. It took industrialisation to expose the enzyme systems with reduced robustness. Without the load of pollution, mineral deficiencies and other stress factors, many of these genetic variants might have caused no problems at all.

Rather than dismissing ailments as genetic, we need to understand how to get the best out of the genetic hand we have been dealt. Whether it is a question of our response to alcohol, or the chance of our 'cancer genes' giving us cancer, the fundamental issue is *what else* is going on in the cell to activate or suppress these genes.

To modify or limit the effects of genes there are three main areas of interest:

- Can the body adjust to a genetic weakness by some compensatory mechanism?
- What affects the expression of our genes?
- How do we avoid mutations (as these are more likely than not to be deleterious)?

Compensatory mechanisms

Toxins include synthetic and natural poisons. Some, such as alcohol, aldehydes and alkaloids, occur naturally. Some are in our food. Some are produced by normal metabolism. Mother Nature has equipped us to deal with toxins.

One example is alcohol, which occurs widely in nature. There are wood alcohols, yeast alcohols, alcohols in ripe fruit, and so on. Retinol, also known as Vitamin A, is an alcohol.

After consumption, ethanol is metabolised to acetaldehyde by enzymes known as *alcohol dehydrogenases*. (There are at least four of these alcohol dehydrogenases, but most detoxification is performed by Class I dehydrogenase, which occurs in the liver.) Then the mitochondria of the liver and muscle cells convert this acetaldehyde to acetic acid, with energy as a by-product. However, about 40 per cent of Japanese, Chinese and indigenous Americans, and a further 10 per cent of other people, lack the necessary enzyme, *aldehyde dehydrogenase*. This results in an accumulation of aldehyde (causing among other things, a red face and reduced alcohol tolerance). Such people are dependent on a much less efficient second pathway to deal with alcohol. This is known as *the oxidising pathway of the endoplasmic reticulum*. We all use this pathway when the first one is overloaded by excess consumption.

The issues here are several. All the dehydrogenases are metallo-enzymes, requiring two zinc atoms (Chapter 3). One zinc is structural and the other is required by the catalytic process. The conversion of acetaldehyde to acetic acid by aldehyde dehydrogenase requires the presence of molybdenum.[12] Both pathways require zinc, one requires molybdenum. They also consume Vitamin C and the B-group vitamins. The degree to which we react to alcohol is determined not only by the kind of enzymes we drew from the genetic lottery, but also by the vitamins and minerals in our diet.

Another example is high levels of homocysteine, recognised as a risk factor for cardiovascular disease. This problem seems to have a genetic base, and to run in families. A similar observation can be made about people with high cholesterol levels, despite low fat consumption. The genetic basis of these problems is well understood.

Raised plasma homocysteine is treatable with folic acid, Vitamin B6 and Vitamin B12. Raised cholesterol can be treated with Vitamin C, Vitamin B3, B5, and a whole range of dietary interventions.

Consumption of alcohol is a challenge to our metabolism, which has to work hard to detoxify it. The refined modern diet also acts as a challenge for those with any vulnerability in one or more of their enzyme systems. The natural consequence of this diet is to effectively ferret out our genetic weaknesses.

Another example is a condition known as spinal muscular atrophy (SMA), which occurs in about one baby in 6000. It is the most common genetic cause of infant mortality worldwide. It causes muscle weakness and wasting, and most victims die before they reach the age of two. Yet some people with SMA live reasonably long lives. The illness is caused by a single mutation in a gene which is responsible for making a protein vital to the function of motor neurones. For this protein to be effective it needs to undergo methylation (Chapter 3). Once again, folic acid and Vitamin B12 are included in the list of important methylators. Current research suggests that the reason that some people live long lives with SMA is that they have diets naturally high in these nutrients.[13]

Even genetic disorders as ghastly as Huntington's chorea appear to affect different sufferers with differing degrees of severity. It has been suggested that both dietary and toxic influences can impact on the expression of such genes.

This is not to imply that the effects of mutations are to be seen only as the result of bad diets. But it is interesting to consider that, if even lethal genes may be affected by good diets, how many defects are defects only in the presence of a poor diet.

Controlling the expression of genes

Do we have control over whether 'bad' genes are turned on in the first place? Are they indeed only bad when turned on inappropriately?

Can they be switched off when their activity is damaging the cells or the organism? Can other genes be switched on to improve the situation? These questions form the focus of much exciting research.

Geneticists distinguish our *encoded* genetic sequences from our *expressed* genetic sequences. Many of our genes require constant expression — such as the genes for energy metabolism — or the function of the cell will simply cease. Sometimes, however, illness is the result of inappropriate expression of genes. This can happen in either direction. Genes may be on when they should be off, or off when they should be on.

The prevailing demands on the cell determine what genes will be 'read' or expressed at any one moment. They may be turned on or off to deal with toxins such as alcohol, prescription drugs or pollution, or to govern minute-by-minute running of the cell.

Genes are switched on and off by elements known as *transcription factors*, which include steroids. Or the triggers can be proteins which bind directly to enzymes (polymerases), and thus increase the rate of transcription. Inappropriate transcription (Chapter 1) can result from a range of influences, including ionising radiation, noxious chemicals, circulating stress hormones or co-enzyme deficiencies.

It is possible that structural stress on the DNA causes it to unfold, resulting in automatic transcription. Even the electrical impact of free radicals may provoke inappropriate transcription.

If we return to our image of DNA as a library, like all libraries, it is only as good as the interpretation of the data by whoever does the reading. Books in any library can get damaged. They can be misinterpreted, over-interpreted, disregarded or lost, or simply irrelevant.

As a doctor I have a sinking feeling when a patient says that they expect to get arthritis, cancer or whatever, because it 'runs in the family'. There is no doubt that genetic weaknesses run in families. But except for particular genes, such as those which cause haemophilia, not all will lead to disease.

Suppose I have been told that I have a cancer gene (an *oncogene*), BRCA1 or BRCA2. What should I make of this? Do I join those women who have prophylactic mastectomies or oophorectomies (removal of both ovaries)? I might ask what evolutionary sense there is to have a gene like this in the population. I might wonder if I had been born at another time, another place, how serious a threat these genes might have posed me. I would certainly want to know what turns these genes on, and off, what influences the transcription factors.

Junk genes

From the description of the genetic code earlier in this chapter, it would be easy to get a picture of base pairs all neatly aligned in a linear sequence. However, while many sequences code for genes, the total amount of DNA coding in this manner constitutes only about 5 per cent of all our genetic material. Traditionally, the remainder has been referred to as 'junk DNA'.

We believed that junk DNA consists of leftovers from our evolutionary past. Now we suspect that this genetic 'debris' is carrying out vital functions, which may include turning the coding genes on and off.

About one-third of our junk genes are known as 'jumping genes' or *transposons*. They are thought to be ancient viral remnants of retroviruses which infected our ancestors. Their DNA can persist as part of the genome. Some of these viral remnants can reproduce themselves and insert themselves into other chromosomes, causing illnesses such as the 'hereditary' leukaemias. Other retroviruses may bring adaptive benefits with them.

Histone codes

The 'beads' in the DNA necklace have turned out to be more complex than we thought. It appears that the proteins in the histone core have a code of their own. This new code may well explain a type of inheritance known as 'epigenetic'.

Epigenetic inheritance

Epigenetic refers to characteristics that appear to be inherited, but do not appear to be encoded in the genome. 'Some researchers even suspect that this might be where nature and nurture converge, the route by which our environment, stress, toxic chemicals and the food we eat can modify and manipulate the message written in our genes.'[14]

There is a disturbing aspect of epigenetic inheritance: genes may be permanently switched on or off by environmental presences or absences, such that future generations will show the effects.

For example, vitamin and mineral deficiency during pregnancy gives rise to a greater risk of diabetes, obesity and cardiovascular disease in the offspring, independent of subsequent nutrition. Has the histone code of the infant been damaged by nutritional depletion? Will this be passed on to his or her children?

We know that there is a greater incidence of congenital abnormalities in babies conceived in test tubes. Cloned animals which appear normal at birth have greater vulnerability to infection; they are prone to dying suddenly from conditions such as organ failure or cardiovascular disease. It is perhaps too early to speculate on the causes of such problems, but it is reasonable to observe that, during the critical phases of fertilisation and embryogenesis, the complex nutrients from a mixed healthy diet might be difficult to duplicate in the culture medium. The embryos have the same set of genes as the mother, but we have to wonder about what is happening to the on-off switches of those genes.

Other evidence has come from work at the University of Sydney, which shows that epigenetic inheritance may be one of the factors involved in the rising incidence of asthma and autism.[15] Another example is a study that has shown that the diet of a mother animal can permanently influence fur colour in the offspring.[16]

The mechanism by which this may occur is through the acetyl and methyl groups attached to the histone core, which can affect whether the gene is expressed or not. Enzymes inside the nucleus (such as *methyl transferase* and *deacetylase*) add methyl groups, remove acetyl groups and so on. Researchers have identified at least 20 or 30 such enzymes with the potential to affect gene transcription in this way. The implication of this is that these dietary nutrients can determine the transcription of individual genes through gene silencing or activation.

Viral infection has been shown to trigger a series of acetylation reactions which turn on the gene responsible for the transcription of beta feron, a powerful anti-viral. Hormones have been shown to trigger gene expression via acetylation reactions. Many illnesses occur when cells act autonomously, or when genes ignore the modifying instructions of other genes. The histones provide a mechanism whereby 'bad' genes can be controlled. The methyl and other groups come from things as simple as the folic acid in leafy green vegetables.

It has been proposed that the gut bacteria may have a role in determining how genes are read. Here, too, the influence may come via modification of the histone code. Gut bacteria, as previously discussed, produce short-chain fatty acids, or SCFAs, including butyric acid. Butyric acid has been demonstrated to be a potent inhibitor of histone de-acetylases.[17] A deficiency of butyrate as a result of a reduction in gut flora may, in theory at least, allow an enzyme to switch on an 'oncogene', which is then inappropriately expressed.

Plant and animal cells seem to be able to block a specific gene by destroying the RNA copies made by that gene. This is called RNA interference, or RNAi. There has been some excitement in the research world about the potential for many illnesses to be treated by blocking the relevant genes in this way. The approach has been to add small matching pieces of interfering RNA (RNAsi) to the cell. So far the results have indicated that there is collateral damage to adjacent genes, which is, of course, undesirable. Perhaps the most reliable technique for the moment is to ensure that the cell has all the nutrients it needs to support its own targeting process.

Avoiding mutations

When a gene is damaged, several things can happen. The cell itself may recognise that the damage is beyond repair and commit suicide. Within the genetic material are genes which contribute to this process.

Often the damage is recognised by the very enzymes the DNA itself has produced, and these enzymes will set about repairing that damage. The enzymes, called *DNA repairase*, are in constant use. Mutations occur when these enzymes fail to do their job. As the enzymes are dependent on co-factors such as selenium and zinc, it is clear that a deficiency of such co-factors compromises the ability of DNA to repair itself.

If repair has not taken place, and the cell has not destroyed itself, then the result is that a permanent change has taken place in the code, and this is called a *mutation*.

A mutation that occurs in a germ cell (eggs or sperm) is passed on to the next generation. If it occurs in a somatic cell (that is, any cell in the body which is not a germ cell), the damage is confined to that cell and its daughter cells. It may be of no consequence at all. On the other hand, it may be the first step in the process of that cell turning into a cancer cell.

Although we have many defences against mutations, prevention is always better than cure. Avoiding cigarettes, radiation, pollution and chemicals is one half of this equation. But we should be quite clear about one thing: 'Most genetic mutations are caused by free radicals scavenging electrons from DNA.' This is nothing more nor less than oxidative damage.[18] Therefore, eating a good diet rich in anti-oxidants and leading a healthy lifestyle is the other half.

We cannot blame our genome, millions of years in the making, for the diseases of Western civilisation. We have significant control over most of our bad genes. Although at this stage much is still in the research phase, we may arrive at the conclusions our grandparents never questioned: that sunshine and exercise are good for us; that we need fresh air and adequate rest; that we are what we eat.

Chapter Four

MACRONUTRIENTS
AND MINERALS

MACRONUTRIENTS

Fats

FAT IS A PART OF A FAMILY OF NUTRIENTS known as the lipid family, one of the most misunderstood areas of human nutrition. This list of some members of the lipid family is only a partial representation, but it helps us to appreciate the intriguing complexity of these nutrients, and it highlights the fascinating array of functions of fat in our bodies:

- hydrocarbons (saturated, unsaturated, cyclic, aromatic)
- specialised hydrocarbons (alcohols, aldehydes, fatty acids, amines)
- waxes
- fats and most oils (fatty acids attached to a sugar-derived molecule)
- glycero-phospholipids
- sphingolipids (e.g. ceramide, sphingomyelin, gangliosides)
- steroids (sterols such as cholesterol, bile acids, cardiac glycosides, sex and adrenal hormones)
- other lipids (Vitamins A, D, E, K; eicosanoids, acyl CoA, acylcarnitine, lipopolysaccharides, ubiquinone).[1]

A no-fat diet would sooner or later prove fatal. It also can create health problems whose early symptoms may be subtle. When we talk about dietary fats, the three most important groups under discussion are fatty acids, fats and oils, and cholesterol. We will look at the first two here; cholesterol is discussed in Chapters 3 and 8.

Fatty acids

Fatty acids are one of the main building blocks of most dietary fats. They consist of hydrocarbon chains, at the end of which is a molecule known as a carboxyl group. This latter has an affinity for water, and is therefore termed 'hydrophilic'. This is an important feature of a fatty acid.

Fatty acids come in three kinds: monounsaturated, polyunsaturated and saturated. The terms refer to the availability of carbons in the chain for binding to something else. This occurs wherever there is a double bond between carbons (Chapter 3). One of these bonds can be broken open, and the molecule can form different structures. Monounsaturates have one such double bond, polys have more than one, and saturated fats have none.

Monounsaturates are found in oils such as olive oil, and are believed to have considerable health benefits. Polyunsaturates provide us with the molecules known as the essential fatty acids. While not all polyunsaturates are 'essential', all essential fatty acids are polyunsaturated. These important molecules are discussed in more detail in Chapter 5. Saturated fats are those commonly found in animal fats.

Fats and oils

Most of the fats in our diet come as fats or oils, complex molecules made up of various components. If we want to measure them in a blood test, we ask for a triglyceride level. A triglyceride consists of a glycerol molecule (derived from sugar), with three fatty acids attached to it. It is also known as a *triacylglycerol*. When we eat oil, cream, fatty meats or foods fried in fat, the fats that we are consuming are largely triglycerides. Numerous combinations of fatty acids, mono-, poly- and saturated, go to make up the end molecule, resulting in hundreds of different complex triglycerides.

If we consume an excess of protein or carbohydrate, the body will readily convert it to fat. Most carbohydrates, along with ingested fat, are stored in this form.[2] Indeed, in contrast to the popular notion that this is a pathological process, it is the normal mechanism by which the body handles its energy supply.

Immediately after a meal we derive much of our energy from the carbohydrates we have just consumed. But the actions of insulin, growth hormone and related factors ensure that within an hour or two of eating, food recently ingested is stored for later use. The liver and fat tissues are two of the main storage sites. Skeletal muscle also plays a significant role in this storage process by removing glucose from the bloodstream and storing it as glycogen.

Glucose, and the other forms of sugar and carbohydrate, are readily converted to fat. Fat is the most efficient mechanism for storing energy, but liver and muscle glycogen are more readily available for use than fat.

So most intermediate and long-term energy is stored as fat. It is tempting, especially in view of the current obsession with body image and obesity, to regard fatty tissue as undesirable. We think of it as providing insulation at best, as inert and sluggish at worst. In fact, it is one of the most metabolically active organs in the body, with a constant turnover of its component parts. In diabetes, it is the inability to store glucose as fat, and convert fat back into energy, which is the key metabolic disturbance. Diabetes is a disorder of fat metabolism as much as a disorder of sugar metabolism.

Proteins

As we saw in Chapter 3, the building block of a protein is an amino acid. This structure resembles the organic acids found in nature, but which are not derived from living matter. (A widely held theory is that, in a primeval soup of these carbon-based acids, some found each other and reacted in such a way that life on earth began.) When two amino acids combine, the result is called a peptide. Neurotransmitters such as dopamine and serotonin are peptides. When several peptides combine, the result is a polypeptide, and these link together to make proteins.

The desired end-product of amino acid is usually, although not always, the production of a protein. Proteins are usually large molecules. The proteins making up intestinal cells, muscle cells, ligaments or blood vessels are examples. The specialised form of protein known as an enzyme was discussed in Chapter 3. Hormones, immune globulins and red and white blood cells are also proteins.

Just to get some sense of proportion here, a 'small' protein contains about 50–100 amino acids. The upper limit of a protein size is of the order of 5000 amino acids. The protein discussed in Chapter 8: Cardiovascular Disease, apo-lipoprotein B, is about this size.

Of the hundreds of peptide/protein compounds found in nature, all are made up of the same basic 20 or so amino acids. One implication of this is that living things can feed on each other. The proteins in plants can be broken down to their component amino acids by the animal which eats them. Those animals can then rearrange the amino acids into the molecules from which they make their own proteins. Likewise, carnivorous species can use the amino acids of other animals, to turn them into their own proteins. The inevitable similarity in proteins between species results in some curious and important medical conditions. These include food allergies and autoimmune disease.

The rearrangement of dietary amino acids to form new proteins is done under the guidance of genes. Indeed, directing this assembly line in protein manufacture is the main purpose of the gene.

Carbohydrates

If proteins provide the components of the living organism, carbohydrates are the primary source of fuel that keeps it running. The glucose molecule is the principal material (substrate) used in the combustion process. Between consumption and combustion, carbohydrates may undergo several transformations, as described in Chapter 8: Obesity. The key point here is that the main purpose of carbohydrate is energy.

Much of that energy is produced through an enzyme-driven cycle known as the citric acid cycle or Krebs Cycle, which takes place in the mitochondria of cells. These are the little energy-producing units found in the cytoplasm of the cell (Chart 3.2). There is a production line known as the electron transport chain, which produces energy in a series of redox reactions. This production line depends on the energy provided by free radicals. Without the free radicals, life would cease. Free radicals demonstrate that 'good' and 'bad' are relative terms in biological systems.

Food produces energy by several other pathways, including the pentose phosphate pathway, which we need not go into. Not all carbohydrate is 'burnt'. Some of it is used structurally in making compounds with such impressive sounding names as N-acetyl neuraminic acid, glycolipid, sphingoglycolipid and globoside. These substances can be found in tissues from brain to cartilage. The one most familiar to the public in recent years is glucosamine, an ingredient in cartilage.

Nucleic acids

A protein sub-unit combined with a sugar molecule gives us a nucleic acid. So we could say that there are only three classes of biological compound, because a nucleic acid is merely a combination of protein and carbohydrate.

It is because of the unique role that nucleic acids play in biological systems (they form the genetic material), that they are afforded a classification of their own. Nucleic acids were discussed in Chapter 3: Genetics.

MINERALS

Minerals are essential to our health, indeed to our very existence. Calcium and magnesium were introduced in Chapter 1 because it would have been impossible to discuss agriculture without them. Imbalance between the two has important biochemical implications. Sodium and potassium also need to be in balance. But questions of balance are not the main reason that these minerals are well known. Like iron, they are well known because medical science has long been aware of their importance, and this has translated into dietary wisdom. This chapter gives a brief overview of minerals that are less well-known.

Trace and 'ultra-trace' minerals are present in tiny amounts. Although they were previously thought to serve no purpose in humans, they may play significant roles in health. This has become particularly relevant now that our food is grown with superphosphate, NPK and other such fertilisers. If the role of minerals such as germanium, vanadium, boron or molybdenum is unknown, then it is hard to assess the damage that may result from their absence.

Molybdenum is one such trace mineral. We have seen in Chapter 3: Genetics that it may be important in detoxifying certain chemicals. Most of what we know is found in textbooks of veterinary medicine and agricultural science. Germanium is another trace mineral. Most of the clinical studies on germanium have been done in rats, where organic compounds containing germanium have reportedly demonstrated anti-tumour activity. Could a lack of germanium in synthetic fertilisers contribute to the rising incidence of various cancers around the world? We simply don't know. An ingredient which might be vital goes unresearched because it cannot be patented.

About 90 elements naturally occur in the environment; most of them can be described as 'minerals', and 20 or so are known to be essential to human life. Some, such as lead and mercury, are regarded as toxic in any amount. Widespread planetary pollution has led to the insidious concept of 'acceptable levels' of these substances (Chapter 6).

Most of the essential elements—sodium, iron, calcium and zinc—are toxic in overdose, but at normal exposure they rarely pose a risk. The body has mechanisms to combat excess, such as vomiting to counter sodium (salt) overload, or purging to counter magnesium overload.

Some elements are widely distributed in the body fluids in what is known as the *ionised state*. This means that they have parted company with one or more of the electrons in their outer shell, or have gained some extras (Chapter 3). They are then usually referred to as *electrolytes*. The principal electrolytes are sodium (Na^+), chloride (Cl^-) and potassium (K^+): the pluses and minuses indicate their ionisation. They are found in the blood, the lymph, the cerebrospinal fluid, and the extra and intracellular fluid of every cell in the body.

Elements such as magnesium, zinc and fluoride are often ionised in bodily fluids and can therefore be rightly regarded as electrolytes. Not all of them are serving a specific electrolytic function; some are simply in transit to somewhere else. Some, such as calcium and magnesium, are an important part of the electrolyte balance *and* serve multiple functions elsewhere.

Minerals and trace minerals play various roles in the body:

- Minerals form the structural part of solid components like bone.
- Minerals can be found floating in fluid, where they maintain osmotic balance and electrical gradients. (In this context the word 'osmostic' simply refers to the density of electrolytes in the solution.)
- Minerals form the structural part of organic compounds. For instance iodine is part of tri-iodothyronine (thyroid hormone), and iron forms the heme part of the

haemoglobin molecule.
- Some minerals act as messengers in one of the body's fluid systems. This is often referred to as 'signalling' or as a 'second messenger system'. The role of calcium and magnesium in this regard will be discussed shortly.
- Minerals can form part of an enzyme or other highly complex protein. They play various roles which can be classified as structural, catalytic or regulatory. The most important elements in this regard are the transition elements (Chapter 3).

The importance of some minerals is well known. Calcium is the most abundant element in the body; we can read about it on the labels of everything from baby food to breakfast cereal, milk to mineral water. Iron, by contrast is present in relatively small quantities. However, because it is so easily measured in the blood, it is also well known. Some soils and some food processing methods are associated with markedly low levels of iodine, and the resulting deficiency can cause spectacular goitres or the congenital condition of cretinism. So iodine, too, has achieved deserved attention.

Doctors learned about these nutrients in medical school. But what of the rest? The assumption is that a normal diet will provide the basic requirements. The measurement of minerals has not been given a high priority in human medicine.

Hospital and standard laboratories can determine the level of various minerals in the blood—whether in whole blood or in serum, plasma or red cells. This is a reasonable approach for, say, iron, because blood is one of the main repositories of iron. But to assess magnesium status, a more representative measure would come from a biopsy of muscle or bone. For obvious reasons, this test is rarely performed.

What makes blood values even more unrepresentative is this: blood is an important buffer solution. Because it is critical to maintain a finely tuned electrolyte balance in the blood, the body will do everything it can to maintain the homeostasis (the medical term for status quo) of the blood. It will leach every last bit of calcium and magnesium out of the bones to maintain serum levels if it has to.

Nowhere is this better illustrated than in the condition of hyperparathyroidism, when an excess of parathormone results in bones demineralising. Severe osteoporosis develops as precious calcium and magnesium are lost in the urine. Meanwhile blood levels remain normal, or even high. Sometimes it takes a pathological fracture or a kidney stone to alert the physician to the fact that this patient's bones are literally melting away.

Zinc is another mineral whose status cannot readily be assessed from blood levels. Asked how best to assess zinc status, a pathologist replied that the only truly accurate method was to weigh the patient, incinerate them, and then sift through the ashes to extract the zinc and weigh it. He added that he had never had a volunteer for this test. The next most accurate method was a biopsy of the retina or gonads (testicles or ovaries), but volunteers were in short supply there as well. The next preference was for a well-done mineral analysis of hair or toenail clippings. Least reliable were blood and serum levels, which were useful only for the extremes of toxicity and deficiency.

Ease of measurement should not determine the emphasis we place on a mineral. Cynics have observed that certain brands of dog food list up to 40 different vitamins and minerals on their labels, but that baby food has less than a dozen.

Zinc

As my interest in nutritional medicine began with zinc, I will start this part of the mineral story with an account of that experience.

After 10 years of hospital and family practice in Australia, I found myself working as a GP in a busy London clinic under the National Health Service in the mid-1980s. It was Thatcher's England, and it seemed that what had been the best health service in the world had disintegrated through lack of funding. Patients who, in Australia, I would have admitted to hospital, had to be managed in their homes for lack of hospital beds.

Particularly worrying were depressed patients. In the underprivileged area where I worked, services for these people were strained to breaking point. In those days the only medications available were the tricyclic anti-depressants, or MAO inhibitors. Both of these are dangerous in overdose, and the risk of patients using them to suicide is high. In an area of mostly single-parent families and widespread unemployment, the addition of depression made for a lethal mix.

The patient who started me on the nutrition odyssey was a young mother with a new baby. She had a past history of post-natal depression and was showing all the signs of a severe recurrence. I had been reading a book on zinc deficiency by Prof. Derek Bryce-Smith,[3] and decided to give some zinc to this patient. It was a normal commercial product which also contained a bit of magnesium and some Vitamin B6. Within a week the patient was transformed. She greeted me with a smile at the door, cradling the baby in obvious affection. By contrast to her earlier complaint that the baby never stopped crying, both were sleeping well and breastfeeding had become established.

Being cynical about miracle cures, I began to doubt the original diagnosis, but the other doctor and the social worker involved in her care confirmed it and noted the remarkable change. I had to accept that it might have been the supplement which had made the difference.

The book by Bryce-Smith is now almost 20 years old, and unfortunately out of print. The ideas it contains are only now starting to creep into mainstream medicine. The author's background was in chemistry, not in medicine. In discussing veterinary practice in Chapter 1, I compared the entries for zinc deficiency in a textbook of medicine and textbook of veterinary medicine, noting that *Harrison's Principles of Internal Medicine* listed only four zinc-deficiency disorders.

By contrast, Bryce-Smith made a cogent case that zinc deficiency is widespread and common, with multiple possible manifestations including depression. He argued that agricultural change, the use of chemical fertilisers such as NPK, and the modern refining of grains and cereals were at the heart of the problem. If the food is depleted, does this explain serious medical conditions? What evidence do we have? Although one patient of mine appeared to have a good response to zinc, we cannot generalise from that.

Unfortunately, proof in this situation is harder to provide than when testing a drug. We know that laboratory rats fed on refined flours do not survive; they must be given whole grains and soy beans if they are to remain healthy. What are the missing ingredients? Vitamins? Minerals? Essential fatty acids? Zinc?

It is probably all of these, and to isolate the contribution of zinc, while not impossible, can be difficult. Level 1 evidence (Chapter 2) is hard to produce. Instead of applying the RCT model to the investigation, we might take the approach of looking at the known roles of zinc, asking how a deficiency might manifest itself, and whether we can test this clinically. But research into the role of minerals is much less popular than research into drugs. The difficulties, and successes, in answering these questions may be seen in the following account.

In his book, Bryce-Smith made the biochemical case for the role of zinc deficiency in conditions as wide-ranging as depression, anorexia nervosa, acne and benign prostatic hypertrophy. Traditional treatments of those conditions, then as now, were either invasive or ineffective. I felt I had little to lose by offering zinc to my patients as an alternative or an adjunct. One patient, a postman with a large prostate, had found urinary frequency to be such a problem that he'd befriended several elderly people on his route who were always at home and happy for him to use their toilet. After a few weeks on zinc he found he had no further need for this service, only to be met by a dear old soul waiting for him. 'I thought you must have died or something,' she said, distressed that he nò longer made his daily visit.

Inspired by this and other happy stories, and with good feedback from some of the specialists who shared the care of these patients, I sought a grant in 1989 from the Royal College of General Practitioners to research the role of zinc in several conditions, citing Bryce-Smith's work on anorexia. Its response was dismissive:

> an eminent psychiatrist [unnamed] … knows of no significant
> current research work on the role of zinc in [anorexia] …
> There does not appear to be good scientific evidence for this
> role for zinc in this disease and most psychiatrists at present
> reject this theory. Illnesses such as post-partem [sic] depression,
> anorexia nervosa and bulimia are uncommon in general
> practice.

I sent the college some well-referenced studies of both humans and animals, supplied by Bryce-Smith, showing an association between zinc deficiency and mood, but there was no further correspondence.

Musing on what might be the medical term for 'closed-mind syndrome', Bryce-Smith also pointed out that, at the time of writing, the *British National Formulary*—then, as now, the college's gold standard of prescription — contained an entry that refuted one of the college's objections: it described a taste test as the most reliable test of zinc deficiency. The zinc taste test consists of giving someone a very weak solution of zinc salts to drink. The expectation is that, if the person has adequate body levels of zinc, the drink will have an unpleasant metallic taste to it. If they are depleted, the drink has no flavour and will be consumed as if it were a glass of water. This can be seen as an 'unscientific' test, and yet it is the principle used by farmers for salt licks. It is probably also the basis of animals' self-medication, discussed in Chapters 1 and 10.

This episode shows that failure to research an idea does not necessarily imply that it lacks merit. For a drug company, research needs to make money; for an academic institution, limited funds need to be well spent. Thus it is hard to get funding for research in an area which is not already being researched. The premise is that 'if this idea were any good, everyone would be researching it'.

The chemistry

Zinc is an important part of various metallo-enzymes (Chapter 3). There are more than 200 zinc-containing metallo-enzymes throughout the animal world, and many of them operate in humans.

Zinc enzymes are involved in virtually all the major metabolic pathways. This includes the replication, repair, transcription and translation of genes, and also the metabolism of proteins, lipids, carbohydrates and certain neurotransmitters. Zinc enzymes are the rate-limiting factor in protein biosynthesis (the manufacture of proteins, guided by genes, from their component amino acids), and have a role in the production of certain hormones such as insulin and testosterone.

To get some idea of the importance of zinc, let us look at protein metabolism. The zinc enzymes involved have names such as collagenase, alkaline phosphatase and gelatinase, and they take part in such vital processes as ovulation, blastocyst implantation, embryogenesis, mammary development, bone remodelling, angiogenesis and macrophage function. In simple terms this means fertility, wound healing, bone and joint health and immunity. Other protein-related zinc enzymes include aminopeptidase, carboxypeptidase A and B, and neutral protease. These are involved in the digestion of protein, and in all cases, the role of zinc is to catalyse, or speed up the reaction.

The *pathological* processes in which these zinc-containing enzymes exert a regulatory role include cancer invasion and spread, liver cirrhosis, gastric ulcer, cardiomyopathy, atherosclerosis and lung fibrosis.

Zinc is also important for the structural integrity of the DNA molecule. Researchers commented that by this means, zinc deficiency could contribute to problems as serious as cancer.[4]

Zinc has a role in redox enzymes called the superoxide dismutases, which are among the most important antioxidant systems in the body. They are an essential part of the mechanism by which we fight cancer, cardiovascular disease, arthritis, and all the diseases of ageing. Zinc's essential role in the enzyme alcohol dehydrogenase was discussed in Chapter 3: Genetics. Without this enzyme even a glass of wine would be toxic to us.[5] Zinc enzymes are also involved in the metabolism of Vitamin A, and its release from liver stores, the metabolism of essential fatty acids and the control of the storage and release of the stress hormones.

It would be wrong to imply that *only* zinc deficiency will account for the aberrations which can occur in any of these processes, but even a minor deficiency has the potential to disrupt their function, and so compromise the health of the individual.

As well as forming a part of vital enzymes, zinc has been demonstrated to combat viruses. Zinc ions disrupt the process by which viral invaders usually reproduce. For a long time it had been suspected that zinc inhibited the replication of rhinoviruses, the causative agents in the common cold. Since then it has been demonstrated that zinc ions behave in a similar manner, known as protease inhibition, against the viruses responsible for polio, foot-and-mouth disease, encephalomyocarditis, herpes simplex and herpes zoster, and human Coxsackie disease.[6] Of course, it would be inappropriate to use zinc as the only therapeutic agent against these viruses. But in Western medicine it is not used at all for treatment, and only rarely for prevention.

Zinc is somehow involved in taste sensitivity and appetite regulation. Rats in an experimental situation fed a diet devoid of zinc kept eating until they became morbidly obese. It was as if their brains knew there was an essential element missing and told them to keep eating until they got it. Farm animals which are known to lack zinc become listless and depressed and *lose* their appetite. In contrast, malnourished Aboriginal children regained their appetite when given zinc supplements (Chapter 8).[7] With the current epidemics of eating disorders and morbid obesity, research into the lack of zinc in the modern diet would seem promising.

Oysters and shellfish, red and organ meats, nuts, whole grains and legumes are good sources of zinc, especially when produced from zinc-replete environments. The reference daily intake (RDI) of zinc in the United States is about 15 mg a day.

Calcium and phosphorus

I will not devote much space to these minerals because there is little need to stress their importance. For both of them the key roles include the function of cell membranes, the maintenance of electrolyte balance within the cell, the structural integrity of bone, and the modifying effects on hormone balance, often referred to as the 'second messenger system'. The importance of calcium for teeth needs no emphasis.

One of the defining characteristics of calcium is the readiness with which it gives up two electrons from its outer shell. This enables it to bind easily to phosphate to form hydroxyapatite — the scaffolding on which bone is built. It binds equally well to lipids and proteins within membranes, and thus has a deciding role in the passage of other ions through the membrane. Permeability to these ions gives rise to the concept of 'ion channels' within the membrane. Ions affected include sodium, potassium, magnesium and calcium itself.

Detailed discussion of ion channels is beyond the scope of this book, but they have health implications as wide-ranging as hormonal dysfunction, hypertension, renal failure, leaky gut, and many other metabolic disorders. Some readers will be familiar with ion channels through the prescription of 'calcium channel blockers' in the treatment of hypertension, angina, and certain cardiac arrythmias.

The biochemistry of 'second messenger systems' is complex, but it comes down to this. Many hormones and neurotransmitters use an enzyme system to interface between the messenger molecule (the hormone etc.) and its receptor site. Calcium and magnesium often act as the go-between, 'deciding' which messages will be allowed to activate these enzymes — hence 'second messenger'.

Phosphorus in biological systems is present in the form of phosphate and is involved in a variety of biochemical reactions.

Magnesium and calcium in particular have a special relationship with phosphate. As part of ATP (adenosine triphosphate) it plays a major role in energy production. The function of many enzymes depends on the presence of phosphate, including, of course, the family of enzymes known as the 'phosphatases'. It has structural roles in tissues ranging from bone through to DNA and RNA molecules.

Control of calcium and phosphate levels is vital. It is effected through various means including the kidneys, the action of the hormones calcitonin and parathyroid hormone (PTH), and Vitamin D.

Food sources of calcium include milk, tofu, sardines, nuts and green vegetables. Phosphorus can be obtained from meat, milk, eggs and cereals.

Magnesium

In clinical practice, magnesium is one of the most useful of all the prescribed mineral supplements. Magnesium is the second-most common mineral in the animal body (calcium being the commonest). It is the fifth-most important element for green plants, and one of the most abundant elements in the earth's crust. It is not surprising that animal systems have developed with a need for it. Evolution would not have got very far if biological systems required things that were in short supply.

Indeed, it is probably the abundance of magnesium which has resulted in its clinical neglect. Most people know that they need calcium for their bones, but few are aware of a similar need for magnesium. About 70 per cent of all our magnesium is in our bones. Although the actual mass of calcium in bone is much greater both in relative and absolute terms (99 per cent of our calcium is in bone), it is function rather than absolute amount which matters. Even doctors don't understand it, as we can see from the number of patients treated for osteoporosis with calcium alone. This practice is not only ineffective: it is actually counter-productive.

The relationship of calcium to magnesium
It is difficult to discuss magnesium without discussing calcium, because their atomic structures are very similar. In the body they often have similar functions and are handled similarly. Both are transported from the gut into the bloodstream, and from the extra-

cellular fluid into the cell, by similar mechanisms. They have a highly interactive relationship.

The clinical importance of this is that the body works constantly to maintain a balance between these two minerals. Anything which disturbs that balance will affect our health. In the plant as well as the animal world the balance is generally maintained. In a broad-based omnivorous diet, the human organism can expect to get both an adequate amount *and* an appropriate balance of these minerals. Problems arise when either or both minerals are deficient, or when there is an imbalance.

In the developed world, calcium deficiency is less common than magnesium deficiency. One of the main reasons for this is that superphosphate, a key fertiliser, is made up largely of calcium phosphate. Right there at the beginning of the food chain, while the need for calcium is addressed, magnesium deficiency is not.

There is another problem: acid soils can reduce magnesium uptake by plants. So magnesium deficiency can result from eating good food grown in acid soils and in soils fertilised by superphosphate. It can also be caused by a high-calcium diet with lots of dairy foods, or by unbalanced supplementation. If the calcium intake far exceeds magnesium, the calcium can 'swamp' the magnesium. (For more on the contribution of dairy to the disruption of calcium and magnesium ratio, see Chapter 10: Funny Diets.)

The chemistry
There are an estimated 300 roles for magnesium. Unlike zinc, it is not part of a metallo-enzyme. It actions are far more diverse.

The biochemical functions of magnesium include:

- regulating cellular energy metabolism with particular importance in cardiac and skeletal muscle
- optimising the actions of the enzyme systems responsible for the transcription, translation and replication of nucleic acids (RNA, DNA), and the synthesis of protein
- participating in the second messenger system, the means by which various hormones and neurotransmitters 'talk' to their target organ
- controlling various ion channels, including that of potassium and calcium.

Clinically, its most important functions are:

- lowering blood pressure and maintaining normal cardiac rhythm (via its action on ion channels)
- forming an integral part of bone
- relaxing smooth and skeletal muscle
- forming part of the energy system in skeletal and cardiac muscles
- continuously repairing all body proteins.

As with zinc, assessment of body status is not easy. More than 99 per cent of all body magnesium is either in the skeleton or is held inside cells.

Gross magnesium deficiency is not difficult to identify. The level in both serum and the red cell levels will be abnormal, and the patient will be in a state of agitation and tetany, have muscle tremors and cramps, and may well be having fits. If they are really unlucky, they may have a cardiac arrhythmia and even a cardiac arrest. These patients will not be sitting in my waiting room—they will be in an ambulance or dead on the floor at home. But it is the much more subtle states which are the concern of this book. How might we identify them? Is it you or me?

Some effects of lack of magnesium
Some of the most common medical problems involve the malfunction of smooth muscle: asthma and migraine, painful periods (dysmenorrhoea), irritable bowel syndrome and high blood pressure. Of course, all these conditions involve other factors as well, but magnesium deficiency is easy to fix.

The muscles in the gut are smooth muscles. The uterus is a smooth muscle. And the tiny muscles circling the arteries and airways, controlling their diameter, are also smooth muscles. If these muscles for any reason have difficulty in relaxing, they may go into spasm.

A muscle essentially has two states: one is resting or relaxed, and the other is contracted. Prolonged contraction amounts to spasm. When the muscles in the uterus spasm, the patient will experience cramps or, if she is giving birth, a prolonged and difficult labour. If the circular muscles of the gut are constantly in spasm, the patient will experience cramps and constipation, and will pass hard, segmented stools. If spasm of the longitudinal muscles of the gut predominates, the patient is more likely to experience intestinal hurry and diarrhoea. Patients with irritable bowel syndrome often experience both constipation and diarrhoea, and both are helped by magnesium.

Asthma involves an inflammatory response which includes spasm of the bronchioles. The ability of the bronchioles to relax is determined by several factors (Chapter 7), one of which is magnesium status. If you are low in magnesium and have asthma genes, inhalation of an irritant may precipitate an asthma attack. When I inhale a lungful of dust or pollen, my airways contract. Thus they can limit the amount of irritant entering my lungs, and at the same time, build up pressure so that I can cough and expel the foreign matter. When those airways cannot relax, coughing and wheezing become pathological and an asthma attack ensues.

A 1994 study which looked at a random sample of 2633 adults successfully tested the hypothesis that high dietary magnesium intake is associated with better lung function and reduced airway hyper-reactivity.[8] The results were highly significant. At doses above 400 mg the benefit on lung function levelled out, but hyper-reactivity continued to improve as the dose went up. They also showed that consuming just one standard deviation (about 68 per cent) below the mean of dietary magnesium was the equivalent—in terms of lung expiratory volume, risk of wheezing and lung hyper-reactivity—to 12 pack years of smoking. (A pack year is one packet of cigarettes a day for 12 years, or two packets a day for six years and so on.) Yet despite the rising epidemic of asthma, we do not find magnesium in the prescriptions for asthmatics.

Similar principles operate in regard to the smooth muscles which surround the arteries and control their diameter. A deficiency of magnesium, either in absolute terms or relative to the calcium load, favours the development of hypertension. Of course, other factors operate, but magnesium status is at least as significant as any of those. Various studies support the role of magnesium supplementation in helping to lower blood pressure.

In 1996 a well-conducted double-blind study showed that chronic migraineurs supplemented with 400 mg daily of elemental magnesium showed a decrease of about 50 per cent in both the frequency and severity of their headaches (Chapter 9).[9] At the beginning of a migraine the scalp arteries contract, causing the sense of tightness across the head so often reported by patients. This vasoconstriction often takes place elsewhere as well—in the brain where it causes visual disturbance and even stroke, and in the gut where it causes cramps. Although such vasoconstriction is triggered by a series of biochemical events, it is easy to understand how low levels of magnesium may prolong the headache or increase its severity.

So far we have been considering the role of magnesium and its effects on smooth muscle, but it should be reiterated that with skeletal muscle, leg cramps and generalised muscle pains can be a sign of magnesium deficiency. Cardiac problems, such as cardiac arrhythmia, will be discussed in Chapter 8.

I have mentioned magnesium's role as a 'second messenger'—a mediator—in various hormonal and neurotransmitter systems. This may be one of the ways in which muscle relaxation, just discussed, is effected. We know that there are receptors throughout the body, including the gut and blood vessels, for hormones and neurotransmitters like serotonin and oestrogen. The levels of, and balance between, calcium and magnesium can determine which messages get through. No matter how much oestrogen, serotonin or dopamine we produce, if those chemical messengers can't activate an oestrogen-receptor site or the appropriate nerve cell, they might just as well not be produced at all. The ramifications of this are significant. Magnesium is vital to both the production and the mediation of such chemical transmitters.

Magnesium has a modifying role on serotonin and nitric oxide levels, and in the production of dopamine. These various chemical messengers are involved both in the spasm of smooth muscle which causes the pain of migraine and period pains, and in the cerebral appreciation of that pain. A deficiency of magnesium therefore, can exaggerate not only the factors producing pain, but also the awareness of it.

Stress hormones are neurochemicals which include catecholamines, such as adrenalin, and corticosteroids. The evolutionary purpose of these hormones is to raise blood pressure, release glucose and fatty acids into the bloodstream, and prepare us for flight or fight. This is still sometimes a necessary response in today's world, as when a car runs the red light just when we step off the kerb, but it is often evoked by mental stressors not requiring a physical response. And that, of course, contributes to the whole spectrum of ills known to be stress-related.

The high blood pressure, the coronary and cerebrovascular constriction, and the increased heart rate are fine as a transitory phenomenon; but when they become sustained or are invoked inappropriately, they become a health risk. A low ratio of magnesium to calcium favours the release of catecholamines, as well as the release and formation of factors that lead to further vasoconstriction and platelet aggregation. A low ratio of magnesium to calcium also favours blood coagulation—a lethal addition.

The patient: Mary

We met Mary in my waiting room in Chapter 1. If we were for the moment to forget that such terms as asthma, dysmenorrhoea and depression had ever been coined, and if human medicine as a discipline had evolved with some of the biochemical understanding now available to us, how might I see a patient like Mary? Just as we might list the problems that go with a diagnosis of scurvy, could she be a 'classic case' of magnesium deficiency? After all, magnesium has roles in asthma, migraine, menstrual cramping, irritable bowel, energy metabolism, mood disorders.

Is it simplistic to say that all of Mary's problems could be solved by the addition of magnesium? Perhaps. But look at some of the other factors.

A US survey found that dietary *intake* of magnesium had fallen below the recommended dietary allowance (RDA) or reference daily intake (RDI) in up to 75 per cent of people (see Appendix 1). Mary is on an average diet; what are her chances of being in that 75 per cent? And independently of her intake, what about her *absorption*? She drinks milk, eats cheese and likes yoghurt. Is this calcium load subtracting from her magnesium status?

Alcohol, the oral contraceptive pill, and some other prescription medications all cause the body to lose magnesium. Mary is on the pill. She drinks alcohol, although not in excess. As for her prescription medications, in some cases the effects on magnesium status of these have not even been quantified.

If Mary wants to correct a magnesium problem with diet alone, she will need to eat such foods as unpolished grains, nuts, legumes, sea vegetables, citrus fruits, green leafy vegetables and the brassicas (cabbage family). But if these foods are not grown in organic or biodynamic soils, they may not contain adequate levels of magnesium.

And although Mary likes all of these foods, do they form a significant part of her average diet?

High levels of magnesium dissolve in hot water and can be absorbed gently through the skin. In a bygone era, Mary would have been told to have a sitz bath or go to a hot spring. It would have worked. Grandma fixed a lot of problems with a judicious dose of Epsom salts. Epsom salts are magnesium sulphate; they were named for the town of Epsom in England, where a natural hot spring was noted for its curative benefits. But for oral administration commercial preparations of magnesium are best: Epsom salts can overdo it, causing an osmotic diarrhoea.

As I look around at the other patients, I see Louise who gets migraine; Sonya who would like a good delivery and wants to avoid post-natal depression; and Mrs Green who wants a smooth transit through menopause. Their stories will be introduced elsewhere in this book, but I am confident that each of them should be taking supplementary magnesium.

The RDA of magnesium is about 400 mg for males and 300 mg for females. As a supplement, it is best absorbed as an amino acid chelate such as magnesium aspartate or orotate. The cheaper preparations containing magnesium oxide and magnesium sulphate are much less suitable.

Selenium

In December 1996 the results of a clinical trial on the effects of selenium should have made headline news around the world, but it barely rated a mention.[10] The trial was unusual in several ways. First, it was being carried out on a natural element rather than a drug. Second, its results were so significant that it gained publication, even though the effect it sought to demonstrate was not present. Third, the results of the treatment were so beneficial that, by internationally agreed ethical standards, the trial had to be stopped prematurely so that the treatment could be offered to the control group. Fourth, medical indifference to a non-drug treatment of one of the most feared diseases of the modern day reached, I suspect, an unprecedented level.

Some outcomes of this trial are discussed in Chapter 7: Cancer, but the main points are these. A group of 1312 individuals with a history of non-melanoma skin cancer were randomised to receive either a placebo or 200 mcg daily of selenium. The aim was to see whether selenium reduced the incidence of non-melanoma skin cancer. It did not. But those receiving selenium experienced 63 per cent fewer cancers of the prostate, 58 per cent fewer cancers of the colon, and 46 per cent fewer cancers of the lung. Of those who were diagnosed with cancer while taking part in the trial, those taking selenium were 50 per cent less likely to die of their cancer than the control group. *There is no known drug treatment with statistics as good as this.* By almost all measures selenium is the ideal anti-cancer drug.

There were too few women in the trial for any statistically significant data on breast cancer incidence to emerge. Another trial is exploring that question. The same researchers are also investigating the effects of selenium in the deadly problem of ovarian cancer, and have shown beneficial results in women who combine selenium with their standard treatment.

The original trial had been designed to run for ten years, but it was stopped after five. Cancer is generally agreed to have a long incubation period. As such, it has always been assumed that preventative measures could not show benefit in such a short period.

Soon after the selenium trial had been reported, Margaret Rayman, a research fellow in the Department of Chemistry at the University of Surrey in England, pointed out that soil selenium levels were falling dramatically, and there was a parallel drop in both dietary intake and blood levels.[11] She quoted a 1994 report by the British Ministry of Agriculture and Fisheries which showed a drop in average daily intake to 34 mcg from an average of 60 mcg a day in the mid-1970s.

Once again, it is instructive to look at the medical bible. In 1991, the 12th edition of *Harrison's Principles of Internal Medicine* listed five entries on selenium but no clinical conditions as such associated with selenium depletion.[12] By the time the 15th edition was published in 2001, selenium entries had leapt to 11.

The story unfolds

Selenium was first discovered in 1817 by a Swedish chemist, Berzelius, who gave it the Greek name for the moon. In 1943 it was noted in *mass* doses to cause neoplasia (growth, usually malignant) in the liver of rats, thus identifying it as a potential carcinogen. In the mid-1950s it was identified as an essential trace element in rats, and by the 1970s evidence was beginning to emerge that it had anti-cancer properties in mammalian systems. Twenty years after it had been shown to be essential for rats and chickens, the first clear evidence was found that it was also essential in humans.

Then in 1979, a New Zealand patient was undergoing total parenteral nutrition—where no food is taken by mouth and life is maintained by what can be fed through a vein. During the course of this treatment he developed cardiomyopathy, a condition in which the heart muscles become weak and flabby. The patient had come from an area in New Zealand which, like many parts of Australia, had some of the world's lowest levels of soil selenium. His doctors thought that they had little to lose by treating their patient as if he had a selenium-deficient cardiomyopathy. His rapid recovery was taken as confirmation of their suspicions.[13]

At about the same time, conclusions were being drawn about an epidemic of childhood cardiomyopathy observed over the previous decade in one part of China. The area was Keshan, which gave its name to the disease. (It, too, was an area known to have low soil levels of selenium.) The condition, it was noted, had similarities to the cardiomyopathy seen in selenium-deficient pigs and mice. A study involving just over 46,000 children was begun. The trial had to be abandoned two years prematurely, because the death rate in the control group was 5.6 children per thousand, compared with 0.08 in the selenium-supplemented group.

Although most patients recovered from Keshan disease on selenium supplements, a few did not. A simple deficiency state should have given close to 100 per cent recovery rate. It was suspected that a virus might also be involved, and what was finally uncovered demonstrates both the complexity and awesome simplicity possible when medical management is based on cause and effect.

By the mid-1990s some researchers from the University of North Carolina were studying the Coxsackie family of viruses, now known to be the mystery virus in Keshan disease. They found that a benign form of the virus could mutate into a virulent form in the heart tissue of mice whose diets lacked selenium. Mice that were given selenium did not become sick, because the selenium not only boosted their immune systems but also prevented the development of a resistant strain in the virus.[14]

This was a new way of looking at host resistance to disease. Traditionally the thinking had been that a virus, bacterium or parasite of fixed virulence invades the host and, depending on the host's ability to mount an appropriate response, it kills or is killed. (Or at least the virus is suppressed, as with chickenpox virus, which re-emerges as shingles only when the host's resistance is seriously compromised.) It was novel to think that the invader might take advantage of a run-down host which can ward off only the weaker germs. The implications embrace not only chronic viral illness such as HIV and herpes, but the actual development of epidemics.

Most of the virulent new strains of influenza sweeping the world seem to originate in China. Could endemic selenium depletion be part of the reason for this? One report of this research certainly raised the possibility. HIV is thought to have originated in northern Zaire, where many people have low blood levels of selenium: could HIV have begun in a similar manner?[15]

The chemistry

The clinical manifestations of selenium deficiency are protean, and its metabolism in the body is still incompletely understood. It is absorbed highly efficiently from the gut, and a constant level is maintained largely through urinary loss. Most selenium in the body appears as seleno-cysteine in protein complexes known as seleno-proteins. These seleno-proteins are widely distributed; and most, if not all, are enzymes.

The most common way for us to ingest selenium is when it is bound to an amino acid called methionine. Its origin lies in plant foods, or in animals which have eaten those plants. By a series of biochemical reactions seleno-methionine is converted to seleno-cysteine. This selenium-containing amino acid is present in both prokaryotes and eukaryotes (primitive cell lines or micro-organisms). This indicates the ancient origin of the amino acid,[16] and perhaps hints at its importance. Certainly the synthesis of the seleno-proteins is as complex as any in biology, requiring, among other things, a unique RNA gene product.

In all, eleven mammalian seleno-proteins have been identified. They include:

- *The glutathione peroxidases:* These vital enzymes protect cells and tissues — that is, they quench free radicals. They occur in the plasma and every cell of all animals. Stipanuk suggests that one of these enzymes may have evolved specifically to maintain milk selenium levels rather than, as has previously been assumed, to prevent the peroxidation of milk.[17] (Lipid peroxidation is a serious consequence of uncontrolled free radical attack on unsaturated fats. When it occurs in cell membranes, a chain reaction can lead to mass destruction of cells. The best defence against it is Vitamin E.)

• *The deiodinases:* For 20-odd years we have known that these enzymes convert inactive forms of thyroid hormone into the active forms. It is possible that the reverse may also be true, and that selenium deficiency can cause thyroid deficiency and may also contribute to thyrotoxicosis (thyroid excess).

• *The muscle and plasma seleno-proteins:* These are not yet fully understood, although depletion of the former is associated with white muscle disease in sheep. It is possible that cramps which do not respond to normal treatment, and the muscle weakness and excess tiredness seen in chronic fatigue syndrome, could be related to selenium depletion.

It is estimated that up to 50 more seleno-proteins await delineation in higher animals. In selenium deficiency the body gives priority to glutathione peroxidase and the seleno-enzymes in the brain, the endocrine glands and the reproductive organs.

The recommended daily allowance

Calculations of the RDI are based on the amount of selenium it takes for all glutathione peroxidase in the plasma to be replete. This is referred to as 'saturation'. The amount of selenium required to saturate glutathione activity, while satisfying the enzymatic or antioxidant role of selenium, appears to be *below* the levels needed to optimise the immune response and reduce cancer risk.[18] The implication is that RDIs may be set too low. Similarly, the amount of Vitamin C required to prevent scurvy is almost certainly not the same as the amount required to *optimise* health.

There is as yet no internationally agreed RDI for selenium (see Appendix 1). The current British value is 75 mcg for men and 60 mcg for women; the American level is 55 mcg. If saturation of glutathione activity in platelets rather than plasma were taken as the criterion, the RDA would be in the range of 80–100 mcg.

In Britain the current estimated intake is 29–39 mcg; France, 29–49 mcg; Germany, 35 mcg; Sweden, 38 mcg; and Poland, 11–24 mcg. Switzerland is the highest at 70 mcg. When blood (serum or plasma) levels of selenium were measured from 26 different regions in 14 European and Scandinavian countries, *not one* mean value reached the level required to optimise glutathione peroxidase activity.

Even more worryingly, not one reached even the top of the *bottom one-third* (tertile) of the range of blood levels at entry in the American cancer trial.[19] In other words, about 66 per cent of the people entering that trial already had blood levels of selenium higher than the average European or Scandinavian. This may be a result of American soils, less intensive farming, or some other factor. As it was the people in the *lowest* tertile who benefited the most from selenium supplements, the desirability of raising blood levels in the European countries should be apparent.

Some effects of selenium

Supplementation with selenium, even in selenium-replete individuals, stimulates the immune system: it enhances proliferation of activated T-cells, increases the activity of natural killer cells, and accelerates the expression of the receptors for interleukin-2.

Selenium deficiency increases vulnerability to Coxsackie virus and possibly other RNA viruses such as polio, hepatitis, influenza and HIV. One study showed that, over three and a half years, selenium–depleted HIV patients were 20 times more likely to die of AIDS-related conditions than those who had adequate levels.[20] 'Depletion' in this study was defined as 85 mcg per litre, a mean plasma concentration attained in few northern European countries.

Selenium plays a role in reproductive health. Miscarriage, where no cause could be found; recurrent miscarriage; and the structural abnormality and poor motility of sperm were all noted to be associated with selenium depletion in animal and/or human studies.

Selenium deficiency altered the turnover rate of some neurotransmitters in some studies.[21] Intractable epileptic seizures in children were reduced with supplementation. Low plasma selenium concentrations were associated with senility and cognitive decline; and, in one study, brain concentration in Alzheimer's patients was noted to be only 60 per cent of that in controls.[22]

Dietary selenium was found to have a clear association with mood. In the above study, dietary depletion over just 15 weeks led to increased depression and hostility. In other studies, either high selenium intake or selenium supplementation were associated with increased confidence and composure, and decreased anxiety and depression.[23]

The seleno-protein glutathione peroxidase protects against the oxidation of lipids. This is a major factor in both the integrity of arterial walls, and the accumulation of damaging low-density proteins in those walls. Selenium depletion tips the balance between constriction and dilation of arteries in the direction of constriction. It also encourages platelet aggregation. Both of these conditions increase the risk of heart attack and stroke.

Selenium also offers protection against oxidative stress and inflammatory conditions including rheumatoid arthritis, pancreatitis and asthma. Rayman quotes studies supporting a role for selenium in all three.[24]

The role of selenium in cancer has already been discussed. The American cancer trial is supported by some equally impressive studies, some of which date back to the 1970s. These include a Finnish study of 9000 people showing a clear inverse relationship between risk of lung cancer and serum selenium levels. A massive study in the Qidong province in China recruited 130,000 people in an area known for a phenomenally high rate of hepatocellular carcinoma. The supplementation dose can be estimated to be about 30–60 mcg (selenium-fortified salt was used, so intakes varied). After six years, although the dose was low and no other supplements such as Vitamin C or E were given, the incidence of the cancer had fallen by 35 per cent in the supplemented township.

How much is too much?
Aware of the toxicity potential of selenium, at one stage I decided to check selenium levels in some of my patients. Unlike zinc, a blood level of selenium is deemed to be a reasonable indication of the selenium status of the individual. I was prescribing within the 200 mcg range of the American cancer trial, in which the absence of toxicity had been a feature despite the fact that local soil levels were superior, and intakes therefore higher, than in Australia.

I was surprised to find that some of the test results, both in patients never before supplemented and those on supplements for a year or two, were asterisked as exceeding the upper limit. When I contacted the laboratory I found I was the only doctor regularly doing this test in the Sydney area. The pathologist himself had queried the normal values, feeling that the given range was too low. The source of the numbers was the chief scientific body in the country, the CSIRO. It turned out that the CSIRO had taken selenium levels from a population of *hospitalised patients* and adapted them to a normal curve. In other words, the values had been normalised on a population consuming a modern Western diet in a selenium-deplete country. And a sick population at that.

This kind of self-referencing, and the assumption that what is common is normal, is sloppy science, and demonstrates how little a substance such as selenium is regarded.

The mean of the Australian 'normal' values did not reach the top of the lower tertile achieved in the American cancer trial. My 'toxic' patients had blood levels of selenium that barely pushed them into the middle tertile for cancer prevention.

One of my patients was advised that he would eventually require a heart transplant for his chronic cardiomyopathy. After six months on selenium his condition had effectively resolved, and he has remained well for several years. He was from a rural area where farmers routinely supplement livestock for selenium deficiency, endemic to the area. Had his cardiologist measured his selenium?

Medical inertia

It is a matter of wonder that doctors do not check selenium levels in patients suffering from cancer, thyroid disorders, endocrine disorders, reproductive or mental problems, not to mention heart disease, arthritis and the whole range of oxidative diseases. Nor do they offer selenium as part of the treatment regime. Doctors know more about prescription medications than they do about these biochemical considerations.

Selenium is not the whole answer to these problems, any more than magnesium or Vitamin B or any other nutrient is. But in the case of selenium it is reasonable to conclude that many people, both in the West and elsewhere, are consuming a depleted diet.

The American cancer trial showed no toxic side effects in a five-year period, so it is hard to comprehend medical resistance to, or neglect of, this safe therapeutic tool. Moreover, if deficiency causes a problem, what other conditions are neglected by failing to address the cause?

Harrison's Principles of Internal Medicine had few entries in 1991;[25] the 2001 edition shows some improvement, as we have just seen. There is a one-line reference to the cancer study but only a few other brief, unrelated entries. Several current oncology books do not even list selenium in their index. These are the textbooks used in universities to educate medical students, the references that specialists have on their desks. These are the books which, updated regularly on CD-ROM, are used to refute 'unorthodox practices'.

At the time of the first edition of this book, the Australian Therapeutic Goods Administration (TGA) approved the sale of selenium supplements in tablets containing up to 50 micrograms per tablet. There were dire warnings about exceeding this as a daily dose. Mysteriously, two years on, tablets containing 150 micrograms are now available in Australia.

The distribution of selenium in the earth's soils is widely variable. Volcanic soils are the richest source. Toxic levels occur where there is industrial contamination, or in irrigation areas where selenium has accumulated. Areas of low rainfall suffer because there is insufficient water to leach the selenium from the soil, even if it is present. The loss of ancient topsoils, the lack of volcanic activity and the low rainfall make Australia particularly vulnerable.

Copper

The theory that a copper bracelet can be beneficial for rheumatoid arthritis is a long-standing piece of folklore. Copper is essential in mammals and most animal species for the formation of the collagen matrix of bone and connective tissue. As this includes tendons, ligaments and joints, it is not surprising that patients with arthritis might derive some benefit. When the patient perspires some of the copper ions go into solution, and like magnesium, can be absorbed through the skin.

Farm animals with arthritis are a significant economic loss. If they are in pain, they refuse to mate. Their appetite decreases, and they lose condition. The collagen matrix is essential not only to joints but also to the strength and integrity of the arterial walls. Animals on copper-deficient feed suffer aortic rupture and cardiac hypertrophy, and show abnormal electrocardiograms. Even a farmer who was silly enough to treat a copper deficiency by putting Celebrex into the feed troughs could not afford bypass surgery to repair cows' aortic aneurysms.

As with most essential elements, the uses of copper are not confined to one system. Copper is part of a metallo-enzyme, and it participates in many reactions: energy utilisation, digestion, detoxification, the production of melanin and haemoglobin, amino acid metabolism and cellular respiration. Copper is an important co-enzyme in the pathway which produces dopamine and adrenalin from tyrosine precursors (Chart 3.3), and along with zinc and manganese, is essential to the group of enzymes known as the superoxide dismutases. Like the glutathione peroxidases discussed under selenium, the superoxide dismutases constitute one of the body's major defence mechanisms against free radical or oxidative damage (Chapter 3)

Copper is necessary for the production of pigment. Dark-coloured animals are recognised to have a greater need for copper, and premature greying is a marker of deficiency. Human patients with coeliac disease are often noted to be prematurely grey, and copper malabsorption may be a cause. The possibility of copper deficiency is rarely investigated in human premature greying, even though it could hint at a weakness to vascular aneurysm, such as aortic and cerebral aneurysms.

Copper status is worth checking in those with abnormal ECGs, and in patients undergoing surgery for aortic aneurysms. Serum levels are a good indicator, but good hair mineral analysis may be better. Liver, shellfish, whole grains, nuts, legumes and black pepper are all good sources of copper.

Copper in excess is toxic, but this is usually the result of industrial or domestic contamination. It is easily established with a blood test. As a supplement, it has the potential to interfere with iron and zinc absorption, and so it is best taken as part of a well-formulated multimineral. The reverse is also true. High intake of zinc or iron supplements can contribute to copper deficiency. This should be borne in mind when we consider that deficiency has been associated with conditions like Alzheimer's.[26] Recommended intake is of the order 1.5–3 mg daily.

Boron

Since the 1960s boron has been used to prevent osteoporosis and osteoarthritis in farm animals. In 2005 it was beginning to make its shy appearance in medical textbooks.

Boron appears to be important for the growth and maintenance of bone, perhaps because of its positive effects on Vitamin D metabolism. It also appears to be significant in the metabolism of oestrogen and testosterone. Patients being treated with hormones for osteoporosis may in fact be suffering a boron deficiency. Boron has been demonstrated to be essential for the normal development and reproduction of frogs. People aren't frogs, of course, but boron is under-researched in the area of human fertility.

Boron has been shown to be important for the development of red blood cells, for the utilisation of glucose for energy (with the subsequent lowering of blood sugar), and perhaps most interestingly, for cognitive changes such as mental alertness and improved psychomotor skills. There is no requirement for its addition to infant formula, and no agreed RDI.

The addition of boron to a supplement regime is often associated with increased bone mineral density. This result is regarded as rare in the absence of pharmaceutical agents, but the actions of boron on bone, Vitamin D and hormone metabolism explain this outcome.

Epidemiological studies have found an inverse relationship between soil levels of boron and the incidence of arthritis. Osteoarthritis responds to supplementation, as does rheumatoid arthritis, including juvenile forms.

Boron is found in fruits, especially pears, leafy and cruciferous vegetables, honey, nuts, legumes, wine, cider and beer. This, of course, will depend on the boron level of the soil in which these foods were grown.

In clinical medicine to date, the main interest has been toxicity. Borax, a commercial product, is toxic in overdose. Toxicity has not been found to be a problem of the supplement preparations available for more than a decade in Europe and the United States. Until 2002, a doctor's script was required for its use in Australia.

Chromium

As with boron and several other elements, epidemiological and animal evidence indicate the role of chromium in human health, yet it is not accepted as an essential human nutrient. On current evidence, chromium seems to be important in glucose metabolism. It increases the sensitivity of cells to insulin, facilitating glucose uptake and thereby lowering blood sugar.

Diabetes in pregnancy has been known to respond to chromium supplements. Studies to establish the place of supplements are being undertaken in various centres around the world. The outcomes of these studies will have implications for the use of chromium in all Type 2 diabetes.

In pregnancy, the foetus makes demands on the mother's mineral stores. If these are insufficient, the foetus may get preference. In this way, pregnancy can be seen as a natural experiment for the effects of mineral depletion. Chromium depletion, it would seem, might increase the risk of diabetes. Pregnancy, after all, is a stress that may induce diabetes. The demand on minerals such as chromium, magnesium, selenium and zinc, all of which are important to a normally functioning pancreas, may be one reason why pregnancy identifies those genetically at risk for diabetes.

The RDI for chromium in the UK is 25mcg whilst the American level is set at 50 mcg, with supplemental ranges of up to 200 mcg suggested. Various studies indicate the American average daily intake to be around 25 mcg, with a significant number of people consuming less than 20 mcg.[27]

Highly refined diets make greater demands on chromium stores, perhaps because of the high glycaemic burden they impose. Yet chromium is in the outer layer of the grain, the very part which is removed during processing. A vicious circle develops: the more nutrient-deplete the diet, the greater the need for the missing elements to make use of it.

Both whole blood levels and hair mineral analysis are useful measures for chromium. It is found in brewers yeast, organ meats, whole grains and nuts.

Molybdenum and friends

Many of the comments made on the preceding elements apply to molybdenum. As an element needed only in small amounts it has been easy to overlook.

In agriculture its importance was established when it was found that it was essential to the azotobacter group of nitrogen-fixing bacteria in the soil. Molybdenum is less available in acid soils, and as acid soils become an increasing problem in Western countries, it is possible that we will learn more about molybdenum by watching deficiency states unfurl.

Molybdenum-dependent enzymes detoxify nitrates and nitrosamines, aldehydes and petrochemicals, sulphites and sulphates in the liver. These toxins include some known carcinogens. If the liver is hampered by molybdenum deficiency in its ability to detoxify these, it is reasonable to say that the deficiency contributed to the cancer. Studies in China on the role of molybdenum in reducing gut cancers go back several decades.[28]

Molybdenum may have a destructive effect on cancer cells as well. It has been shown to 'switch off' cancer cells by inhibiting angiogenesis, the means by which cancer cells grow. It is also important in the activation of folic acid.

Molybdenum is also important in the metabolism of histamine. So if my patient Mary finds that her asthma is triggered by drinking wine with metabisulphite preservatives, should she blame her asthma genes, or is she suffering from a molybdenum deficiency? Perhaps the superphosphated soil in which her food is grown is as deplete in molybdenum as it is in selenium or magnesium.

Molybdenum has a buffering effect on other minerals—it helps to maintain the delicate balance needed between iron, zinc and copper. Sometimes iron deficiency is resistant to iron therapy. The addition of molybdenum can make the difference.

Australia and certain other countries do not have an RDI for molybdenum. It has been estimated that the minimum should be around 25 mcg. The best-known sources include dairy products, pulses and legumes, organ meats and whole cereals, again with the proviso that the soil from which they were produced had appreciable levels, and was not acidified.

There are other elements such as vanadium, nickel, lithium, arsenic, fluorine, germanium, silicon, aluminium, cadmium, bromine and even lead, which in very tiny (ultra-trace) amounts are suspected of playing some essential role in animal biology. Lead deficiency, it would seem, is sometimes described in rats. Certain elements such as fluorine and lithium have been shown to have strong medicinal effects in humans when used in pharmacological amounts. While these medicinal values are not proof that the element is essential, a substance that is not essential to life may still have a role in maintaining optimal health.

Iodine and bromine

Earlier in this chapter I commented that iodine deficiency, because of its association with goitre, had been given due attention by the medical profession. Most doctors think about iodine in relationship to thyroid problems, and we know that neurological disorders as severe as congenital cretinism can result from deficiency. In Chapter 9: Multiple Sclerosis, a link between thyroid disorders, multiple sclerosis and Parkinson's disease is noted, with iodine deficiency the common factor.

But has this non-patentable element been given its full due? The work of people such as Guy Abraham and Jorge Flechas has opened up new and dramatic cause for concern.[29] Could diabetes, insulin resistance, fibrocystic breast disease, PCOS—and cancers of the breast, uterus, ovary, prostate and thyroid—all be linked to iodine deficiency? As at June 2008, a vigorous debate, mainly about the safe upper limit for iodine supplementation, is to be found online in the Townsend Letter—a body that styles itself as 'The Examiner of Alternative Medicine'.[30]

Under scrutiny, too, are mood and psychological disorders. An Australian study published in 2006 showed that half of Australian primary school children were iodine deficient[31] and studies in the UK found that 40% of women across the UK consume less than half of the recommended levels of iodine. Perhaps iodine deficiency should be added to the list of factors discussed in Chapter 9: Outrage: the changing picture of mental health in children.

Flechas and others have explored the toxic association between iodine deficiency and bromine excess. Bromine is added to bread in place of iodine, and is to be found widely in processed food—and the implications of this association certainly warrants further study.

Abraham suggests that the RDA of iodine should be 12.5 to 100 times the US level, which he gives as 125 mcg. The estimated daily intake of iodine in the Japanese diet is 1300–1400 mcg.

Chapter Five

VITAMINS AND ESSENTIAL FATTY ACIDS

VITAMINS

A VITAMIN IS USUALLY DEFINED as an organic compound, essential to life, which cannot be made in the body and therefore must be eaten. As it is not broken down for the production of energy, nor used as a building block for bodily tissues, it is required in only tiny quantities.

There are limitations to this definition. For example, Vitamin D is classified as a vitamin because people who don't get enough of it can develop rickets. However, this is one of the vitamins which well-nourished bodies can make for themselves, so long as they have adequate exposure to sun.

Another vitamin which humans can produce is niacin (Vitamin B3), which can be made from the amino acid tryptophan. As with Vitamin D, the definition 'cannot be made and must be ingested' does not apply strictly. However, as deficiency states can occur easily, and can be corrected by either diet or supplements, it is not unreasonable to regard it as a vitamin. Another way to see this is to assume that in the ideal state our needs are met by dietary means, but that we also have a back-up mechanism.

Over time it is possible that the definition of a vitamin may change. Co-enzyme Q10 behaves like a vitamin, but we make it ourselves. As we age we make less of it, and supplements have been shown to benefit certain medical conditions. A new definition might also include those dietary elements not strictly necessary to life, but potentially capable of promoting health and prolonging life.

Vitamins are *elaborate* structures made up of *common* elements. The plant, animal or bacterium which manufactures the vitamin uses raw materials such as carbon, nitrogen, hydrogen and oxygen, arranged in carbon chains and rings. The delicate structure is carefully built in a series of enzyme-driven steps, and once this structure breaks down in any way, it loses its usefulness. Heat, freezing, ultraviolet light, irradiation, microwaving, chemical additives, even the passage of time, may disrupt the delicate bonds holding these molecules together.

Some vitamins are more vulnerable to particular stresses than others. Vitamin C is largely destroyed by cooking, but the yield of Vitamin A is greater from cooked than raw carrots. Heat in the latter case breaks down the cell walls, making the vitamin more available to its human or animal consumer.

Once in the body, the vitamin may be 'consumed'. This means that as it serves its biochemical purpose it irrevocably changes its structure and is no longer a vitamin. It is the nature of vitamins that there is a high attrition rate, and new vitamins must constantly be ingested.

The body has some mechanisms to protect its precious vitamin stores. The process by which Vitamin C is recycled has been discussed in Chapter 3. There are also means to ensure maximum efficiency in the work the vitamin does. This is known as 'sparing'. Thus, adequate supplies of selenium have a sparing effect on Vitamin E, assuring maximum conservation of the value derived from Vitamin E.

Patients often ask about the difference between a vitamin and a mineral. If a *mineral*, such as magnesium, is in food, it stays there until it is eaten. It may be lost to the cooking water; or, if it is volatile, like selenium, it may be lost by evaporation, but careful cooking methods will usually conserve its content. The main requirement is that the mineral be there in the first place.

Vitamins, as we have just seen, are easily broken down. Freshness is of the essence. Doctors and dieticians tell people that they will get all the vitamins they need from a healthy diet. The assumption is that this diet will consist of fresh food. 'Fresh' does not encompass packaged, bottled, canned, frozen or dried.

Some history and background

We now have a detailed understanding of the biochemistry of vitamins, but knowledge of their function goes back a long time. Stipanuk observes that writings as far back as 1500 BCE record the consumption of liver as a cure for night blindness.[1] Embedded in the folk wisdom of many cultures is evidence that food was used as medicine because of its vitamin content. The most dramatic evidence that factors other than mere victuals were required for survival came when humans began to make long sea voyages. Then the signs of scurvy and beriberi began to manifest themselves, only to resolve when fresh food supplies became available.

The first of the vitamins to be identified was Vitamin B1; the work was done by a Polish biochemist called Funk, working at the Lister Institute in London. He coined the term 'vitamin' because B1 is a chemical structure known as an 'amine' and it is 'vital' to life. By 1912 he had expanded the concept to embrace other complex molecules that appeared to be essential in the diet.

The next to be unravelled were Vitamins C, D and B3, the deficiency of which causes scurvy, rickets and pellagra respectively. The 'e' was dropped from the end of 'vitamin' as it came to be realised that the structure of a vitamin was not typically an amine.

In all, 13 nutrients have been identified as vitamins in human biology, and many of them play similar roles in other animal species. The human vitamins include eight B-group vitamins, and A, C, D, E and K.

In extracting vitamins solvents were used, and this led to the appreciation that some vitamins are water-soluble and others are fat-soluble. The water-soluble vitamins were found to be distributed through the aqueous compartments of the body such as the fluids in and around cells, and last only a short time in the body because of their excretion in the urine. As a result, they are unlikely to be toxic when taken as supplements. The fat-soluble vitamins, by contrast, are stored in fatty tissue and are not so easily disposed of. Excess amounts, although often over-emphasised, do therefore have potential for toxicity. The fat-soluble vitamins are A, D, E and K. All other vitamins are water-soluble.

It was also realised that, even among mammals, vitamin requirements vary from species to species. The human need for Vitamin C is well known, but humans and other primates are unusual in this need. Along with guinea pigs and the Indian fruit bat they are among the small minority of animals which cannot manufacture their own Vitamin C. One assumes that these animals evolved in an environment in which there was an abundance of dietary Vitamin C.

Some species can take advantage of their gut bacteria to do some of the manufacturing for them. For instance ruminants such as cows get their B-group vitamins from their gut bacteria. It is not necessary for the animal to eat food containing those vitamins. When for some reason the gut bacteria are destroyed, as in the oral administration of antibiotics to farm animals, the animals can develop deficiency disorders. Doctors are just beginning to appreciate this function of the gut bacteria in humans.

Vitamins are not single entities. They can exist in different states, each of which has different functions. Thus, Vitamin B3 can exist as niacin or niacinamide. Vitamin C can appear in several forms, including ascorbic acid and dehydroascorbate. There are whole families of retinols (Vitamin A) and tocopherols (Vitamin E). This has important implications for the interpretation of vitamin trials where single forms are used.

The functions of the vitamins can be classified into three broad categories. Some vitamins fit into more than one category.

- *Co-enzymes:* This is by far the commonest function of vitamins. All of the B-group vitamins, Vitamin C and one form of Vitamin K serve this function. They have a regulating role in the action of enzymes, which are the means by which most biochemical reactions in the body take place, including the production of energy from food (Chapter 3). The vitamin itself is not used for energy, but it catalyses the reactions that produce energy. Other co-enzyme roles include lipid metabolism and detoxification by the liver of substances toxic to the body.
- *Anti-oxidants:* Vitamins C and E are the most relevant in this regard, as described below.
- *Miscellaneous:* Vitamins A and D are required in the synthesis of some hormones. Vitamin A acts as a pigment in the retina, supporting visual function by regenerating bleached rhodopsin. Under this heading is an unusual role for Vitamin B3, which is discussed below.

We will now look at each of the vitamins in more detail.

Vitamin A

An important distinction is made between the plant-derived forms of Vitamin A, which are the *carotene* forms, and the animal-derived forms (liver, oily fish), which are referred to as *retinols*.

About 600 carotenoids occur in nature. Approximately 50 of these behave like Vitamin A and are known as provitamin A. The word retinoid is used to describe any compound which has a structural similarity to retinol, the alcoholic form of Vitamin A. In the body Vitamin A undergoes many metabolic changes, and the various forms serve a wide range of functions.

Vitamin A is important in vision and as an anti-oxidant. Its role (as 11-*cis*-retinal) in vision is well known to most lay people. Wartime night blindness was the early warning of more permanent visual loss.

Some of the cancer-protective effects of the carotenoids come from their anti-oxidant properties. Patients with exercise-induced asthma are thought to be benefited by beta carotene, an effect attributed to the protection afforded by the vitamin against the oxidative stress of exercise. Less well known is this vitamin's role in reproduction, immune function and gene transcription. For normal functioning in these areas, adequate supplies of Vitamin A are essential.

Vitamin A helps the immune system to resist such diseases as measles and malaria. The conclusion of one study was that mortality was significantly reduced when Vitamin A supplements were given periodically to children at a community level. The recommendation was that they should be given to all measles patients in developing countries, whether or not clinical deficiency was in evidence.[2] A double-blind trial published in *The Lancet* showed that high-dose supplements of Vitamin A protected children in Papua New Guinea against *P. falciparum*, the nastiest of the malaria parasites. As we saw in Chapter 3, malaria is estimated to have killed half of all people who have ever lived. That a vitamin could make such an impact shows that nature provides solutions for illnesses we customarily think of as amenable only to pharmacological treatment. There was no clear impact on the *prevalence* of malaria in these children — that is, they did not seem any less likely to contract the disease. Once they did get it, however, there was a significant change in the immune response of children over the age of one, including a 68 per cent reduction in parasite load, compared to the unsupplemented group.[3]

Vitamin A is also important for cellular differentiation, proliferation and signalling. In plain speak, this means that when cells divide, mature and grow, Vitamin A regulates the process. Nutrient deficiencies can cause errors in the reading of the genetic code, or in the ability of the cell to follow the gene's instruction. As an embryo develops into a baby, mistakes can result in structural abnormalities. Vitamin A is essential to embryogenesis.[4] The retinoid forms of Vitamin A play an important role both in the maturation of primitive or young cells and in the switch that tells the cells when to stop reproducing themselves. This is known as 'signalling'. Cells that don't know when to stop reproducing, or proliferating, produce inflammation (as in acne lesions) or are on the way to becoming cancer cells.

Retinoic acid has been successfully used in the treatment of one kind of human leukaemia, and in epidemiological trials has been shown to help in the prevention and treatment of other cancers.[5] Japanese people have a tendency to develop gastric cancer, but only in some regions. Researchers considered many possible causes including the high-salt diet and the consumption of pickled vegetables. Epidemiological studies indicated that the disease might be explained by the differences in 'plasma levels of beta-carotene and alpha-tocopherol, and possibly alpha carotene, lycopene and ascorbic acid, [which] may partly account for the regional difference in gastric cancer mortality in Japan.'[6]

Despite the many benefits of Vitamin A, it is an unfortunate fact that the public will most frequently hear about it in a negative context. It is true that it may cause birth defects. Both animal studies and human observational studies suggest that large doses of Vitamin A early in pregnancy can be teratogenic (responsible for birth defects).

But of more concern is its undeserved reputation for causing cancer. Indeed, as early as 1925 researchers noted that when Vitamin A was *deficient*, organs actually resembled cancerous tissue. It is ironic but entirely predictable that the reference most commonly cited in relation to Vitamin A is the beta carotene study discussed in Chapter 2, which *appeared* to demonstrate that patients taking the vitamin were actually more likely to develop lung cancer than the control group.

It is generally agreed that pregnant women should not exceed a daily intake of 2500–3000 mcg of Vitamin A. There is no restriction on the consumption of carotenoid vegetables, but intake from animals forms such as liver should be taken into account in this safe upper limit.

The B-group vitamins

There are eight B-group vitamins: thiamine (B1), riboflavin (B2), niacin (B3), pantothenic acid (B5), pyridoxine (B6), cobalamin (B12), folic acid (folate), and biotin. Their numbers are neither sequential nor particularly informative, but I have used them here because readers are likely to know them better than the names.

We will look at them in groups, based on their metabolic functions:

- *B3, B2 and B1* are important in the pathways which produce energy from food.
- *Folic acid, B6 and B12* are involved with the metabolism of amino acids, the building blocks of protein, in which they have several specialised roles.
- *B5 and biotin* are involved predominantly, though not exclusively, in lipid (fat) metabolism.

Vitamin B3 (niacin)

Deficiency of this vitamin gives rise to the disease known as *pellagra*, the classic features being the 'three Ds', diarrhoea, dermatitis and dementia. Although pellagra is rarely seen in its extreme form, it should be considered when elderly people or those on poor diets display any of these symptoms, especially dementia.

The names often cause confusion. B3 has several aliases. As 'niacin' it is sometimes called nicotinic acid, which means the same thing. Slightly different chemistry gives us 'niacinamide', sometimes known as nicotinamide. Collectively, they are all referred to as Vitamin B3. The 'amide' form is different in function, side effects and toxicity to the acidic form. Generally speaking, even in large doses, the B vitamins are not toxic. Some people experience a flushing effect when they take multi-B vitamins because of the B3.

This is unpleasant but it is not an allergy and is not dangerous; it soon wears off.

Functions

Vitamin B3 is vital in breaking down glucose, fatty acids, ketones and amino acids to produce energy. For those familiar with the Krebs Cycle, niacin in its amide form is the N of NAD and NADH. One molecule of NADH entering the electron transport chain produces up to three molecules of ATP, the major energy source in the body. This is ultimately expressed as the complete oxidation of glucose to carbon dioxide and water, with the release of energy for the maintenance of life.

It is this function of B3 which puts it into the 'miscellaneous' category. Its role as a *substrate* — that is, a substance acted *upon* — is most unusual for a vitamin. Normally vitamins regulate the action of something else. (While of more interest to the biochemist than the average reader, this is worth a mention because it highlights the versatility of vitamins, and because the use of B3 in this way forms the basis of the body's single most important means of energy production.)

There are other energy-producing pathways in the body and the niacinamide or nicotinamide enzymes (also known as pyridine nucleotide co-enzymes) are involved in these pathways as well.

Niacin is thought to be part of the chromium-containing structure known as *glucose tolerance factor* or GTF. GTF is thought to increase the body's sensitivity to insulin and protect against diabetes. Syndrome X, discussed in Chapter 8, involves the diagnosis of raised lipids *and* diabetes, raising the possibility that B3 and chromium deficiency have a role in this epidemic.

Pregnant women and those on oral contraceptives appear to have an altered tryptophan metabolism. As we saw when discussing the definition of a vitamin, tryptophan can be used as a source of B3. While the nature of the alteration is not fully understood, it seems that these women, along with lactating mothers, may be making greater demands on their B3 supplies, and may therefore need foods rich in B3.[7] While some pregnant women become diabetic, many become very tired. B3 and chromium status (Chapter 4) may help explain the problem. Pregnant women also often develop widespread itch. As B3 inhibits mast cell degranulation, (Chapter 6: Hypersensitivity; Chapter 7: What you can do), then itch in this case—as well as in the elderly, the allergic and those generally under stress—may also warn of B3 deficiency.

In the days before cholesterol-lowering drugs, niacin or nicotinic acid was the only cholesterol-lowering medication we had. This was an example of a natural dietary component being used in unnatural or pharmacological doses. B3 is absorbed from the gut and reabsorbed by the kidneys. Chronic diarrhoea or high alcohol intake, poor renal function or a low-protein diet (tryptophan comes from protein)—any of these can contribute to low levels of B3 and, thus, raised cholesterol levels.

Vitamin B2 (riboflavin)

The natural colour of Vitamin B2 is a fluorescent green-yellow, so the urine of people taking B supplements has a startling glow. Vitamin B2 is found in liver, dairy products and green vegetables. Because many people live on a refined cereal diet, manufacturers enrich flour and breakfast cereals with B2. This prevents illness, but it is a sad comment on the modern diet. B2 in acidic foods is relatively stable, but in alkaline environments and when heated or exposed to light it breaks down, with subsequent loss of activity. Picked green vegetables turning yellow may reflect a loss of riboflavin.

Deficiency produces sore mouth (angular stomatitis), tongue (glossitis), anaemia and neuropathy. Elderly patients, alcoholics and those on poor diets are at risk of deficiency. These clinical signs are quite common in general practice, and B2 prescription should be routine in such cases.

Vitamin B1 (thiamine)

Severe deprivation of Vitamin B1 is known as beriberi. It has been a major problem in wartime, and is seen among alcoholics in casualty departments. The cardiovascular and nervous systems seem to be the most affected as patients develop heart failure, muscle weakness, peripheral neuropathy (loss of feeling in the hands and feet), confusion, psychosis, ataxia (staggering gait) and finally death.

Due to the peculiarities of the ruminant physiology, beriberi is not uncommon in farm animals. In a manner different from, but analogous to, the disturbance of gut flora in the human, an overgrowth of a normally benign bacterium, in this case *Bacillus thiaminolyticus*, causes the destruction of B1 in the gut. *Polioencephalomalacia*, also known as 'staggers', develops. This occurs in sheep, goats and alpacas. Both the human and the animal forms respond rapidly to the intramuscular injection of B1.

During World War II, prisoners fed white rice developed beriberi. Thus the essential nutrient (as with zinc, chromium, selenium and Vitamin E) was found to be in the brown outer part of the rice or wheat grain. For every cup of white rice and every slice of white bread that we eat, there is a cup of brown rice and a slice of wholemeal bread that we did not eat.

In 'fortified' products the manufacturers are not giving us something extra: they are replacing something that has been taken away. Perhaps one day modern diseases such as diabetes, dementia and heart disease will be seen as the consequences, amongst others, of chronic deficiency disorders.

Folic acid (folate)

Folic acid is found in vegetables, especially leafy green vegetables, strawberries and citrus fruits, meat and fish, fortified cereals and breads. It would seem to be so widespread as never to be in short supply. However, folic acid is unstable, easily destroyed or leached out by food preparation and heating. It is lacking in many junk and highly processed foods. At a symposium for doctors on the relationship between folic acid deficiency and birth defects, less than half of the doctors in a large audience were confident that they would have met the minimum daily requirement in their meals of the previous day.

The word folate is a generic name for the active metabolites of folic acid, and is technically the better term. However, for simplicity I use 'folic acid' in this book. Folic acid metabolites are part of co-enzymes which are involved in the metabolism of amino acids and the synthesis of DNA precursors. In these reactions, folic acid co-enzymes act as single carbon donors or acceptors, the process already discussed as methylation (Chapter 3). The main pathways involving folic acid co-enzymes include the methionine (or SAM) cycle, the thymidylate cycle and the purine cycle.

Some effects of deficiency

Folic acid deficiency has received publicity in connection with birth defects. Among the other conditions linked to deficiency are heart disease, stroke, depression, dementia, neuropathy and a whole range of cancers.

The inadequate metabolism of homocysteine is one of the most important consequences of folic acid deficiency, with raised levels increasing the risk of a wide range of disease (Chapters 3, 6–8).

One of the earliest known functions of folic acid was in the treatment and prevention of one type of anaemia, megaloblastic anaemia. Named for the large red cells that are typical of this condition, the size of the cell merely reflects its immaturity. Young red cells are very large; as they mature they become smaller. Both Vitamin B12 and folic acid are required for their normal development. A lack of either of these vitamins gives rise to megaloblastic anaemia, and another more serious condition affecting the nervous system, *subacute combined degeneration of the spinal cord* (see below, Vitamin B12). When anaemia is due to folic acid deficiency, the red cells fail to mature because the folic acid-dependent thymidylate cycle is disrupted. This leads to the toxic accumulation of a metabolite called *uracil*. The greater the pool of uracil, the greater the risk of it being mistakenly incorporated into the red cell's DNA. This error, if it occurs on both strands of the DNA, can exceed the cell's ability for repair, leaving the cell in a defective state. These cells are removed from the circulation by the spleen, and a constant supply of immature blood cells is formed.

Outside the circulation, it is suspected that such damage to DNA could account for some of the folic acid-related cancers. For some time it has been suspected that folic acid deficiency contributes to the development of some cancers, and evidence has begun to accumulate. Anything which interferes with the repair of DNA is certainly a suspect in the aetiology of cancer, and so the accumulation of uracil in cells other than red cells is a cause for concern.

In Chapter 3 we saw that individuals who have not one but two copies of the defective gene involved in the methionine cycle are at risk from increased plasma homocysteine. In addition the consequent *reduction* in the amount of remethylated methionine carries its own risks. Folic acid donates a methyl-group to homocysteine, which is then converted to methionine. The methionine in turn acts as a methyl donor (hence the word cycle, as this system keeps regenerating itself in the presence of folic acid). It donates its methyl group is to both the synthesis and repair of DNA.

Thus folic acid deficiency could be a cancer risk factor through several mechanisms. In 1997 it was demonstrated that the increased cancer risk in people homozygous for the *methylenetetrahydrofolate reductase* (MTHR) variation (Chapter 3) appeared to be reduced when these people were supplemented with folic acid. As this constitutes between 5 per cent and 25 per cent of the population, it is an important finding.[8]

Large trials are currently in progress at Tuft's University and elsewhere after pilot trials suggested that extra folic acid may be beneficial in preventing colorectal cancers and also breast, cervical, stomach and pancreatic cancers. There is also evidence that childhood leukaemia appears to be reduced in those children whose mothers took folic acid supplements in pregnancy.[9]

The Nurses' Health Study (begun in the United States in 1979 and still going) has followed 88,818 cancer-free women. Over a 15-year period, although dietary folic acid had some impact on lowering cancer risk, the most significant impact was made by folic acid supplements. And the effect was dose-related: women who took 200 mcg daily derived less benefit than women taking 400 mcg. The benefit was most significant after long-term supplementation, but the estimate was that at the higher doses, colon cancer in a 15-year period could be reduced by up to 75 per cent. The effect seemed to be independent of the consumption of Vitamins A, C, D and E.

The overall trend did not support a reduction in the risk of breast cancer, except for one very interesting group. It is often quoted that women who drink as little as two standard drinks a day significantly increase their risk of breast cancer. An analysis of these results showed that for women who drank *and* took folic acid their excess risk was effectively reduced to baseline. These results raise the question of what constitutes 'normal' values.

Supplementing

The current RDI for folic acid is 400 mcg, and 600 mcg for pregnant women. High-risk pregnancies are often treated at 10 times that dosage; that is, 5000 mcg or half a milligram (0.5 mg). Folic acid is used rather than the natural folate form, because it is more chemically stable. There are no known toxic side effects, although the complications of masking B12-related megaloblastic anaemia exist (see above). The curious side effect of possibly raising twinning rates has recently been raised by a Swedish study.[10]

Folic acid is normally absorbed from that part of the small intestine known as the jejunum, and deficiency states sometimes occur as a result of malabsorption syndromes such as coeliac disease and tropical sprue. Chronic alcoholism and severe debility can also give rise to measurable deficiency. By contrast, low-grade ongoing depletion does not attract the attention it deserves.

One point should be made in conclusion. All growing and dividing tissues require folic acid. Cancer cells, as the most rapidly growing and dividing cells in the body, consume a lot of folic acid. In the treatment of cancer, anti-folates such as methotrexate are given to starve the cancer cells of folic acid and slow their growth. In *no way* should this be taken to imply that folic acid supplements can contribute to the *development* of cancer. And while it is usual practice for nutritional doctors to stop the folic acid while a patient is undergoing anti-folate therapy, at the end of therapy it should be resumed.

Vitamin B12

Vitamin B12 is usually discussed in context with folic acid because deficiency of either produces megaloblastic anaemia. This is because B12 co-enzymes are necessary in the same cycles as folate for DNA synthesis and repair, and deficiency results in a functional folate deficiency.

The commonest sources of B12 are animal foods such as meat, eggs and seafood. A lot of nonsense is spouted about vegetarians being at risk of B12 deficiency, but the average vegetarian rarely has abnormal blood levels. Of more concern are vegans, but they mostly get an adequate supply from fortified cereals and supplements. Vegans should have their B12 levels monitored during pregnancy.

Another source for vegans is algae and seaweed which contain B12,[11] and some is thought to be found on the surface of fungi such as mushrooms, or attached to the surface of root vegetables. As anaerobic micro-organisms produce B12 for their own use, it may be present in fermented foods such as miso, or even manufactured by gut flora in healthy individuals. Moreover, as one of the main functions of B12 is in the metabolism of meat, vegetarians require much less of it.

B12 deficiency can arise from failure to eat foods containing B12, and chronic diarrhoea of any origin will reduce B12 absorption. But clinically there is a more insidious cause: something known as *intrinsic factor* may be lacking. Intrinsic factor is a glycoprotein secreted by parietal cells in the stomach which binds onto B12 and facilitates its absorption. Parietal cells are often lost in autoimmune disease and advancing age. It is not uncommon for patients with an undiagnosed autoimmune disease like coeliac to present with pernicious anaemia, even though the coeliac problem is further down the gut. (The lack of parietal cells of any origin also results in declining levels of gastric acid, further compounding the problem, as gastric acid is necessary to split the vitamin from its dietary protein binders.)

Some effects of deficiency

When megaloblastic anaemia is the result of dietary deficiency of B12 or folic acid, it can be simply corrected. When it is the result of the lack of intrinsic factor, it is known as pernicious anaemia. Oral replacement of the missing vitamin does not fix the problem; it has to be treated by injections. Megaloblastic anaemia, however, is not the most serious consequence of severe B12 or folate deficiency.

A condition called *subacute combined degeneration of the spinal cord* is far more dangerous. Fortunately the anaemia usually alerts the treating physician to the possibility that this more serious condition might be present. Unfortunately, however, treatment of the *anaemia* caused by one of these vitamin deficiencies—either folate or B12—corrects the anaemia, even if it was the *other* vitamin which was lacking. Thus, the true deficiency is masked and the nervous system disease progresses unchecked. This is a potential problem with consuming fortified foods or taking *single* B vitamin supplements.

Sub-acute combined degeneration results in loss of the myelin sheath around nerve tissue (comparable to multiple sclerosis), loss of function of peripheral nerves, memory loss and dementia. Lost trekkers who have gone without food for long periods and then eaten high-protein meals when found have been known to develop a nasty form of this condition. This results because the metabolism of the protein makes an acute demand on their low B12 stores, and irreversible nerve damage, even blindness, can ensue.

B12 deficiency should always be considered in patients diagnosed with dementia. A level that prevents an extreme disorder—such as megaloblastic anaemia or subacute degeneration of the spinal cord—may not be sufficient to prevent a more insidious but just as devastating condition such as dementia.

Many patients seek B12 injections for fatigue and chronic fatigue syndrome, despite normal B12 blood levels. Considerable benefit often ensues, probably because our 'normal' values are too low. Also, blood levels do not accurately represent levels in the central nervous system. The use of methylated B12 can be very effective. In this form B12 more easily crosses the blood–brain barrier. From personal experience, methylated B12 can be a very effective treatment in relapses of multiple sclerosis.

Vitamin B6

Vitamin B6 is the last in our second group of B vitamins. B6 acts as a co-enzyme for more than 100 enzymes, including amino transferases, decarboxylases, aldolases and others—a critical vitamin, in short. Improvement in conditions as wide-ranging as asthma, insomnia, and nausea and vomiting of pregnancy has been noted with the use of B6 supplements.

The RDI for B6 is given as 1.3 mg for adults, and 1.9 mg for pregnant women. B6 is found in meat, fish, cereals and non-citrus fruits. There are six major forms of B6 with vitamin activity, and these are all absorbed passively and well from the small intestine. The plant and supplemental forms undergo a process in the liver known as phosphorylation. Plasma levels of one of these forms reflect both liver and body stores, and are therefore a good test of overall B6 status.

Although the wide distribution of B6 in foods and fortified cereals should ensure ready supply, deficiency states do occur. As usual, highly processed flours and polished grains have little, as does most junk food. B6 is light-sensitive and supplements are often sold in dark glass or opaque containers. Significant losses can occur with heat or leaching into cooking water.

People with malabsorptive states such as coeliac disease and chronic diarrhoea can suffer deficiency. People with a high alcohol intake can have low plasma levels independent of dietary status. Metabolism of B6 can be disturbed by liver damage. This is thought to be due to the toxic effect of acetaldehyde, the product of alcohol metabolism. Supplements with B vitamins are important for people who drink a lot.

The list of conditions associated with B6 deficiency includes seborrhoic dermatitis, microcytic anaemia, depression, mental confusion and convulsions. The neurological symptoms listed here are the result of malfunction of the B6-dependent carboxylase enzymes. These are required for the metabolism of tryptophan, one of the most important neurotransmitters in the brain. An outbreak of convulsions in formula-fed infants in the 1950s was traced to a formula low in B6. Increasingly, doctors are prescribing B6 for patients with depression and those suffering from premenstrual tension.

The role of folic acid and B6 in lowering homocysteine has been mentioned.

Excess B6 is excreted in the urine, and toxicity is rarely a problem. Massive daily doses of 1000 to 6000 mg (that is, 1–6 grams) have been associated with a type of peripheral neuropathy. This is slowly reversed after discontinuation.[12] No toxicity has been reported at daily doses of 300 mg and below.

Vitamin B5 (pantothenic acid) and biotin

Vitamin B5 occurs in liver, meat, milk, whole-grain cereals and legumes. There is considerable loss in processed foods. Although extreme deficiency states are uncommon, volunteers on an experimentally depleted diet became listless and complained of fatigue. In an earlier experiment more extreme deprivation produced insomnia, personality changes, impaired motor co-ordination and gut disturbances.[13] These descriptions would fit any number of my patients. Is it possible that they have a B5 deficiency?

Pantothenic acid is metabolised to Co-enzyme A. Most of it is transported into the mitochondria of the cell, where it plays a vital role in the oxidative combustion of fats for energy. The highly complex chemistry of the various forms of Co-enzyme A in the mitochondria gives rise to the citric acid cycle, and the production of energy from keto acids during glucose deficits and starvation. In the fluid part of the cell, the acyl Co-enzyme As are also the basis of the body's own production of cholesterol, all of the steroid hormones, and a class of substances which includes Co-enzyme Q10.

Marginal deficiencies have the potential to disrupt these finely tuned cycles. Vitamin B5 is an important tool in the reduction of the levels of 'bad' cholesterol, as it helps convert cholesterol to these important metabolites.

Biotin is less well known than B5. Deficiency was identified as a cause of dermatitis, hair loss and neurological abnormalities in rats as early as the 1920s. It is an essential part of four enzymes. Three of these are carboxylases, involved with various stages of the cycles just described. Genetic disorders involving the ability to handle biotin result in problems ranging through skin rashes and alopecia (severe hair loss), through to developmental delay, hearing loss, optic atrophy, seizures and death.

Biotin is readily available from liver, egg yolk and cooked cereals, but raw egg white binds biotin in such a way that a diet high in this substance can induce deficiency, as can an extremely-low-protein diet. Long-term use of anti-convulsants (with the exception of sodium valproate and perhaps some of the new agents) has been associated with lowered plasma levels of biotin. The biotin content of processed and junk food is predictably poor.

Vitamin C (ascorbic acid)

Vitamin C is important, safe and the most controversial of all the vitamins. In the space available it is impossible to do justice to any of these aspects, but there is a wealth of literature on Vitamin C, and can be found in various books listed in Further Reading.

Animals unable to synthesise Vitamin C must ingest it to survive. Most species manufacture their own from a glucose precursor. Four steps are involved to transform this precursor into ascorbic acid, each requiring an enzyme.

Humans and other primates lack only the terminal enzyme. Interestingly, it would appear that our distant forebears once made their own Vitamin C, but the DNA is now so mutated that it cannot code for the enzyme.

Enzymes
Electron donation by ascorbic acid is used to drive or catalyse several important human enzyme systems.

- *Dopamine beta-hydroxylase* is essential for the conversion of dopamine to the neurotransmitter norepinephrine (nor-adrenaline) in the central and peripheral nervous systems and in the adrenal gland (see Chart 3.3). This helps explain why major symptoms of scurvy and even mild Vitamin C deficiency are fatigue and depression. The term 'adrenal exhaustion' is sometimes used.

- *Peptidylglycine alpha-amidating monoxygenase* involves the production of hormones relating to the thyroid, gonads, digestive juices, bone metabolism and neuropeptides (neurotransmitters). Symptoms relating to all these systems have been observed in deficiency states.
- Three *hydroxylases* relate to the synthesis and repair of collagen. This is probably one of the most studied and best understood of all areas of ascorbic acid biochemistry. Repair of damaged knee and ankle joints of footballers, ballet dancers and other elite athletes responds well to Vitamin C supplements. Elderly patients often live on a low Vitamin C diet (known as a 'scorbutic diet'), and also have a beneficial response to supplementation.
- Two enzymes, also *hydroxylases*, help to synthesise a substance called carnitine. Carnitine in turn is involved in the transport of long-chain fatty acids into the mitochondria where they can be burnt (oxidised) for energy. A nutrient-dense diet including adequate meat, fish and eggs normally meets the body's need for carnitine. A low-protein diet does not, and here the ability to synthesise it becomes important. The symptoms of fatigue and muscle weakness that occur early in scurvy could be related to lack of carnitine. Low carnitine levels have been observed in scurvy, renal failure, diabetes, malignancy, alcohol abuse and myocardial ischaemia.
- *Tyrosine* metabolism has a relationship to Vitamin C both in the synthesis of adrenalin from tyrosine, and of dopamine from tyrosine. The conversion of tryptophan to serotonin also utilises Vitamin C.

Redox

Vitamin C has various other important anti-oxidant applications.

- *DNA:* Oxidative damage to DNA occurs continually, with significant implication for the development of cancer and other degenerative disorders. Cells have specific enzymes for the repair of DNA but these enzymes do not effect all repairs. *In vitro* studies indicate a role for ascorbic acid in the protection of DNA and the mRNA transcription of certain genes. Definitive roles await further investigation. Much epidemiological evidence points towards a high Vitamin C diet being protective against cancer, especially gastric cancer.

- *In the cell:* Ascorbic acid seems to protect intracellular proteins from oxidative damage in, for example, white blood cells, lung and eye, where exposure to oxygen is high. This is difficult to establish in living tissue, but epidemiological studies support a protective role against cataract, for example, in people taking Vitamin C supplements.[14]

- *The 'bad' fats:* Protection against *extra*cellular oxidative damage has been widely studied in relation to the oxidation of low-density lipoproteins (LDL) or 'bad' fats. (See 'Vitamin E', and Chapter 8). *Oxidised* LDL is responsible for the increased risk of cardiovascular events in people with high levels. Vitamin C seems to reduce the absolute level of LDL, and the arterial damage done by the oxidised form of it.[15]

- *Clot formation:* Experimental evidence supports a role for Vitamin C in reducing white cell and platelet aggregation, another major factor in the development of atherosclerosis. It is hard to prove this in real life, but it seems reasonable on current evidence.

Safe quantities

Because Vitamin C is water-soluble and readily excreted, it is hard to understand the controversy surrounding its use. On its own, Vitamin C is unlikely to cure cancer or any other condition except scurvy. In combination with other micronutrients it is a powerful tool with which to prevent and treat many deadly Western diseases. It is highly probable that our current RDIs are far too low—a fact under consideration by the Institute of Medicine in the United States.[16]

One test-tube experiment demonstrated that an intermediary in Vitamin C metabolism, in highly abnormal circumstances, had *pro*-oxidant properties.[17] It is odd that this made world headlines, when scores of other studies demonstrating a benefit never rate a mention. Bad news sells. Millions of people became afraid to take supplements. The inability of the public to judge these stories is both understandable and excusable. For the medical profession, it is not.

Daily doses of Vitamin C of 1000 to 5000 mg (1–5 grams) are usually recommended. Animals which produce their own make something like 1 gram per 7 kilograms of body weight per day. Under stress, that quantity can rise fivefold or tenfold. Thus, if humans could produce Vitamin C, an average adult would be producing around 10 grams (10,000 mg) daily. This may seem a ridiculous amount, but to people living on fresh berries in a rainforest it would not be a difficult quantity to consume. The Kakadu plum eaten by Australian Aborigines provides quantities like this with just a handful of fruit.

Seriously or acutely ill patients are sometimes injected with up to 15 or 30 grams of intravenous Vitamin C. This should be done only by trained doctors in appropriate circumstances. When I first began giving this treatment I consulted my professional indemnity organisation and found that they had established that thousands of such treatments had failed to produce even one serious or life-threatening event. There are no other treatments with safety records as good as this. The use of aspirin or paracetamol, which can be purchased over the counter by minors, can result in a hospital stay even when guidelines have been followed.

Or contrast this to the widespread use of cholesterol-lowering drugs. These agents topped the list in *cost* of drugs prescribed to the Australian public during 1998–99, accounting for 3.9 million one-month scripts at a cost of $200 million to the Australian health budget. In *frequency* of drug prescribed, cholesterol-lowering agents were second and eleventh on the list while in the US cholesterol-lowering drugs were the most commonly prescribed drugs from 2000–2006. These pharmaceutical agents have short-term side effects, and by lowering cholesterol disrupt some of our most important metabolic pathways. Chart 3.6 shows many of the hormones for which cholesterol is a precursor. The long-term effects of limiting the availability of this building block are unknown.

An Australian story

Archie Kalokerinos worked with Aboriginal children in remote towns in Australia in the 1950s, encountering white, medical and bureaucratic arrogance. The title of his book, *Every Second Child*, refers to the infant mortality rate which confronted the idealistic young doctor when he ventured into outback Australia.[18] The diet consumed by these hapless folk was similar to the diet of most native populations anywhere when displaced by white invaders. Having lost both the opportunity and the skill to pursue their traditional diet, they were subsisting on refined white flours and carbohydrates. Their rations were tea, sugar, white flour and a little meat. It took only a generation or two for such people, forcibly removed from their families into mission stations, to lose all their inherited food wisdom.

As the only doctor in town, it fell to Kalokerinos not only to nurse a child through a terminal illness, often the result of a simple childhood infection, but to perform the autopsy as well. Repeatedly he observed blotchy white patches throughout the liver, a sign of clinical scurvy. He noticed an upsurge in this kind of death after health authorities made routine visits to vaccinate children in outlying areas. His multiple attempts to convey his concerns to the authorities met with little response.

Kalokerinos later co-authored a book about Vitamin C with Glen and Ian Dettman and Nobel Prize–winning Linus Pauling.[19] Pauling, who was ridiculed for his personal consumption of large doses of Vitamin C, died at the age of 93, having worked in his laboratory until a few weeks before his death.

Vitamin D

Vitamin D is not, strictly speaking, a vitamin because our bodies can make it from a cholesterol precursor. This process requires the action of ultraviolet light from the sun on the skin.

Dark skin absorbs less than fair skin. Dark-skinned people who live in far northern countries have an increased risk of Vitamin D deficiency, especially when they cover up against the cold or for religious reasons.

By contrast, with the growing awareness of skin cancer, some fair-skinned people are covering up so much, and using sun block, that they risk Vitamin D deficiency. In my practice in Sydney I am currently diagnosing Vitamin D deficiency at the rate of one to two patients *a week*.

As people age, the skin loses some of its ability to manufacture Vitamin D. The housebound elderly, especially those with poor diets, are at particular risk.

The biochemistry

The precursor for Vitamin D, 7-dehydrocholesterol, moves from the liver to the cells of the skin. On exposure to ultraviolet B radiation, it is transformed to pre-vitamin D3. After a few hours at body temperature, this converts to Vitamin D3 and enters the bloodstream. As Vitamin D is exquisitely sensitive to degradation by sunlight, and enters the bloodstream at a limited rate, the amount made in the skin is never toxic.

The liver takes up both ingested and skin-derived Vitamin D, and uses an enzyme to add a hydroxyl group to form 25-hydroxy-Vitamin D. This is the form most commonly measured in the blood to assess Vitamin D status. Most of it is bound to a protein which acts as a store. The unbound form goes to the kidney where it undergoes a further hydroxylation to produce the active form. This form is known as $1,25(OH)_2D$, and in complex cases this also is measured. During the latter stages of pregnancy the placenta also has the capacity to produce this active form, in order to promote the mother's intestinal absorption of calcium.

A hormone from the parathyroid gland determines how much is converted to the active form. Knowing all this, we can see that skin, parathyroid and kidney conditions all have the capacity to affect the amount of active Vitamin D in the body. So do gut disorders that limit the amount of the vitamin absorbed by the body. Thus considerable potential for deficiency exists.

The process is somewhat different in cats and other animals whose thick fur prevents sunlight getting to the skin. In this case the oil glands secrete the precursor onto the fur. When the cat sunbakes, the transformation takes place, and the cat ingests the Vitamin D thus formed during its vigorous grooming procedures.

Vitamin D is best known for its role in maintaining a healthy skeletal mass, keeping serum levels of calcium optimum for bone mineralisation. This it does by increasing gut absorption of calcium. A steady level of calcium is also essential for normal metabolism in many cells, particularly those relating to neuromuscular function.

Cancer

Vitamin D may have a significant impact on the development of cancer. A wide variety of cells in the brain, skin, gonads, breast, gut, mononuclear cells, B and T lymphocytes and other tissues are found to have receptors for Vitamin D. Many of these cells are not tissues which need calcium as such, implying a more complex role for Vitamin D. It has now been established that the active form of Vitamin D inhibits the proliferation and induces differentiation in a wide range of both normal and tumour cells.[20]

In 2002 an American researcher, William Grant, examined the link between Vitamin D and cancer. Controlling for factors such as socioeconomic status and environment, and comparing cool climates such as Boston with the warmer American south-east, he estimated that about 70,000 people a year in the United States develop cancer through lack of Vitamin D. He also proposed that about 23,000 died prematurely from one or other of the effects of Vitamin D deprivation. His analyses of cancer mortality data and exposure to ultraviolet B showed an inverse relationship between 13 different kinds of cancer, including gut, breast and reproductive organ cancers. Trials to investigate Vitamin D as treatment in breast and ovarian cancer are under way.[21]

A 1990 study indicated that Vitamin D deficiency gave a 200 per cent increased risk of dying from colon cancer. Michael Holick, a professor at the Boston University School of Medicine, cites this study and refers to others that replicate it. The study has now been replicated with regards to prostate cancer. Holick's own research indicates that Vitamin D deficiency increases the risk of some common cancers, Type 1 diabetes, cardiovascular disease and osteoporosis.[22] Metastatic cancer is very aggressive in Vitamin D-deficient animals, but this activity can be suppressed on supplementation with Vitamin D.

Indoor work in a climate such as Boston was sufficient to induce clinical Vitamin D deficiency by the end of winter in 40 per cent of the doctors and nurses studied by Holick. He argues that many elderly people diagnosed as having fibromyalgia are in fact suffering from Vitamin D-deficient osteomalacia, and that the currently accepted lower limit of 'normal' values could be as little as one-third of the true value on the units used in the United States. He also remarked that food was a poor source of Vitamin D; that fish liver oil was the only reliable source; and that salmon and milk were not particularly reliable sources. Humans he said, evolved to be exposed to sun.

Vitamin E

Vitamin E is a fat-soluble anti-oxidant vitamin and it exists in several forms. The family is known as the tocopherols, from Greek *tokos*, 'childbirth', and *phero*, 'to bring forth'. Rat experiments as far back as 1922 showed that diets lacking Vitamin E gave rise to spontaneous abortions.[23] Subsequent experience has indicated a role for Vitamin E in other areas of reproductive health, including the relief of symptoms of premenstrual tension and menopausal symptoms.

The biochemistry

As the biochemistry of Vitamin E has been unravelled, it has become clear that most of its important biological activity lies in its ability to act as an anti-oxidant in lipid environments. It is found in plasma, red cells and various tissues. After passive absorption from the gut, it is taken to the liver where it is either stored, or incorporated into very low-density lipoproteins (VLDL, a 'bad fat'; Chapter 8). From there it moves into the bloodstream or some of it moves into the bile.

In the bloodstream VLDL is converted to LDL (the other well-known 'bad fat' or 'bad cholesterol'). Some of the Vitamin E remains in the LDL and some is transferred to HDL, or 'good cholesterol'. Although the chemistry is somewhat more complex than this, the nett result is that LDL and HDL then distribute Vitamin E to all tissues throughout the body.

A crucial function of Vitamin E is to protect membranes from oxidative damage. Membranes are mostly made up of lipids and are vulnerable to lipid peroxidation (Chapter 4: Selenium). It has been established that lipid peroxidation is probably one of the most significant events leading to the degeneration of individual cells and indeed, entire organs.

It has been said that we are only as old as our mitochondria, the powerhouse of the cell. People who age prematurely, do so because their mitochondria age prematurely. Oxidative processes, where food is burnt for energy, continuously generate free radicals. The protection of mitochondrial membranes from oxidative damage depends on Vitamin E.

Lipid peroxidation, on a microscopic scale, is what all fats do on exposure to oxygen. They go rancid. The hapless rats in the 1922 experiment had been fed rancid oils. Oil goes rancid when time and exposure to air exceed its capacity to protect itself from further oxidation. The Vitamin E in it is consumed by the process of acting as an anti-oxidant, and becomes an inert metabolite. Rancid fat has no Vitamin E available to act as an anti-oxidant in the body.

There are about six classes of anti-oxidant defence mechanisms. Some of these, such as selenium-dependent enzyme systems and Vitamin C, have already been discussed. In its location on the cell membrane, Vitamin E is on the frontline of the whole redox war. In terms of mass, one 'unit' of Vitamin E can protect 1000 'units' of lipid membrane molecules.

A good proportion of the lipids in membranes are made up of polyunsaturated fats, to be discussed shortly. The structure of unsaturated fats is such that they are particularly vulnerable to lipid peroxidation. By eating a lot of polyunsaturated fats you increase the proportion of membrane polyunsaturates even further, and make even greater demand on your Vitamin E stores. The current trend to buy polyunsaturated oils, both for cooking and as a component of snack foods, is a cause for concern. These oils are often heat-extracted, kept too long, left exposed to the air in the bottle, left in sunlight, and worst of all, heated in cooking to high temperatures. Every one of these actions increases the risk of oxidation of the fat, and hence the formation of lipid peroxides and destruction of its Vitamin E content.

Mother Nature ensured a high Vitamin E content in oilseeds and grains, no doubt to prevent their fats from undergoing lipid peroxidation. Whole foods and cold-pressed oils do not contain much in the way of dangerous lipid peroxides or spent Vitamin E. Deep-fried potato chips and potato crisps, fried snack foods and the like are another matter. Even though they are cooked in sunflower or canola oil, they are not a healthy choice.

Some effects of deficiency

If we are to understand *why* the Western diet increases our risk of disease, we need to understand that the rancid oils and the loss of Vitamin E are connected to the prevalence of cardiovascular, arthritic and malignant disease.

Membranes cover the surface of every cell, and they form the outer and inner boundaries of every organ. There is a membrane around the heart and kidney, the arteries and veins. Membranes also line the inner surfaces of these structures. The outer membranes are called the *epithelium*, and the inner, the *endothelium*. A cancer that arises in one of the membrane layers is known as an endothelial or epithelial cancer. Some of the most common bowel, breast and lung cancers are of this nature. Oxidative damage is thought to be a key initiating event in these processes.

Endothelial damage is a key initiator in the development of atherosclerosis. Wear and tear as a result of the constant pressure of the circulation makes the arterial lining vulnerable to tiny breaches. Free radical attack by unpaired electrons increases this risk enormously. The surface of a lipid membrane has a positive charge, providing an ideal means for a negatively charged electron to discharge its unstable energy. In 'grabbing' at the membrane it can actually rip it open and begin the process of inflammatory response, repair, lipid deposition and finally scar formation. This may be the start of the full catastrophe of atherosclerosis and thus damage to organs such as brain, heart and kidney dependent on those arteries.

Joints are lined by a synovial membrane, and rheumatoid arthritis occurs when that membrane becomes inflamed. Vitamin E can be an effective part of the treatment of this condition.

More recently Vitamin E has been identified as one of the essential nutrients to impact on the immune system. This includes the production of antibodies and the cytokine, interleukin 2. It also seems to have activity against the immune suppressor, prostaglandin E2. The significance of this is that drug companies spend many millions trying to develop drugs to have just these effects.

Every so often the media report on the 'harmful effects' of a vitamin, and Vitamin E has not escaped this trend. In 2005, reports emerged that taking more than 400 IU daily increased one's risk of death by 10 per cent. In response, Koyamangalath Krishnan of the University of Texas Cancer Center pointed out that most of the trials used the less effective synthetic alpha-tocopherol. Ronald Watson in the College of Public Health of Medicine also objected: 'We have carefully reviewed almost 100 articles about Vitamin E, its benefits, activity, etc. There is almost no evidence of toxicity or adverse effects in doses used by the average American. In fact, multitudinous animal and human studies proclaim it has limited toxicity and significant benefits.'[24] The parallels to the beta carotene study (Chapter 2) are depressingly familiar.

Vitamin K

This vitamin is best known for its role in the clotting of blood. Warfarin, a rat poison, exerts its lethal effect by interrupting the action of Vitamin K, inducing haemorrhage. (Tight controls are necessary when it is used as a human medicine.)

The main dietary sources of Vitamin K include spinach, broccoli, brussels sprouts and some oils, such as olive and soybean. The brassicas (cabbage family) have up to ten times as much as peas and beans. Liver and some fermented foods are a source, but the main human intake is from plants. It is possible that Vitamin K is not strictly speaking a vitamin, as a healthy gut contains considerable amounts of it, believed to be produced by the gut flora.

The most significant risk of Vitamin K deficiency appears to be in babies, where it is responsible for a fatal condition known as haemorrhagic disease of the newborn. This is a special risk in breast-fed babies, as there is little Vitamin K in human milk. Most formulas are fortified. Babies in Western countries are usually injected at delivery with a one-off shot of Vitamin K, which has effectively eliminated the disease. A few years ago, there was a scare when babies thus injected appeared to have a greatly increased risk of childhood leukaemias, but this is no longer thought to be the case.

Did dietary deficiency cause haemorrhagic disease? And if so, what else is missing? The diet that decreases the mother's risk of premature or assisted delivery (both of which increase the risk of infantile haemorrhage, strangely enough), also provides enough Vitamin K. And yet frozen peas are still the commonest green vegetable, often the only one, that many people eat.

Vitamin K deficiency is rare in adults, probably because intestinal bacteria maintain the supply. One form *is* seen after the administration of antibiotics. It may be produced by the combination of poor diet in the sick person, the effects of the antibiotic on the ability of the liver to handle Vitamin K, and reduced production by gut flora after their exposure to antibiotics.

ESSENTIAL FATTY ACIDS

Essential fatty acids (EFAs) are mostly derived from plants. They occur in the simplest of life forms, such as algae, and are also in tiny seeds, nuts and green vegetables. The various food sources of the essential fatty acids are listed in Chart 5.4. These are foods that many people do not eat.

Snake oil

Animals whose flesh is rich in EFAs include reptiles, wild fish and wild animals. Next time you are driving in the country and see a freshly killed snake on the road, stop and sniff it. (Make sure it's dead first.) It will have a very fishy smell, and this is because it's full of omega-3 fatty acids. The dismissive meaning of the term 'snake-oil medicine' did not evolve because snake oil didn't work. I hope to show you how many things it cured. It got its bad name from the charlatans who replaced it with cheap vegetable oils.

The omega-3s are derived from the diet these wild animals eat. Once domesticated, these animals are fed a commercial diet and the omega-3 content is no longer assured.

Biochemistry of the EFAs

Fatty acids are just one of the many kinds of biological fats listed in Chapter 4. There we saw that the were three kinds of fatty acids: saturated, monounsaturated and polyunsaturated. It is the polyunsaturated fats that we focus on here.

The essential fatty acids are one special group within the class of polyunsaturated fatty acids. All polyunsaturates have more than one double bond in the carbon chain, but not all are 'essential'. This is because either they are not necessary to mammalian biology, or they can be made as needed. For example, the omega-9s are important polyunsaturated fats, but we do not call them 'essential' because they can be synthesised by us from a monounsaturated precursor.

There are two reasons for invoking the word 'essential':

- Although we have the capacity to rearrange some EFAs into others, we cannot manufacture the raw materials: we have to ingest them.

• EFAs are essential to life and we cannot function without them. Just why this is so is the subject of this section.

The two main groups of essential fatty acids are called omega-3s and omega-6s. The numbers refer to the site of the carbon atom at which the first double bond occurs. The distribution of hydrogen atoms at the double bond between the carbon atoms classifies the fatty acid as either *cis* or *trans* (Chart 5.1). Most unsaturated fatty acids which occur in nature have the cis form.

Collectively, there are about six or seven omega-3 and omega-6 fatty acids. They make up the bulk of the EFAs to be found in human tissues. They cannot replace one another, and this especially refers to the *classes* of 3s and 6s. While some *within* a series can be made from another in that series, the necessary precursors for each series must be in the diet.

As in most biochemical reactions, the transformation from one fatty acid to another depends on the action of enzymes. Some of these enzymes, such as delta-5 and delta-6 desaturase, in turn depend on the presence of various co-enzymes. If these co-enzymes are missing, then the reaction will proceed inefficiently, if at all.

In the 1970s, when medical science was just beginning to appreciate the health benefits of the polyunsaturated fats, people were

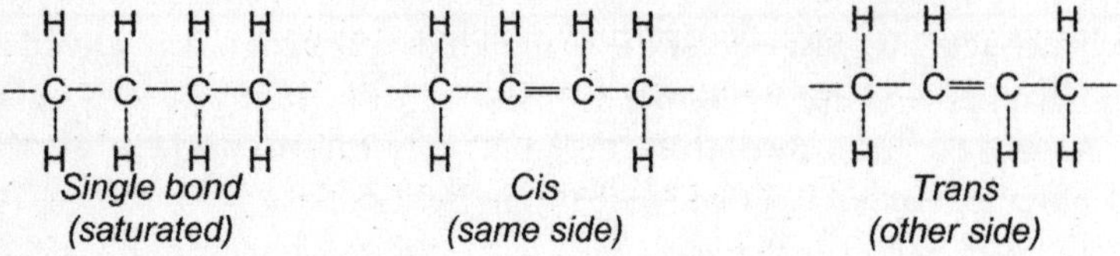

Chart 5.1: Single and Double bond formations

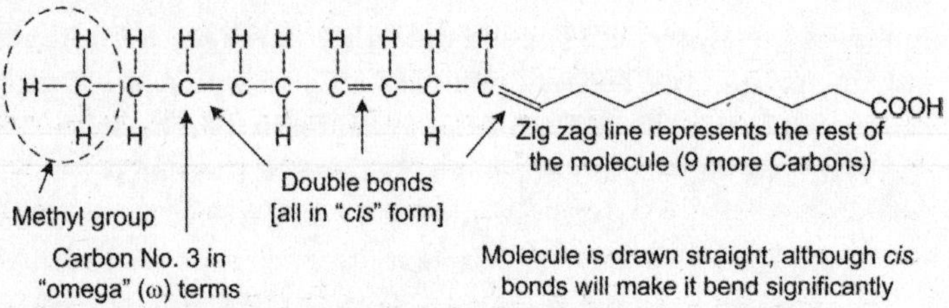

Chart 5.2: Alpha linolenic acid—a typical essential fatty acid

advised to switch from butter to margarine. Not only were people avoiding eggs because cholesterol was seen as a fast track to heart disease, but butter was off the menu too. Years later, the synthetic unsaturated fats used in the manufacture of margarines were found to contain large amounts of trans fatty acids (Chart 5.1). Margarines sold as 'olive oil' and 'sunflower' were so far removed from the natural product as to qualify as deceptive advertising. There were two problems. They were often hydrogenated to firm them up, so they became — in part at least — saturated fats. And, more worryingly, the unsaturated parts had 'trans' bonds. Far from being beneficial to health, these fats were to become linked to a wide range of medical disorders, including heart disease, diabetes and cancer — the very conditions they were supposed to help prevent.[25]

Chart 5.2 shows the structure of an important omega-3 fatty acid, and illustrates the terminology used to describe the family.

Functions

The need for the EFAs was first shown in 1929 when it was noted that laboratory rats required dietary fats to thrive and reproduce. After it was established that an omega-6 fatty acid, linoleic acid, was the essential ingredient, it was observed that this was also essential in human biology. The main clinical manifestations of deficiency were dermatitis and poor wound healing. The difficulty the rats had in reproducing when deprived of linoleic acid should be ringing bells for anyone experiencing fertility problems today.

Generally speaking, the functions of EFAs fall in three main categories. They are important structural components of membranes and brain tissue; they act as chemical messengers; and they make fats fluid rather than solid.

Structure

In the discussion on Vitamin E, we saw that a significant part of a membrane is made up of lipids. About 25 to 35 per cent of these lipids are polyunsaturated. This is important in terms of the flexibility of the membrane. In some regions or 'domains' of the membrane, flexibility is not so critical. In others, it determines how the fatty acids (some of them essential, some not), interact with protein components of the membrane.

In naturally occurring EFAs the double bond which occurs in the *cis* position causes a rigid bend in the fatty acid chain. This reduces the tightness with which the fatty acid molecules can 'pack', and produces a substance that is generally more fluid. This chemistry results in a lowered freezing point. It also explains why dietary polyunsaturates remain liquid in the refrigerator (or even in the freezer). A saturated fat, such as butter, readily sets in the cold. The effect holds true whether the fat is in a jar in the refrigerator, or in a living tissue such as a membrane in the body. To fully appreciate the importance of membrane fluidity, we need first to understand more about the physiology of membranes.

Membranes are everywhere, as we saw in the discussion on Vitamin E. The gut, urogenital tract, lungs, ducts in the breast tissue, arteries and veins—these are all covered by, and lined with, membranes. Within an organ, each cell is separated from each other cell by a membrane. Within the cell, the *internal* structures are likewise compartmentalised. Thus, inside the cell, there is a membrane around the nucleus, the mitochondria, the lysosomes, the endoplasmic reticulae and so on. The myelin sheath around nerve cells is a series of stacked membranes. The brain is a mass of nervous tissue packed in membranes.

Thus the understanding of illnesses as diverse as multiple sclerosis, mental illness and coronary artery disease becomes the understanding of membrane physiology.

The membrane not only compartmentalises the cell, but it also acts as a gatekeeper. It allows nutrients, waste products or the specialised substances produced by the cell to diffuse, or be actively 'pumped', across the membrane into another compartment, or out of the cell and into the circulation. The integrity of the ion channels discussed in Chapters 4, 8 and 9 is another example of gatekeeping. The *structure* of the membrane determines whether all goes to plan. That structure depends entirely on which fats are available for incorporation into it.

EFAs are important structural components of the brain and retina. The retina of the eye is, anatomically speaking, an outgrowth of the brain. (EFAs also have a role in the *metabolism* of the brain—Chapters 3 and 9.) EFAs, the omega-3s in particular, are concentrated in the brain and retina in a way that is equalled in few other parts of the body.

Chemical messengers

Polyunsaturated fats have a significant role to play in transcription and expression of many of the genes connected with fatty acid metabolism. There are still many unknowns in this area, but research is vital because of the prominence of lipids in the spectrum of Western disease. Many lipid disorders are blamed on heredity. As is true of so many 'genetic' disorders, the role of the genes depends not only on the genes we inherit, but how and when those genes are 'read'.

The EFAs are used by the body as the basis of a subset of hormones and hormone-like structures. These include a group known as the *eicosanoids* and a group called the *inositol phosphoglycerides*. These terms do not lend themselves to casual conversation, but the concepts are straightforward.

- The *eicosanoids* are derived both from the omega-3 and the omega-6 families of the EFAs. They are sourced from the membranes of individual cells, and from the free fatty acids (triglycerides) circulating in the bloodstream. They are used to make *prostaglandins* (Chart 5.3), the main function of which is cell-to-cell communication. That is to say, prostaglandins are one of the many ways in which cells throughout the body can talk to each other. The communication can be between cells (and organs) at distant ends of the body, or it can be between adjacent cells, co-ordinating the actions of a particular tissue. Prostaglandins have important functions in the reproductive system (Chapter 7) and the cardiovascular system (Chapter 8).
- The *inositol* group, which in a large measure is derived from *arachidonic acid*, appears to have a regulatory role in the interaction between a hormone and its receptor. The letter is sent, but is it delivered to the right address? And if it is, does it get opened, does it get read, is it understood?

As with many other hormones, neurotransmitters and chemical messengers within the body, the action of the prostaglandins is varied, complex, and may alter according to the particular receptor site at which they act. There are thought to be at least 16 different prostaglandins and at least eight different receptor types. Further

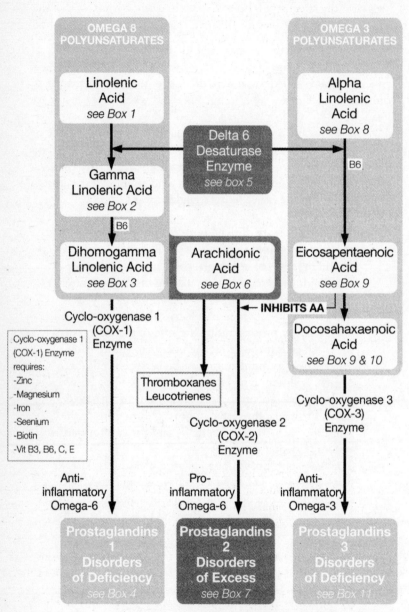

Chart 5.3: Pathways of essential fatty acids

analysis of the chemistry is beyond the scope of this book. The point is that with so many roles for EFAs, dietary deficiency or imbalance cannot fail to have significant health consequences.

Acting as 'anti-freeze'
As we have seen, the addition of the double bond to the carbon chains in a fat makes the fat more fluid. In some ways, EFAs act like anti-freeze. The addition of a small amount of anti-freeze to a car radiator prevents water freezing, or solidifying, in cold weather. Similarly, if butter is melted down with the addition of even a small amount of unsaturated oil, the blend will remain relatively spreadable when refrigerated. Many of the secretions in our bodies, such as wax and sebum, rely on this liquefying action of the EFAs, as we will soon see with the patients Mike and Sanjiv. (See also Chapter 7.)

The appeal of margarine derived from this anti-freeze characteristic; the trans fatty acids were an unfortunate, and dangerous, side effect.

EFA deficiencies: a question of balance

Although fish contains omega-3 fatty acids, canned fish may not be a good source. If they are 'skinless and boneless', the vital ingredients may be missing. A study of asthmatic children in Australia shows that fresh fish had a clear protective effect, but the effect of canned fish was variable.[26] Sardines are probably the best of the canned options. They are low in the (fish) food chain and therefore least likely to be contaminated with mercury. And mostly, they retain their skin and bones.

The loss of omega-3s from canned products is another result of commercial food production. It is easy to extract some fish oil in the canning process and make an extra profit by selling it for fish oil capsules. Even though the resultant product is a bit tasteless, it will still have a market. People often try to get their fish quota from canned tuna because it doesn't taste like fish. But without the oils, they may as well not bother. For those who like flavour, chillies, lemon or pepper may be added, and the label reads 'salmon plus'. Surely the more honest term would be 'salmon minus'.

But it is not only canned fish we need worry about. Remember that animals do not make their own omega-3s; they must obtain them from their diet. When fish are wild, algae is at the bottom of their food chain and they get their intake that way. But in fish farms, how do we know what they are fed? Feeding fish to fish is not efficient when the world's fish stocks are in decline, and the diet of farmed fish gives cause for concern. The antibiotics and other chemicals to which they are exposed hardly bear thinking about. Unfortunately, contamination and deficiency are not our only problems: the EFAs must be in correct proportion. A builder cannot simply substitute one material for another and end up with the same result. If he has a surplus of timber and a short supply of glass, he must make the windows smaller. If he has a surplus of glass, a feature wall will provide a great view, but it will not support a heavy iron and timber roof. And finally, if twice the amount of roofing iron has accidentally been delivered, he can't just stack it on top without putting unsupportable stress on the whole structure.

When it comes to the essential fatty acids, we require an adequate supply of each of them; they cannot be substituted for each other; and an oversupply of one kind can actually produce a functional deficiency of another. Or in the terms of our builder, if he *does* decide to put the extra iron on the roof, he had better shore up the walls with extra bricks and timber to hold the whole thing up.

At first, Chart 5.3 looks daunting, but it contains some of the most exciting biochemistry covered in this book. We can also see that there is limited ability to turn one EFA into another. Chart 5.4 shows a whole range of illnesses which can be targeted by these simple dietary ingredients.

If we look at the various food sources shown in Chart 5.4, we can see why the Western diet favours the production of the inflammatory PG-2 mediators over the anti-inflammatory PG-1 and PG-3. And although the foods in the left-hand column give rise to *anti*-inflammatory mediators, the omega-6 fatty acids of both kinds, taken collectively, are likely to swamp or overwhelm the omega-3 fatty acids. Our diets simply do not contain enough omega-3s to withstand the onslaught. This is made even more likely by the fact that DGLA can be converted into arachidonic acid. The nutrients required to complete it on its pathway to becoming PG-1 are often deplete; so it is shunted across to form arachidonic acid, and thus increases the pro-inflammatory PG-2.

Thus, we can characterise the Western diet as inflammatory, because of its lack of omega-3s and its over-abundance of omega-6s.

This should also clarify another point. There is no such thing as

Box 1
LINOLEIC ACID (LA)
Sources: oils of:
-Safflower (75%)
-Evening primrose (72%)
-Grape seed (71%)
-Sunflower (65%)
-Corn (60%)
-Hemp seed (60%)
-Walnut (51%)
-Soy (50%)
-Pumpkin seed (50%)
-Wheat Germ (50%)
-Sesame (45%)
-Olive (8%)

Box 2
GAMMA LINOLEIC ACID (GLA)
Sources: oils of
-Evening primrose
-Blackcurrant seed

Box 3
DIHOMOGAMMA LINOLEIC ACID (DGLA)
Source:
-Human Breast Milk

Box 5
DELTA 5 DESATURASE ENZYME
Requires:
-Vitamins B3, B6
-Zinc, magnesium, iron
Blocked by:
-Alcohol
-Saturated fats
-Trans fats
-Some chemicals
-Some viruses
Enzymes not as effective in:
-Allergic families
-Diabetics
-Advancing age (over 40)

Box 6
ARACHIDONIC ACID (AA)
Sources:
-Meat
-Milk
-Egg
-Shrimp
-Seaweed

Box 8
ALPHA LINOLEIC ACID (LNA)
Sources: oils of
-Flax seed (58%)
-Horse milk (39%)
-Hemp seed (20%)
-Pumpkin seed (0-15%)
-Wheat germ (5%)
-Rice bran (1%)
-(linseed)
-Chestnut
-Walnut (7%)
-Canola (0-10%)
-Seaweed
-Algae
-Soy (6%)

Box 9
EICOSAPENTAENOIC ACID (EPA) AND DOCOSAHEXAENOIC ACID (DHA)
Sources: oils of
-Cod liver
-Salmon
-Trout
-Mackerel
-Herring
-Sardine
-Wild game
-Kangaroo

Box 10
DOCOSAHEXAENOIC ACID (DHA)
Functions:
-Reduce blood clotting
-Reduce APO & fibrinogen in arteries
-Reduce blood triglycerides

Box 4
PROSTAGLANDINS 1 PG1
Deficient in:
-High cholesterol
-Eczema
-Hyperactivity
-Hypertension
-Pre-menstrual syndrome
-Thrombosis
-Vascular spasm

Box 7
PROSTAGLANDINS 2 PG2
Excessive in:
-Angina
-Arthritis
-Crohn's disease
-Diabetes
-Depression
-Cancer
-Food allergy
-Menstrual cramps
-Multiple sclerosis
-Thrombosis
-Schizophrenia

Box 11
PROSTAGLANDINS 3 PG3
Deficient in:
-Acne
-Asthma
-Dandruff
-Depression
-Elevated blood
-triglycerides
-Learning impairment
-Auto-immune diseases
-Thrombosis
-Schizophrenia

Chart 5.4: Foods, co-factors and conditions affected by essential fatty acids (EFAs)

a 'bad' EFA. Inflammation is part of our immune defence system. PG-2 hormones help destroy the 'bad guys', including germs and cancer cells. They relax coronary arteries (Chapter 8) and they help initiate labour. The problems arise when there is no means to counter the pro-inflammatory pathways. The majority of the conditions which threaten you and me with a reduced quality or length of life are inflammatory disorders.

The patient: Mike

In the waiting room is a teenager. His expression says that he would rather be almost anywhere else. He is Mary's younger brother Mike, and he has asthma. (He was also thought to have ADHD in primary school, and for a while was on Ritalin. However, he is reasonably bright, quite good at sport, and has reached high school relatively unscathed.) Now, at 16, his asthma bothers him only occasionally, although he can become quite sick with it and it always occurs at the worst times.

Today, though, he is here for a bad case of acne. His parents are worried about him and his mother has phoned before accompanying him to the doctor. Mike used to be very sociable, but now he is moody and less likely to accept invitations to join friends. Is he depressed? Could it be the acne? Could he be on drugs? Should he try antibiotics for his acne?

The honest answer to all these questions might well be yes. Acne is associated with an increased risk of depression in young people, attributed to the social stigma of bad skin. Indeed, Mike would probably not have agreed to come today were it not for the school social next week, which, after a lot of deliberation, he has decided to attend. Mike is at an age when drug experimentation is common. Kids with acne are known to be more likely to be depressed. Kids who are depressed are more likely to try drugs. If acne results in low self-esteem, the use of antibiotics to control the acne might be a sensible idea.

But let us stand back from this a bit. Mike is a loved, well-educated person from a 'normal' home. He has not, we will assume, been either abused or neglected. Both his parents, Doug and Fran, are non-smokers. Yet, in his young life, he has been on Ventolin, Atrovent, steroids, and a short course of Ritalin. The Ritalin was stopped because his parents felt uncomfortable about it.

At 16, he is facing long-term antibiotics for his acne. He may even be prescribed Roaccutane (a Vitamin A analogue). If the family doctor agrees that he is depressed, he may end up on Prozac as well. Mother Nature has certainly stuffed up here! Or is it Doug and Fran? They have never suffered depression. They don't understand where they have gone wrong with Mary and Mike.

Let us take another look. Is Mike's acne really due to the fact that he doesn't have enough antibiotics in his system? Perhaps it is a marker for something else. Could it indicate EFA deficiency? If it does, what else might EFA deficiency explain about Mike's health?

We know that the total amount of saturated fat in the diets of youngsters like Mike has increased since industrialisation. A lot of this saturated fat is a result of commercial processing, re-use, and high-temperature cooking. The oxidised state of these saturated, and non-essential fats in his diet will make a great demand on Mike's anti-oxidant reserves. Selenium, zinc, and Vitamins A, C and E, are the mainstay of such reserves. From earlier chapters it can be deduced that he is likely to have deficiencies in all of these areas.

Let us turn now to his intake of EFAs. The importance of the ratio of the omega-6 to omega-3 has just been discussed. Fran has read in the press about the role of fish oil in various conditions, from asthma through to ADHD. Mike dislikes fish, but Fran has persuaded him to eat tuna and 'salmon minus', canned in unspecified vegetable oils.

Mike, let us say, has inherited his asthma genes from his paternal grandfather, Herb. Herb was a recreational fisherman who supplemented the family meals with freshly caught fish. Sometimes, during the Depression, he also shot wild rabbits. Both the fish and the rabbits were good sources of omega-3s. When neither were available, the family often ate sardines on toast, the 'poor man's steak'. They were canned in sild oil, the omega-3 rich oil from the sardines themselves. (Sardines in sild oil have not been seen on supermarket shelves for over a decade. No doubt the surplus oil has found its way into expensive supplements instead.) Herb had the occasional bout of wheezy bronchitis as a child. He never had an asthma attack. He didn't know he had asthma genes. He and his family still wonder where Mike's asthma has come from.

If Mike is on a typical Western teenage diet, he is consuming an excess of saturated fats over the EFAs. Fran cooks well at home, but Mike likes fast food for lunch and when out with friends. This will contribute to his risk of obesity. If the saturated fats are oxidised, arguably they will contribute to a later risk of cancer, arthritis, diabetes and heart disease. But for the moment, we are concentrating not on the saturated fatty acids but on the *essential fatty acids* in his diet. Our concern is whether Mike is getting enough EFAs, and in what ratio.

To answer this, we have to look at food trends. During the long boom after World War II, people began to find they could afford cream, butter and red meat. Until the consequences of a diet of affluence became apparent, little thought was given to the consumption of the 'good oils'. On the other hand, sardines were still on the menu for most people, junk food was in its early days, and commercial food processing was still a new science.

In the 1960s and 1970s, the belief that cardiovascular disease was due to over-consumption of saturated fat led to promotion of oils and margarines rich in polyunsaturated fat. That trend has continued to the present, and it is probably reasonable to assume Mike's *total* intake of EFAs is reasonable. Salad oils are likely to have replaced the creamy mayonnaise that used to grace his parents' and grandparents' salads. Even his chips and burgers are now more likely to have been fried in corn or soybean oil than in tallow. At home, his family cooks everything in the 'good oils', such as safflower, sunflower or olive oil. Olive oil won't cause Mike a problem, because it is a monounsaturate, not a polyunsaturate like the EFAs, and olive oil is therefore out of this discussion. So probably Mike, even more than his parents or grandparents, is growing up on a diet rich in essential fatty acids. But *which* essential fatty acids, and what is the *ratio* between the two kinds?

If we refer back to Chart 5.3 we see that even these good oils may end up as a source of the inflammatory leukotrienes implicated in asthma. They may remain as precursors to the PG-1 series, and therefore protect him with their anti-inflammatory action, or they may be converted to PG-2, and make his problem worse. But the main question is, where does Mike get PG-3? Regardless of the amount of EFAs Mike consumes, the *balance* between the omega-3s and omega-6s will determine whether his genetic predisposition towards asthma will be expressed.

And what about his acne? A diet high in saturated fat causes increased viscosity in secretions such as sebum. Sebum is largely made up of branched-chain fatty acids that require the 'anti-freeze' action of EFAs to remain liquid. A high ratio of omega-6 to omega-

3 favours inflammation. The combination of thick secretions and an inflammatory response increases the risk of acne. (The treatment of Mike's acne is followed in Chapter 7.) But isn't a pattern emerging here?

Omega-3 fatty acids are one of the ingredients implicated in behavioural disorders (Chapter 9).[27] So has Mike become anti-social and withdrawn because he has acne, or do his acne, depression, asthma and ADHD all have a common cause? Mike has not offended against the law, but he comes from a supportive middle-class family. If he had come from a depressed socioeconomic background, his childhood ADHD and his teenage sullenness and low self-esteem might have ended badly.

This may seem far-fetched, but it is no more far-fetched than the idea that the human genome has such faulty biochemistry that young people must depend on the pharmaceutical industry to lead normal, responsible lives, to breathe normally and have healthy skin. Yet this is what we doctors suggest, in effect, every time we multi-prescribe acne medication, Ritalin, Ventolin and Prozac.

Mike is in no way unusual. To repeat, up to one-quarter of Australians will be diagnosed with asthma at some stage in their lives. A significant number of young people are being treated, or are treating themselves, for acne. Depression is known to be one of the commonest health problems, and 11 per cent of Australian children suffer from ADHD. The laws of chance ensure that it is not unusual to suffer from all these problems, as Mike does. In considering the clustering of these conditions, shared genes, shared diets and shared socioeconomic factors all must be considered.

Suppose Mike inhales some pollen which triggers the secretion of inflammatory mediators. These will produce some mucus to trap the pollen, and some smooth-muscle contraction to help him cough out the offending material. But as we know, Mike probably has low levels of PG-3. If there are other factors against him, such as low selenium and low magnesium, the chances are that this inflammatory response goes unchecked and may become an asthma attack.

Mike could, of course, depend on the anti-inflammatory actions of the PG-1s. After all, just about everything is cooked in sunflower oil these days. But PG-1s are much weaker anti-inflammatories than PG-3s, and are also at risk of conversion to arachidonic acid (Chart 5.3).

Arachidonic acid is not only a source of the inflammatory prostaglandins; it is also a precursor of the inflammatory leukotrienes.

Leukotrienes are targeted by the asthma drug Singulair, which was introduced a few years ago. It works by antagonising the leukotriene receptors. Its side effects include headache, abdominal pain and gastrointestinal upset. If Mike is prescribed Singulair, it is drug option number 8, for those who are counting. Despite its problems, it is not a bad drug. But it would be simpler to encourage Mike to eat more fish, walnuts, linseeds and essential micronutrients.

Who else in the waiting room needs some EFAs?

If we take Mike as representing asthma, acne, depression and ADHD, we have looked at the typical manifestations of the young end of the age spectrum of EFA problems. As we move up the age scale we find some other typical disorders.

Sitting across from Mike is David, who is in his late 30s and has had several attacks of rheumatoid arthritis. We learn more about David in Chapter 7, but at the moment, we focus on one of the drugs he has been prescribed—Celebrex.

Like Singulair, Celebrex works directly on the prostaglandins pathways. Both asthma and arthritis are inflammatory disorders, mediated by inflammatory pathways such as PG-2. Until now, arthritis drugs have worked by blocking enzymes such as the cyclo-oxygenases, which convert EFAs to the various prostaglandins. These drugs included steroids, aspirin, and the non-steroidal anti-inflammatories (NSAIDs) such as Indocid and Brufen. The problem with these drugs is that they are indiscriminate. Not only do they block the conversion of arachidonic acid to the inflammatory PG-2s, they block the formation of PG-1 and PG-3 as well. In other words, they are blocking the body's own natural anti-inflammatory defences.

So it might seem that treatment should start with an increased intake of fish and fish oils prior to starting anti-inflammatory treatment. David has tried taking fish oil but was unsure that it made a difference. It is not hard to see why. The benefit of the eicosapentaenoic acid in fish oil is limited by the blocking action of his NSAIDs on the formation of PG-3.

However, fish oil can still be of benefit even if the NSAIDs are being used. This is because one of the main actions of eicosapentaenoic acid is to directly block the conversion of arachidonic acid to the PG-2s. And this is why fish oil is so effective. With no conversion necessary, it becomes an anti-arthritis, anti-asthma, anti-inflammatory medication in its own right.

Next to David sits Sanjiv. Sanjiv's parents still eat a traditional diet, but his mother despairs of his wholesale adoption of Western junk food. His name is Hindi for 'long-lived', but she is not so sure about this any more. He isn't actually sick, but he has become increasingly deaf of late. Whenever this happens he comes in to get the wax in his ears suctioned or syringed. He used to clean them with a bobby pin, but once he made a hole in his eardrum doing this, so now he submits himself to more professional care.

Surely Sanjiv doesn't have an EFA deficiency? Look back at the list of fatty substances in Chapter 4. Wax is a fat, but it needs 'anti-freeze' to stop it sticking up. The fact that the wax has become stuck ('inspissated' is the medical term) may be warning Sanjiv of an EFA problem.

Patients like Sanjiv sometimes ask their doctors what people did in the past. Did they all have holes in their eardrums from employing fingernails and sticks? No. The hairs lining the ear canal are designed to beat in a rhythmic manner, rather like the fronds of a jellyfish. This clears the ear canal of wax, along with the debris it has gathered. Provided the component oils in this wax have a modest amount of EFAs in their structure, the wax remains fluid and clears easily without intervention.

As we look around the waiting room, it becomes difficult to find anyone whose condition might *not* be helped in some way by ensuring adequate EFA intake and balance. Even Sonya, waiting patiently for a routine ante-natal visit, will reduce the risk of allergies in her unborn child if she consumes sufficient EFAs. We will meet some of these people in later chapters.

Clinical applications

For some perspective, here is a list of medical conditions associated in some way with EFA deficiency or imbalance:

- impaired cholesterol transport
- mental ill health, including depression, schizophrenia and Alzheimer's disease
- specific learning defects
- autistic spectrum disorders
- visual defects
- autoimmune disorders
- asthma

- pre-term delivery and babies with low birth-weights
- infertility
- diabetes
- arthritis
- food allergies
- chronic inflammation
- neurological disorders such as multiple sclerosis
- cancer.

The good oils supply EFAs, but mostly in the form of omega-6s. Even then, the consumption of these oils can in no way be equated with the consumption of the whole food. If we want walnut or safflower oils, we should obtain them from walnuts or safflowers.

The lack of dietary omega-3s seems by far the greatest problem. Wild game plays a very minor part in today's diet. Herb and his rabbits are becoming a distant memory. If a youngster like Mike has ever tasted rabbit, it is likely to have been farmed. The diet fed to farmed animals typically does not raise the omega-3 level in their flesh. Fish are the one remaining wild animal that we are likely to consume, and now even they are often farmed, as we have discussed.

Maybe it is even worse than we think. The source of omega-3s is right at the bottom of the food chain. Algae, tiny seeds, the foundations upon which higher animals depend. If one of the largest sources of omega-3s in the human diet is ocean fish, what are we to make of a recent report that the ocean's plankton has fallen by *70 per cent* in the last 50 years.[28] This is thought to be a side effect of rising levels of carbon dioxide. So now, as well as overfishing, does climate change pose a threat to the world's already diminishing fish stocks? What happens to the food chain, to us, when change as profound as this occurs?

Chapter Six

A SYSTEMATIC APPROACH TO DISEASE

Our only health is the disease
If we obey the dying nurse
Whose constant care is not to please
But to remind of our, and Adam's Curse, And
that, to be restored, our sickness must grow worse.

T. S. ELIOT, FOUR QUARTETS

SIR DENIS BURKITT, who gave his name to the disease Burkitt's lymphoma, once famously declared that doctors were involved in a disease profession, not a health profession. He referred to hospitals as 'disease palaces' and claimed that the size of the British medical budget could be halved by doubling the size of the British stool.

Perhaps Burkitt was oversimplifying, but we could argue that it was not by much. We can approach disease by looking either at the end result or at the multiple processes that may have contributed to the end result—either symptoms or systems. By drawing attention to something that most people would prefer not to think about, Burkitt was dramatically highlighting the contribution of dietary choice to the national disease burden.

This chapter deals with the benefits of a systematic approach to disease. Later chapters examine various 'end-point' or 'fixed-name' diseases, demonstrating the benefits of the systematic approach. By looking for system designs, 'alternative' medicine challenges evidence-based medicine. Many of us remember sitting in school trying to disprove the obvious—drawing diagrams to show that Pythagoras was wrong, or that the shortest distance between two points was not a straight line. When we got it right, it was because we had discerned the natural order, the natural 'laws'.

KISS: keep it simple, stupid

Sometimes the simple is as far as we need to go. A solution is not better just because it is ingenious. The absurdity of ingenuity is represented by these examples:

- The rise in conditions such as asthma and peanut allergy is thought to be a result of lack of germ exposure in infancy. We have already discussed the idea that that when the immune system is unable to hone its skills on everyday germs, it develops those skills by reacting to pollens, animal hair or food (Chapter 3). One solution is to pass Junior around a bit more, allow him to be coughed on by siblings, and worry less about Mogsy's furtive visits to his cot. But it has been seriously proposed that a vaccine could be developed to do the same job.[1]
- Scientists have discovered the mechanism by which 'bad' cholesterol is converted into 'good' during exercise. With a link established, you would think that people would be told to hop on their bikes and leave the car at home. But no — the good men and women of science 'are working on a drug that could perform the same function'.[2]
- In 2003 the introduction of a 'polypill' was proposed. This drug would break new ground in that it would be prescribed for *healthy* people. It would combine a number of prescription medications in a single pill intended to prevent diseases largely caused by poor diet and lack of exercise. As one cardiologist remarked: 'When I first heard about it, I thought it was a joke!'

DEFICIENCY DISORDERS

Most people in the Western world generally get enough calories and protein to sustain health. Most of their deficiency problems, however, are the result of micronutrient deficiencies. It is a central thesis of this book that these deficiencies are common, low-grade, and usually unrecognised. Also, they rarely occur in isolation: a diet producing one deficiency is likely to produce multiple deficiencies. I mention them here because they are important for a systematic approach, but they have already been discussed in detail in Chapters 4 and 5.

GENETIC DISORDERS

Again, genetic disorders are mentioned here for completeness. For a full discussion see Chapter 3. To summarise, look after your bad genes, and you may never know you've got them.

TOXICITY DISORDERS

The chemical leak in Bhopal, India, which killed many thousands and seriously injured even more, was catastrophic. The use of Agent Orange in Vietnam and the bombs which fell on Hiroshima and Nagasaki, likewise. Far more difficult are the questions of everyday poisoning, low-level poisoning, toxic mixtures, and individual sensitivity.

The Plimsoll line

Samuel Plimsoll, born in 1824, was known as the Sailor's Friend. Until the 1870s, British ship owners had complete control over the loading of their ships. Many a sailor drowned because his overloaded ship was not fit to weather a heavy storm. Plimsoll's agitation in Parliament led to the passage in 1876 of the Merchant Shipping Act, which compelled every merchant ship to carry a loading mark on either side. This legislation had to be redrafted more than once,

212 THE GOOD BODY GUIDE

because without clear guidelines some wits painted the mark around the funnel. In the final Act the level was specified, and varied for different seasons and localities.

Discussing toxicity in medicine is sometimes easy and sometimes impossibly complex. The moral obligation to impose a Plimsoll line all too often gives way to political and commercial interest.

Fran and Doug go out for the night with some friends and have some wine with dinner. As they drink, the gene for the manufacture of *alcohol dehydrogenase* (Chapter 3) is switched on. If they are regular drinkers, the DNA is more 'geared up' and their tolerance of alcohol is greater than that of someone who normally does not drink.

If they drink excessively, they will overwhelm the capacity of the cell to produce this enzyme. If they do this often enough, damage to liver and muscle cells may ensue. If they combine a moderate amount of alcohol with some other drugs, even simple pharmaceutical products such as painkillers, they may compromise the ability of the liver to detox the alcohol. As we saw in Chapter 3, some people and some racial groups are genetically less able to produce this enzyme. Also, the detox enzymes need co-enzymes. These include vitamins such as A and B and C, and minerals, like zinc, selenium and molybdenum.

Let us imagine that Fran has genetically lowered alcohol tolerance. As a female with a lower muscle mass than a man, her tolerance is further reduced. She doesn't eat junk food, but when she is very busy her diet is less than optimal. She sometimes gets headaches and takes paracetamol, perhaps more frequently than she would like. She has had mild hypertension which has not needed medication yet, but which must be watched.

Their friends, Alice and Sam, have come to stay for the weekend. They are teachers who live in the country, grow their own vegies on a few acres and are trying to live close to nature. Most of the time they eat organic food, avoid fumes and have an aversion to medication of any kind. As luck would have it, they have both inherited robust detoxification enzyme systems. The soil they are growing their vegies in is volcanic, part of an ancient basalt cap. It is rich in selenium, molybdenum and other trace elements.

Everyone has a nice night out. As no one has to drive, they drink a bit more than they usually would: two bottles of good red wine between them. Next morning, Alice, Sam and Doug are up for a morning jog, followed by a swim. Fran is in bed, nursing a headache.

Was her hangover inevitable? Is she genetically doomed to get sick every time she drinks alcohol?

This example highlights some of the most interesting problems in human health. Here we are not only dealing with the effects of poisons such as alcohol, of which we have at least a measure of understanding. There is also the question of the literally thousands of chemicals which have been produced by human technological activity over the last century. Fran is unlucky enough to have inherited one or two sluggish detox enzymes. This makes her more prone to headaches, and the medication she takes adds to the burden of substances to be detoxed. As she lives in the city, under the flight path of an international airport, she is exposed to aviation fumes as well as those from cars and trucks. Then there are the office and household poisons. Even a perfect diet supplemented with additional vitamins and minerals may have an uphill battle supporting her vulnerable enzyme systems.

So do we paint the Plimsoll line to suit her metabolism or her friends'? Or even that of her neighbour Fred, for whom no amount of bodily insult seems to cause effect? Who is the odd one out, Fran or Fred?

Poisons—then and now

Throughout the history of life on this planet, there have always been toxic substances. One of the first, in fact, was oxygen. Slowly, life forms evolved which not only could tolerate oxygen, but actually depended on it. Even then, however, the balance was delicate and the adaptive process was millions of years in the making. Reactions involving oxidation underlie many of the diseases of civilisation.

Plant poisons, animal venom and volcanic gases are just some of the sources of other natural noxious agents. But in the past, with the exception of massive volcanic eruption, avoidance was usually possible. All it took was to make the association between the toxin and its effect. Today, chemicals so permeate the air, water, soil and food chain that it is no longer possible to avoid them.

The cryptic nature of today's toxins means that we rarely know they are there. And since exposure is ubiquitous, it is not easy to establish cause and effect. It is sometimes argued that plants and animals will adapt to these challenges. But if the time scale involved in the adaptation to oxygen is anything to go by, things do not bode well for the species alive today. As for control, mostly we have to rely on government regulation for the setting and implementation of rules concerning 'safe' levels. Herein lie many paradoxes.

Measuring safety

There is no reason to believe that there is any 'safe level' of substances such as lead, mercury or dioxin. Yet as they permeate the environment and the food chain we have invented 'allowed limits', a neat way of side-stepping the issue. The allowed limit implicitly admits that the substance *can* cause harm, but it also implies that at this level it is unlikely to do so. Like the Plimsoll line, the value of this control depends on who does the 'allowing'. Standards vary from region to region, country to country. Here are some commonly used safety criteria:

- *Acute toxicity:* This is sometimes expressed as the LD50. The letters stand for 'lethal dose', and it measures the amount of a substance required to kill 50 per cent of the animals exposed to it. This criterion assumes that the substance is toxic: the only question is how much is required to cause death. Acute toxicity may, of course, produce effects which do not result in death. Vomiting, diarrhoea, headache and skin rashes are examples of acute toxicity reactions.
- *Carcinogenesis:* Does the substance cause cancer?
- *Teratogenesis:* Does the substance cause birth defects? If so, at what dosage?
- *Mutagenesis:* Does the substance cause genetic damage (mutation) which can be passed down through the generations?

On the face of it, these criteria seem comprehensive. However, they fall short by a long way of ensuring safety.

Animal experiments

Many of the substances mentioned above are tested on animals. Ignoring for the moment the whole ethical question, it has to be emphasised that while animals share a lot of their biochemistry with humans, there are also critical differences between species. The thalidomide tragedy occurred because it was assumed that the safety of thalidomide demonstrated in animal experiments could be applied to humans.

Long-term effects

Many safety assurances are to do with acute toxicity. Yet this is the aspect of safety that probably concerns us least, simply because it is the easiest to establish.

Under the commercial pressures of a competitive marketplace, the long-term effects can tick like a time bomb. Cancer, for example may take decades to develop. New drugs or industrial chemicals certainly are not withheld for decades before release. In fact, they are ushered in at an alarming rate. The US Environmental Protection Agency in 1985 recognised the existence of more than *4 million* toxic compounds. Of these, 60,000 were produced commercially, with another three coming onto the market every day.[3]

Fatal time lags have produced the tragedies of asbestos and DES (diethyl stilboestrol). These substances did untold damage before they were identified as the causative agent of lung and urogenital cancers. Women born to mothers who took DES in pregnancy developed cervical cancers, or learned that they were infertile, only decades after the original exposures. In some cases, cause and effect are never established because of such time lapses.

It is now over 40 years since Rachel Carson wrote *Silent Spring*. Carson herself died of breast cancer, which has become an epidemic. Hormones, pesticides including DDT, heptachlor and atrazine, and toxic chemicals such as PCB, PAH and polycarbonate, have all been linked to it.[4]

Scope

Industrial toxins and even prescription medicines have a clear association with the development of autoimmune and inflammatory disorders. These conditions too can take years to develop. It will be of little comfort to the sufferer to hear that a substance that initiated such an illness was found not to have any *acute* effects, or to have caused cancer, in a group of genetically selected laboratory rats 20 years previously.

Teratogenesis is usually measured by gross physical deformity of a child, recognisable at birth. What of more subtle defects? There is an association between the season in which one is conceived and the risk of becoming schizophrenic. Dopamine metabolism is associated with mental disorders such as schizophrenia, addiction, anxiety and depression. PCBs have been shown to interfere with the dopamine pathway and thereby affect psychomotor, cognitive and intellectual functions.[5] How many families affected by these disorders have any idea of the PCB exposure during pregnancy?

Many drugs, both recreational and prescription, affect the dopamine pathways. We are told that certain substances are 'safe', yet there are no relevant studies. Chemicals which can cause disruption of neurotransmitters abound in the environment. Subtle alterations to brain function are not visible in the newborn.

If it is difficult to see damage which affects such hidden variables as brain function, it is even more difficult to detect genetic damage. This is because we usually get two copies of each gene. If one is damaged, we may not see an emerging pattern until a couple of generations have elapsed. So much for establishing mutagenic potential.

Dose–response relationships

Throughout the debate on the safety of chemicals, conflicting results have been cited by opposing sides. The connection between dose and response has usually been assumed to be simple, but new studies indicate that these ideas may need to be revisited.

Lead is an interesting case in point. Research into IQ in children in relation to blood lead levels found that it was *at the lower levels that proportionally the most damage was done.*[6] When the lead burden increased, only a small extra loss of IQ performance was observed. The effect increased with the dose, but the curve flattened such that past a certain point, little extra damage was done. This is contrary to the previous notion that we really only needed to worry as levels reached the upper end of the 'allowed limit'. And, of course, lead contamination may be affecting other areas besides IQ, such as depression, addiction and anti-social behaviour.

We can take little comfort from a recent study on the chemical atrazine. It has long been banned in many European countries as an endocrine disrupter, or gender-bender, with a 'profound effect' on the risk of breast, uterine and ovarian cancers.[7] In 2003, atrazine accounted for more than 40 per cent of all herbicides applied in the United States. Chromosomally male frogs become hermaphrodites at a dosage which is just *one-30th* of the 'safe' drinking water level, as set by the EPA.[8]

A study of an over-the-counter weedkiller containing phenoxy acid derivatives found that pregnant mice miscarried significantly at levels just *one-seventh* of the level allowed by the EPA. (Phenoxy acid derivatives are discussed further below under Pesticides.) Despite the risks of extrapolating from animals to humans, it is known that women exposed to phenoxy acids take longer to get pregnant.[9] And once again, it seems that it is at the *lowest* levels that the most damage is done.

Atrazine and the phenoxy acid weedkiller present a startling contrast to lead. At higher doses, the effect seemed to be *less* than at the lower doses. One explanation is that the endocrine system operates on a feedback loop which can be turned off by excessive hormone levels. Alternatively, a massive dose may evoke an immune response which suppresses the toxic effect. Either way, this low-level effect could explain why in some studies a chemical appears to be safe when workers or experimental animals exposed to large doses do not become sick. The message is that we should be very wary of 'safe limits'.

Synergism

The interaction of chemicals is one of the most perplexing and important issues of all.

It was customary, until a decade or so ago, to assume that the effect of toxic mixtures was additive. That is to say, if chemical A gave a 10 per cent risk of a particular side effect, and chemical B gave a risk of 5 per cent, then the risk of illness on exposure to *both* chemicals was 15 per cent. Now the thinking is that it may well be a *multiple* of both risks.

This concern may also apply to prescription medications. Sometimes pharmacological mixtures are preferable because small doses of several drugs do less harm than a larger dose of just one of them. An example of this effect is provided by the combination of salicylic acid and acetophenomenin, in which the toxicity of one is actually *subtractive* from the other.

In some better-known examples, such as the 'fen–phen' crisis (when the anti-obesity drugs fenfluramine and dexfenfluramine were both withdrawn in 1997) and aspirin-phenacetin-caffeine, the serious risk of combination therapy was identified only after much harm was done. The second cocktail, known as APC, was the commonest cause of death from renal (kidney) failure in Australia in the 1960s and 1970s.

Certain antibiotics, when combined with over-the-counter antihistamines, can cause fatal cardiac arrhythmias. There are regular reports about combinations of anti-depressants or cholesterol-lowering drugs with other common medications, indicating that gold standard RCTs do not alert us to the real-life situation. And not all people taking these combinations of drugs will suffer, for genetic and other reasons already discussed.

In terms of industrial poisons, the idea that the toxic mixture may be more harmful than the sum of the component parts has seen the growth of a branch of toxicology known as synergism. An example of this is the incidental production of bis(chloromethyl) ether (BCME) from the mixing of two common industrial chemicals, hydrochloric acid and formaldehyde. BCME is a potent carcinogen in the development of lung cancer. Textile workers sometimes use formaldehyde in making permanent-press fabrics, which are then treated with an acid wash. The result is a toxin greater than the sum of the parts.[10]

Nor is it reasonable to artificially separate the effects of, say, prescription medications from the effects of other insults such as recreational drugs and environmental toxins. All three groups are potentially inter-reactive, and they often share common detoxification pathways.

Yet synergism is rarely discussed. There is a feeling that if it were a problem, then surely everyone would know about it, and someone would do something about it. Such confidence is remarkable. In one study in Britain adverse reactions to medicines *while in hospital* were estimated to number 10,000 annually and cost the NHS £500 million a year in extended hospital stays. And they were the lucky patients. The number of deaths was estimated at 1000 in the year 2000. This report does not include those harmed outside hospital.[11]

Individual sensitivity

The question of individual response takes us back to Fran's story. With the unravelling of the human genome it will be possible to design drugs suited to individual genetic makeup. However, we already know enough to tailor our use of drugs and environmental poisons to prevent harm to individuals. I argue that this happens minimally.

Take pollen as an example of a non-drug noxious agent. It doesn't matter how much pollen you expose some individuals to, they will never have an asthma attack; they simply do not have those genes. Toxicology can work like this too. Some individuals have enormous resistance to certain illnesses. This explains people like Fred. Many people when confronted with the need to stop smoking recall someone like Fred, who lived down the street from them as a child. He started smoking when he was eight years old, had a two-pack-a-day habit for most of his adult life and lived to be 103. Whatever contribution the personality and diet of the Freds of this world make to their remarkable survival, they simply do not have 'lung cancer genes'.

Human susceptibility, like most natural phenomena, occurs largely along a normal distribution curve. At one end sits Fred. At the other, there are those who are chemically sensitive. Where do we put the Plimsoll line for them? Chemical sensitivity often runs in families and, like Fran's ability to tolerate alcohol, depends to a large extent on the robustness of various enzyme systems.

Classifying chemicals
The poisons or chemicals which the body has to deal with can be broadly classified into three groups.

The first group is those which we produce ourselves but which must be handled appropriately lest they become toxic. The feminisation often observed in male alcoholics is one such example. Men normally produce oestrogen, but in lesser amounts than women. When alcoholics sustain sufficient liver damage, they are no longer able to degrade or conjugate oestrogen. Such men have a higher level of circulating oestrogen and often develop high-pitched voices and show a degree of breast development. Similarly, serotonin is a neurotransmitter which is toxic in overdose. The body continually produces and destroys serotonin to a very fine balance. It is this balance which is manipulated by the anti-depressant drugs known as SSRIs. Over-dosage on one's own serotonin by the use of these drugs, especially when combined with certain other medications, can cause the dangerous 'serotonergic syndrome'. There are several unpleasant features to this condition, which include anxiety, gut cramps and headache. Most worrying can be a severe rise in blood pressure.

The second group includes substances which are ingested and are then used by the body as a nutrient. Some of these nutrients are toxic in excess, and the body must have a means of eliminating that excess. Some compounds of nutritional value must first be metabolised if they are not to have toxic effects. (Ethyl) alcohol is an obvious example, but there are many compounds in the plant world that would be toxic if we did not have the appropriate detoxifying mechanisms.

Finally, there are the *xenobiotics*. These are foreign chemicals that have no role in normal physiology. Xenobiotics further divide into two groups:

- *inorganic chemicals* such as lead, mercury, cadmium, nickel and aluminium
- *organic chemicals*, which include 13 classes of potentially toxic compounds: acids, nitro compounds, thio compounds, aromatic hydrocarbons, phenols, alkyl halides, aryl halides, aldehydes, alcohols, ketones, esters, ethers, amines.

Enzymes are involved with the degradation of many organic chemicals. Some xenobiotics are also dealt with by the immune system. Sometimes this results in damage to the immune system by the chemical.

Biotransformation: how the body deals with chemicals

The subject of toxins and detoxification is vast. Here I will highlight just some of the more interesting aspects.

The term biotransformation describes the *non*-immune means by which foreign threats are dealt with. The biotransformation pathways that degrade toxic environmental chemicals are often shared by substances which are of food value. As part of a chemical classification system, many of our daily nutrients are also organic compounds, like acids or esters. The process of biotransformation allows us to detox nutrients or eliminate toxins. There are four kinds of biotransformation reaction:

- oxidation
- reduction
- degradation — for example, by hydrolysis
- conjugation.

The first three of these are the predominant means by which *nutrients* are incorporated into the body. Conjugation is more important for the *elimination of (foreign) chemicals*. As conjugation is also the means by which *hormonal balance is maintained*, hormonal disruption is a common sequel of toxic exposure.

Before these foreign chemicals can be conjugated, they first are changed into one of six less toxic compounds by one of the first three biotransformations (that is, oxidation, reduction or hydrolysis). Thus, all four of these systems may overlap, and important nutrients and xenobiotics may use them simultaneously. Moreover, any one toxic chemical can use several biochemical pathways. Toxic overload can lead to breakdown of the major pathways, and the process is then shunted to an inferior pathway. The toxic chemicals may persist undegraded in the body, and normal metabolism may be interrupted. This in part explains why patients who have been exposed to an excess of toxic chemicals may develop food allergies and hypersensitivity. It is also thought to explain many of the symptoms of the Gulf War syndrome and chronic fatigue syndrome. The foods, animals or pollens to which they now react have never in the past caused them any concern.

The first line of defence against toxic compounds comes from the barriers provided by skin and mucous membranes. Many solvents break down these barriers. Examples are chloroform, trichloroethane, tri- and tetra-chloroethylene. In this case, not only does the *solvent* gain easier access; so too do other foreign invaders like toxic chemicals, undigested food particles, pollens and pathogens. In Chapter 2: Vaccination, we saw an example of this when cigarette smoke damages mucous membranes and enables the meningitis organism to invade.

The battlefield extends to include all bodily cells. Particularly affected are liver cells (hepatocytes), because they are especially evolved to deal with toxic insults. Vulnerable, too, are kidneys, skin and lung. While excretory organs such as these have been specially 'designed' to reduce the total body burden of toxic chemicals, the survival of any one cell is dependent on its individual ability to detox itself.

Vulnerability is increased when an organ has been weakened by previous health problems. Kidneys that have undergone previous episodes of infection, or a gut damaged by antibiotic usage or chlorine, are more likely to succumb to the effects of a toxin. It is common, therefore, in patients exposed to a toxic assault, to witness the development of irritable bowel or recurrent cystitis, even when these organs would not seem the most vulnerable to the chemical. It also explains why symptoms arising from the same chemical can vary from individual to individual.

The outcomes can be surprising. The correlation between atherosclerosis and pollution turns out to be as significant as the correlation between atherosclerosis and raised cholesterol levels.[12] Also affected are the lipid components of the arterial linings. Membranes again. Pollution also damages the cholesterol transport systems, the lipoproteins. The end result is an increased burden of 'bad' cholesterol, and an accumulation of it at the sites of wear and tear in the arteries.

The role of enzymes

The most important part of biotransformation is carried out by the enzyme systems. Of the thousands of enzymes that the human genome codes for, many are there for detoxification. As a medical student I used to wonder at Mother Nature's luck in having provided enzymes to detox Valium and pesticides, thousands of years before they were invented. Gradually it dawned on me that most compounds, whether synthetic or naturally occurring, fall into one of the classes of organic molecule listed above as xenobiotics. Expressed another way, these chemicals fall within the natural limits of possibility, and are defined by the natural 'laws' of organic chemistry.

In fact, the means by which many chemicals, drugs, pesticides and herbicides exert their effects *is* their ability to mimic biological molecules. They were created to do just that.

We have already seen in Chapter 3 that genes which code for enzymes can exist in multiple forms (exhibit polymorphism). In the past, the enzyme variants which caused problems for their human owners were mostly those which we now know as 'inborn errors of metabolism'. Many of these variants are incompatible with normal life. Sometimes it is a normal nutrient which becomes the toxin.

Examples of these diseases include 'maple syrup disease' and phenylketonuria (PKU). In the case of PKU the amino acid phenylalanine has damaging effects because the body cannot detox it.

Nowadays, enzyme variants are making their presence felt in people like Fran. They are not defective enzymes. These enzymes served our species until the industrial age. Unfortunately, in this polluted world, even those with genetically robust enzyme systems are not spared. One of the effects of some xenobiotics is to damage the very enzyme systems 'designed' to detoxify them.

The enzymes involved in biotransformation are further classified in this way:

- *Phase I enzymes:* represented by the multi-gene cytochrome P450 family — that is to say, aldehyde and xanthine oxidases, and, the peroxidases. They are responsible for oxidation, reduction and degradation. Many prescription medications are detoxified by this family of enzymes.
- *Phase II enzymes:* primarily involved in conjugation reactions, they include the glutathione s-transferases, the glucuronosyltransferases, and the sulfotransferases.
- *Mixed function enzymes:* to demonstrate that little in biochemistry is simple, some enzymes, such as epoxide hydrolase and the P450 oxidases, operate within both systems.[13]

Enzyme variants

Some enzyme variants have been identified, either because their very existence is incompatible with normal life, or because modern drugs and poisons have dramatically highlighted them. I will discuss a few of these in detail because this subject is both fascinating and important.

The first example of a 'defect' relates to an enzyme called *pseudocholinesterase*. About 4 per cent of the population makes this aberrant form of the enzyme acetylcholinesterase. Under normal circumstances the variant causes few problems, and most people who carry it are not even aware of the fact. But, with the advent of anaesthesia, some healthy individuals would stop breathing when the drug succinyl choline was used. One in 2500 has a double dose of this gene. This (or another genetic problem known as malignant hyperthermia) is why the anaesthetist asks whether you or your relatives have ever had a bad reaction to an anaesthetic.

'Defects' relating to oxidation, reduction and degradation
Defects may occur in the enzymes relating to oxidation, reduction and degradation of toxins. Some examples are :

- *Paroxonase polymorphism:* The pesticide parathion is metabolised to Paraoxon by one of our inbuilt detox enzymes. The advent of pesticides has identified a group of people who do not handle the pesticide well. The pesticide has thus lent its name to the enzyme. People who are homozygous for this autosomal recessive gene may have difficulty handling not only parathion, but other organophosphates as well. (The term 'autosomal recessive' means that the gene needs to be in a double dose to cause problems, and that it does not sit on the sex chromosomes.)
- *Sulphate oxidase deficiency:* A significant percentage of the population reacts to sulphur-containing drugs and to inhalation of sulphurous gases. The reaction varies from mild discomfort to life-threatening conditions such as severe asthma. An autosomal recessive gene is suspected of being involved in these reactions.
- *Hydroxylation:* About 9 per cent of the population of Britain have been demonstrated to be slow at hydroxylation (one of the means by which xenobiotics are oxidised), resulting in exaggerated or adverse reactions to drugs and toxic chemicals. They have a defect in the cytochrome P450 system which results from an autosomal recessive gene. They may also have difficulty in metabolising phenformin, nortriptyline and phenacetin. The first of these was a notorious component of a diet pill, and the last was a popular over-the-counter painkiller. The English worker J. Monro found up to 66 per cent of chemically sensitive people had this genotype.[14]

'Defects' relating to conjugation

Conjugation can take place by various means, all of them involving enzymes. It should be remembered that conjugation is the process by which the body rids itself of most drugs and pollutants.

- *Sulphonation:* Up to 20 per cent of the population are slow sulphonators. Sulphonation is part of the conjugation process which handles naphthalol, oestrogen and other steroids, aliphatic alcohols, various amines and bile salts. Pollution places a heavy burden on this system. If the enzymes are occupied in dealing with pollution, the threshold of tolerance leading to food sensitivities, steroid-dependent cancers and other such medical conditions is lowered. These people metabolise sulphur slowly and become ill while doing so. They may become ill when they consume sulphur-based food additives, or are exposed to gases from certain refineries.
- *Acetylation:* Up to *half* the population of Europe are believed to be slow acetylators. Patients with this genotype are vastly over-represented among lupus patients. The full name of this disease is systemic lupus erythematosus (SLE). *Lupus* is Latin for 'wolf', and like a wolf in sheep's clothing lupus can appear in many guises. Environmental factors are suspected in the rising incidence of lupus, and indeed of many of the other autoimmune disorders. Slow acetylators react to several known drugs, including isoniazid and procainamide.

Vulnerability

The pathways revealed by variant enzymes were intended to deal with normal toxins in the food chain, or by-products of normal metabolism such as oestrogen. They were never designed to deal with the burden imposed by industrial pollution. For those like Fran, who clearly have several of the vulnerable variants, things are even worse. Menstrual, fertility and menopausal problems are so common today that we almost take them for granted. Oral contraceptives and their derivatives are widely used to correct the symptoms of these 'imbalances'. These are man-made solutions to man-made problems, and often place a further burden on conjugation systems.

Furthermore, in processes such as conjugation, intermediate

metabolites are produced that are more toxic than the original substance. In a non-polluted world, this did not matter. Oestrogen, for example, when being metabolised, produces some intermediate products which are thought to promote cancer. Under ideal circumstances, these would be only *intermediate* products. However, in a system stretched to capacity, they accumulate. Worse still, some of the intermediates of *xenobiotic* metabolism are also thought to be more toxic than the original substance. This is thought to be the basis of many carcinogenic events, and it reveals how misleading it may be to declare a product 'safe' on the basis of laboratory tests.

Those patients who seem to react to all chemicals and medications, or who suffer chronic fatigue syndrome, are not making it up. In all probability they just got more than their fair share of these variants, which are defects only in a polluted chemical world. They and Fran are the canaries down the mine.

Many of these genetic conditions can be tested for in specialised laboratories, but many patients *and their doctors* are unaware of the effects of this genetic variability. These conditions do not appear in the medical school curriculum; they are *not* routinely checked; and tests for them are *not* available from most regular laboratories. They are rarely taken into account when prescribing medications or assessing the effects of toxins.

So how does the genetic hand that each of us has been dealt translate into our everyday lives? Which is the greater threat—the germ and the cockroach, or the chemicals used to attack them? Where do we meet these chemicals, and how can we avoid them?

Most classification systems are a compromise. Above I classified chemicals as they might be seen from the body's point of view. They can also be classified according to other characteristics:

- *their chemical properties:* polychlorinated biphenyls, organochlorines, benzenes
- *their commercial use:* pesticides, herbicides, petrochemicals, aviation fuel, food additives
- *the damage they do:* carcinogens, teratogens, mutagens.

I will focus on carcinogens because data are readily available and because cancer is a clear diagnostic category. However, it is an overriding theme in this book that the biological malfunction which gives one person cancer may give another asthma and yet another, arthritis. Although the actions of some chemicals are specific and the effects predictable, the outcome also depends on each person's genetic makeup, their nutrient defences, and the myriad other factors that influence health and disease.

The workplace

Certain occupations have been associated with increased cancer and other health risks. Here is a partial list:[15]

- Tanners, smelters, vineyard workers and plastic workers have an increased risk of liver cancer. The identified carcinogens are arsenic and vinyl chloride.
- People working with glass, pottery, linoleum, nickel, and in electrolysis, have increased risks of *nasal and sinus cancer*. The carcinogens are fumes of chromium, nickel and isopropyl oil.
- Vintners, miners, tanners and those working in smelters, glass and pottery, coal tar, iron foundry, chemical and electrolysis industries, are all at increased risk of *lung cancer*. Radiologists also have this risk. The identified carcinogens are arsenic, asbestos, chromium, iron oxide, mustard gas, nickel, petroleum, bis(chloromethyl) ether and ionising radiation.
- People working in industries involved in the production and usage of gas, asphalt, coal tar, dyes, paint, leather and shoes have all been found to be at increased risk of *bladder cancer*. Coal products and aromatic amines have been identified as the carcinogens.
- People working with benzene, explosives, rubber and cement, distillers, dye users, painters and radiologists have higher risk of *bone marrow cancers*. The identified carcinogens are benzene and ionising radiation.
- Anaesthetists have an overall increased risk of *cancer, lower fertility* and a greater risk of producing *children with congenital defects*. This raises the question of the safety of anaesthetic gases.
- Beauticians and hairdressers have a greater risk of *ovarian cancer* and *autoimmune disease*.

Consumer products

Many products are accepted unquestioningly by the consumer on the grounds that they will have been tested before being released into the marketplace. I believe that such confidence is misplaced.

Tobacco

It is hard to imagine a human in the Western world who is not aware of the risks associated with smoking. They extend beyond lung cancer to bladder and bowel cancer. There is also an increased incidence of cardiovascular disease, ear, nose and throat infections, fertility problems and birth defects. It is probably easier to list the conditions which are *not* worsened by smoking.

Ulcerative colitis appears to be less common in smokers. The mechanism seems to be that of immune suppression which, while retarding this disease, is just as injurious to the rest of health as we might expect.

Many schizophrenics are smokers. Rather than smoking contributing to the condition, the current thinking is that the patients may be self-medicating by altering the dopamine pathways.

Food additives

Epstein estimates that the average American eats about 1500 pounds of food a year containing about 9 pounds of chemicals (or 680 kg of food and 4 kg of chemicals).[16] The chemicals come in two categories, depending on whether their presence is accidental or intentional. Accidental additives include residual insecticides and rodenticides, plastigens from the packaging, and even axle grease from mixing machines. The 'allowed' level of cockroach parts in chocolate has reached the status of urban myth. Maybe the cockroach parts are preferable to the chemicals used to combat them, but in all probability we are getting both.

Intentional additives include colours, preservatives, flavours and stabilisers. The role of food additives was highlighted by the American physician Ben Feingold, who felt that hyperkinetic behaviour in children could be controlled by the elimination of unnecessary additives from the diet. The perception within mainstream medicine is that Feingold was proved wrong. This is far from true.

Some examples of the 'proof' include a trial using only *10* of the 3000 additives discussed by Feingold, in doses of 2–26 mg a day. Yet the US Food and Drug Administration acknowledged that the estimated daily consumption of colourings was between 59 and 76 mg, depending on age. The application of the normal distribution curve indicated that some people were consuming 121–146 mg, and the upper limits of consumption were around 312 mg.[17] Moreover many of the trials used chocolate as both the control substance and the vehicle for the test colourants. Chocolate is highly reactive, totally unsuited as a control substance.

Two of the commonest food colourings are the red dye erythrosine (E110) and tartrazine (E102).

- *Erythrosine* is a xanthine dye like the luminous fluorescein. In fact, it *is* a fluorescein molecule, with four iodine atoms attached. It is also a molecule which resembles thyroxin. Animal experiments have shown an increased level of thyroxin and thyroid iodine retention in animals fed erythrosine. There was also a reduction of uptake by brain cells of dopamine in the presence of this dye. If such animal experiments can be extrapolated to humans, we would expect some children on high doses of junk food to behave as if thyrotoxic. (Thyrotoxic patients are restless, agitated, and in extreme cases known as 'thyroid storm' seem psychotic with serious disturbances of heart rhythm.) The added insult of dopamine deficiency completes the picture.[18]
- *Tartrazine* has been unequivocally associated with hypersensitivity reactions, anaphylaxis, skin rashes and migraine.[19] Banned for many years in some Scandinavian countries, it is still to be found in foods from coloured sweets through to savoury crisps and custard powder in Australia, Britain and the United States. It has only recently been removed from medications — including, ironically, migraine tablets and anti-histamines for skin rashes! About 15 per cent of people with aspirin sensitivity cross-react with tartrazine, so its contribution to asthma attacks in some people is significant.

Sweetening agents have caused as much concern as food colourings. The best-known are saccharin, cyclamate and aspartame.

For many years the debate has raged as to whether saccharin is carcinogenic. Various studies in mice and rats have shown an increased risk for bladder cancer. International animal studies have also demonstrated an increased risk of lymphomas, lymphosarcomas and malignant tumours of the breast, ovary and uterus.[20]

Human studies have been equivocal. One published in *The Lancet* in 1977 indicated that men who used saccharin were 65 per cent more at risk of developing bladder cancer than those who didn't.[21] In 1972 saccharin was removed from the American list known as GRAS (that is, generally recognised as safe), but it remains in use today. The concern lies with the number of young people regularly consuming soft drinks and even toothpastes sweetened with saccharin.

Aspartame has been promoted as safer than saccharin, although the accumulating literature seems set to provide similar levels of controversy.

Another group of food additives that may have toxic effects is preservatives. They include:

- *Nitrites:* Their main usage is in cured meats for protection against the deadly organism *Clostridium botulinum*. They have been strongly linked to childhood cancer.[22]
- *Sulphites:* These are usually present as sulphur dioxide and other sulphites. The ability to handle them depends on the genetic factors discussed above. Their presence is associated with asthma, irritable bowel and migraine.
- *Benzoates:* These are used to control the growth of yeasts and moulds. They are linked to behavioural disturbances and to the same illnesses caused by the sulphites.[23]

Food containers

A substance called *acrylonitrile* became a matter of public concern when Monsanto started to use it in the manufacture of plastic bottles for the Coca-Cola company. After cases of excess cancers among workers were revealed, strict safety standards were set in 1978. Epstein cites this as an example of 'inadequate pre-market testing of a food and soft drink container'.[24]

Bisphenol-A is found in baby bottles and other containers, and is discussed shortly.

Cosmetics

Many cosmetics are based on petrochemicals. There are associations between perfume and migraine, nail polish and endocrine disruption (hormone imbalance), and cosmetics and autoimmune disorders such as lupus.

A report from the United States shows how easy it is for some things to slip through the safety net.[25] Some hair shampoos, particularly those marketed to black people, contain small amounts of oestrogen. American black girls are reaching puberty significantly earlier than their white counterparts. About half of all American black girls have begun to develop breasts or pubic hair by the age of eight, compared with 15 per cent of white girls, and earlier than their black counterparts in Africa. Puberty at such a tender age, by any standard, is precocious.

We should also ask whether the powerful insecticide lindane is appropriate as a shampoo to control head lice in children. lindane is a highly toxic central nervous system stimulant, and has been associated with the development of the leukaemias.[26]

Recreational and prescription drugs

This topic is mentioned here for completeness, but it is dealt with throughout this book.

Solvents

Solvents include chemicals known as toxic volatile chlorinated aliphatic hydrocarbons, and toxic aromatic hydrocarbons. Common names include benzene, toluene, xylene, styrene and chloroform.

Symptoms on exposure include cardiovascular (vascular spasm, bruising and cardiac arrhythmias), respiratory (runny nose, wheezing and bronchitis), musculoskeletal (pain and swelling) and neurological (headache, memory loss, vertigo and paraesthesia), as well as effects on the bowel, genito-urinary tract, skin and eyes.

Chloroform is no longer used as an anaesthetic because it is too dangerous. Yet we can readily buy pens, glue and nail varnish that are made from the same family of chemicals. Many people go through migraine and asthma clinics without inquiry into basics such as these. Patients sometimes report overwhelming depression which can be traced to something as simple as office equipment or a cosmetic.

The insidious thing about solvents is the speed with which they access the brain. While many foreign insults have to get across the lining of the gut or pass through the liver, a solvent goes straight from the nasal cavity through a delicate bony mesh (one of the most beautiful structures in the whole skeleton) called the cribriform plate, and into the brain. Solvents do to the barriers of the body what they do to paint, nail varnish and years-old grease. It's a pity that the brain is little more than sophisticated grease!

Environmental poisons

Pesticides

There are generally accepted to be three generations of pesticide. The first generation was based on naturally occurring organic compounds such as pyrethrum, and inorganic compounds such as copper, zinc, mercury and lead salts and arsenates. The second generation began with the production of synthetic organic compounds such as DDT in about 1940. Third-generation or modern pesticides include the release of sterilised insects and 'natural' and modified viruses.[27] While these methods avoid the hazards of poisoning, the spectre of genetically modified organisms remains.

It is the second generation of pesticides which has created the most adverse publicity. There are three main groups of compound in this category:

- organophosphate insecticides
- organochlorines such as DDT, chlordane, heptachlor, aldrin and dieldrin
- phenoxy acid herbicides: including 2,4,5-T and 2,4-D (constituents of Agent Orange), and chlorophenols, used in wood preservatives and herbicides.

Organophosphate insecticides act by blocking the enzyme cholinesterase, an action which first overstimulates and then blocks nerve transmission. It is used with the assumption that the dose required to kill insects is not harmful to humans when properly handled. These insecticides include dichlorvos (used in pest strips), malathion and parathion. Parathion has been responsible for more suicide and accidental deaths than any other pesticide. Healthy people usually metabolise these pesticides within 24 hours. Unfortunately, some people do not. The relevance of enzyme variants mentioned earlier in this chapter cannot be over-emphasised. Alzheimer's disease, tardive dyskinesia and Huntington's chorea have all been linked to organophosphate exposure.[28]

The organochlorines and phenoxy acid herbicides are commonly, but not always, members of the class of chemicals referred to as PCBs, which have applications beyond pesticide usage. Related chemicals are vinyl chloride, polyvinyl chloride (PVC), and dioxin. We will look at the health effects of these chemicals, whether used as pesticides or in industry, and put them into context.

Some history and some chemistry

There are various ways to classify environmental poisons. A bit of history may help to explain the connections between some seemingly unrelated chemicals.

The place of carbon in biological systems was discussed in Chapter 3: Chemistry. Among the early identified carbon compounds, of course, was coal, 'manufactured' in some past era by plants. In 1859 petroleum first gained commercial significance, but it wasn't until about 1913 that large-scale processing of hydrocarbons (compounds containing hydrogen and carbon), saw the birth of the organic chemistry industry as we know it today. Before 1900 most organic raw materials came from coal tar or the distillation of wood. The catalytic cracking of petroleum after World War II made possible the exponential growth of the petrochemical industry. Crude oil is the source from which most of the raw materials now come.

Chlorine belongs to the group of elements known as the halogens, which are all strong oxidants and highly reactive elements (second-last column in the Periodic Table of Elements, Chart 3.1). They readily form compounds with most other elements, and the carbon-based molecules are no exception. Other members of the halogen group include bromine, fluorine and iodine.

Interesting things began to happen when chemists put hydrocarbons and halogens together. The production of halogenated hydrocarbons became the basis of both the plastic and pesticide industries. The PCBs are a particularly interesting subset.

PCBs (polychlorinated biphenyls)

PCBs were first introduced in 1929 when some chemical engineers found that, by adding some chlorine atoms to a carbon-based molecule consisting of two benzene rings (a biphenyl), they could create a class of compounds which had no equivalent in nature. The PCBs were non-flammable and extremely stable, making them attractive compounds to the growing electrical industry.

The Swann Chemical Company, soon to become part of Monsanto, marketed them as cooling compounds in transformers. Soon they were being used in lubricants, hydraulic fluids, cutting oils and liquid seals. From there they became an indispensable part of the production of plastic, paints, varnishes, inks, wood preservatives and pesticides. They even made possible the first carbonless copy paper.

The very stability of halogenated hydrocarbons became the problem. Once manufactured, they did not degrade. It was a Danish scientist, Sören Jensen, who first noticed that whenever he tried to measure DDT in human blood, he found odd chemicals. When people started *looking* for PCBs, they found them everywhere—in soil, air, water, mud, fish, birds, wildlife, humans. On the continents, at the poles. Nothing, and nowhere, it seemed, was spared.

In 1976 the United States banned the manufacture of PCBs. Other countries gradually followed. By then, however, approximately 3.4 billion pounds (1.5 million tons) had been produced. All of this that was not still in active use was, and still is, contaminating the environment. More worryingly, an investigation funded by the European Union, led by Kevin Jones from the University of Lancaster, has indicated that only about 30 per cent of PCBs are accounted for.[29] Many are still waiting to *enter* the environment from factory and farm stores, or 'sitting in old electrical equipment', according to Jones.

All have adverse health effects which include both gender-bending and carcinogenesis. It is not easy to separate out the respective contribution of each chemical to these—and other—diseases. The interaction between the various compounds at the manufacturing level, during use, during natural degradation and during the active incineration of waste products, makes separation impossible. The formation of dioxin illustrates this complexity.

Contamination: the story of dioxins

Although the organochlorines are all toxic in their own right, it is an inadvertently produced contaminant that is the most toxic product of all. This contaminant is usually known as 2,3,7,8-TCDD or dioxin. Although it tops the toxicity list, dioxin is only one of a family of 74 dioxins, all problematic. Moreover, the same type of process which produces the dioxins also produces a family of 135 furans, with structures and toxicities similar to the dioxins.

These chemicals can be released by the burning of fossil fuels, by forest fires and by volcanoes. By far the most common exposure nowadays, however, is through the industrial production of chlorine-containing chemicals such as plastics, paper, pesticides and wood preservatives. The incineration of these 'disposable' products often occurs after as little as one use. Once, you had to be near an erupting volcano to be exposed to dioxin; nowadays, living near the city dump will probably suffice.[30]

Health effects of the organochlorines

The PCB or pesticide molecules pose danger because they are:

- toxic in their own right to nerves, the brain and other organs
- toxic to genetic material, and therefore potentially cause cancer and genetic mutation
- toxic to enzyme systems either through direct damage or overload, as already discussed
- gender-benders which can result in both malignancy and infertility.

With regard to the first three points, there is extensive literature on the cancer-causing properties of all the organochlorines, and it is largely because of their potential carcinogenic and mutagenic effects that further manufacture has been banned. Some other conditions associated with PCBs, pesticides and herbicides include Parkinson's disease, leukaemias and birth defects, which are discussed in this book where relevant.

It is the gender-bending role of PCBs that has added to their notoriety in recent years. Sometimes gender-bending chemicals are referred to as 'xeno-oestrogens', although oestrogens are not the only hormones affected and PCBs are not the exclusive culprit. ('Xeno' in this context means simply that the molecule is foreign to biology; it is an imposter. A phyto-oestrogen is not a xeno-oestrogen because it is part of a natural diet.)

Of the 50-plus chemicals which have been identified as gender-benders, a significant proportion are PCBs. This is because since their creation in 1929, an enormous scope and quantity of them became readily available. In the manner that was to become depressingly familiar, enthusiasm for their production was little tempered by questions of the safety, the disposal or the longevity of the product. Indeed, durability, as we have seen, was one of their defining characteristics.

Gender-benders or endocrine disruptors can work in several ways. They can mimic hormones, or they can block them. They can influence the degradation of natural hormones, favouring one pathway (such as aromatisation) over another. They can have direct toxic effects on germ cells (egg cells and sperm). They can affect 'signalling' in the developing embryo, leading to ambiguous sexual differentiation. And they can affect other organs such as the hypothalamus or the liver, which in turn affects the gonadal hormones.

A look at a couple of these mechanisms gives an idea of how significantly such molecules can affect every one of us.

Mimicry: PCBs have an affinity for the oestrogen receptors in both males and females. This is odd because the various molecules involved have only a passing resemblance to sterol molecules like oestrogen. However, it is not without reason that the oestrogen receptor has earned for itself the description 'promiscuous'. While many receptors in the body are highly selective and will accept only structural 'lock and key' matches, this cannot be said of oestrogen receptors.

Attention was first drawn to *androgen* mimics when some female fish, which lived downstream from a paper factory in Florida, showed signs of masculinisation. It appeared that sterol chemicals from wood pulp were being converted by bacteria in the water into androstenedione, the precursor to both testosterone and oestrogen (Chart 3.6). Once scientists became aware that foreign chemicals could mimic naturally occurring hormones, a spate of research ensued. Alligators with penises too small to achieve effective copulation;[31] hermaphrodite cubs born to Arctic polar bears; the world's disappearing frogs—all these puzzles have been linked to PCBs.[32]

Most of us, of course, do not experience huge loads of PCBs. But hormones and their inter-relationships are a matter of delicate balance. These relationships are not easily measured in blood samples, and therefore the contribution of any disturbance to a subsequent cancer or fertility problem is difficult to establish.

Research has found that the average German consumes about 7.5 mcg daily of nonyl phenyls (an oestrogen mimic). Formula-fed infants were consuming 1.4 mcg. In the case of the infant, this is about seven times as much as when it is entirely breast-fed.[33]

Blockade: The other side of mimicry is blockade. Rather than substituting for a hormone, the interloper looks enough like the original to be accepted by the receptor, but not enough to effect the desired response. Then it is known as an *anti*-oestrogen, or *anti*-androgen. It is like a key that will slip into a lock but cannot turn it.

Hormones often have natural mimics in the plant world. This is no coincidence. Many hormones are made up of sterol rings, a common natural structure. Co-evolution between plants, and the animals which ate them, provided an adaptive benefit (Chapter 10).

Some of these naturally occurring molecules can behave as both *anti*-hormonal and *pro*-hormonal substances. In this way, an ideal diet provides a buffer system. Women on diets high in the so-called phyto-oestrogens (a better term is phyto-sterol because oestrogen is not the only hormone thus mimicked) suffer less breast cancer and fewer menopausal problems. We can postulate a scenario in which plant sterols act as oestrogen mimics when the woman's reserves are down, or as *blockade* molecules when there has been a surge in her own hormones.

Unfortunately, people who find this kind of 'natural' logic challenging tend to lump plant foods in with the xeno-oestrogens. Every so often a report emerges that soy products cause infertility and cancer, or feminise males. There is virtually no evidence to support this, as upwards of 125 million Japanese bear witness to. As already discussed, many of our metabolic pathways have developed specifically to deal with dietary inputs. Food and humans go back a long way together. The xeno-hormones, by contrast, are molecules never before seen in nature.

A report from *New Scientist* paints a bleak picture:

> On the current list of known anti-androgens in the environment are the fungicide vinclozin, phthalates (from plastics), and DDE, a breakdown product of DDT. These

products are also listed carcinogens. In the Western world the number of cases of testicular cancer has doubled since the 1960s and infertility has also increased. Hypospadias, which, in its extreme form, presents as ambiguous genitalia, has more than doubled in the United States since 1968, such that 1 in 125 boys born in that country have some degree of it.[34]

Could the 'low dose' of these chemicals really cause so much mischief? Fred vom Saal, a biologist at the University of Missouri who has long been involved in the low-dose debate, feels the evidence is clear: even doses in the parts-per-billion range can cause reproductive and developmental abnormalities. He claims to have demonstrated such effects in mice using bisphenol-A, a polycarbonate that appears in everything from plastic wrap to baby bottles (mentioned above under Food Containers). 'This is the next tobacco,' he says.[35] As to the adequacy of testing, *New Scientist* comments that 'very few of the 15,000 chemicals produced in the highest volume in the United States have been tested for any endocrine-disrupting effects'.[36]

Although this knowledge is critical to the work of the field biologist and environmental scientist, it receives barely a mention in the fertility clinics (and cancer clinics) of First World medicine. Somehow the fascination for the high-tech of IVF and gene technology overrides any need on the part of the doctors to engage with the question of causation.

'Safeguards'

Lest one think that all the dangerous chemicals have been banned and safely contained, a brochure current in May 2003 from the Schedules Waste Management Group in Australia should lay such thinking to rest. Labelled 'Safe handling of organochlorines on farms', it points out that some organochlorines listed as registered may not be registered for use in all states, or may be subject to specific controls and codes of practice. These chemicals are not banned; they are not subject to immediate confiscation and collection by the government. It is left entirely to the discretion and the ability of the farmer to interpret the rules. And what do the recommendations include? I quote:

> Wear elbow-length PVC or other chemically resistant gloves
> when handling any chemical containers. ... After handling
> pesticides, always wash your hands with soap ... and water
> before eating, drinking, handling children or pets, smoking or
> going to the toilet. ... Ask for a Material Safety Data Sheet
> from the supplier or manufacturer of the registered pesticide
> that you plan to use. These data sheets contain information on
> the proper handling and use of the pesticide, as well as toxicity
> and first aid information.

What does the farmer do with his PVC gloves (which he is advised to change frequently), now soaked in organochlorines, a dioxin time bomb? He is advised to dispose of them 'properly'. What if he decides to toss them into the incinerator, near where the kids are playing? What if he is a market gardener who barely speaks English, and cannot read the labels on the containers?[37] And if he follows the instructions and washes his hands, where will the water go?

These are not rhetorical concerns. In a medical journal recently I read that US researchers had found 'an average of 200 industrial compounds, pollutants and other chemicals in the umbilical cord blood' of 10 randomly selected newborns. A total of 287 chemicals were identified, including seven pesticides that had been banned for 30 years.[38]

Some other problem chemicals

Formaldehyde

It is appropriate to begin this list with formaldehyde because Hans Selye, the early-20th-century physiologist best known for studying the 'general adaptation syndrome', used formaldehyde as the toxic stressor in his experimental animals. Selye was famously able to demonstrate all of the parameters we would now recognise as 'adrenal exhaustion' (Chapter 5).

The addition of water to formaldehyde produces *formalin*. It is an efficient antiseptic and disinfectant and, being soluble in water, is effective as a preserving agent and embalming fluid. It is also a major component in chipboard and plywood, rubber, paint and plastics. As a synergistic chemical, it can produce the potent carcinogen bischloromethylether, simply by coming into contact with hydrochloric acid.[39]

Some facts about formaldehyde:

- It is recognised as a potent irritant, a carcinogen, and a triggering agent for chemical sensitivity. The World Health Organisation sets guidelines for exposure at about 10 ppb for sensitive individuals and 80 ppb for others — an amazing discrepancy.
- Australian guidelines, worryingly, are set at 100 ppb.
- In the United States serious health problems arising from urea-formaldehyde foam insulation (UFFI) led to a partial ban on this substance. (In Australia, the American problems resulted in a ban on UFFI in schools and private residences from August 1992.)
- Formaldehyde is detoxified via the aldehyde pathways, largely in the liver. The enzymes involved require zinc, iron and molybdenum. Due to the deficiencies in a typical Western diet, few people reach the RDI for any of these elements except iron.
- Formaldehyde has been associated with the triggering of autoimmune disease, notably Hashimoto's thyroiditis.

Aldehyde detoxification enzymes are required to detoxify alcohol and other environmental poisons. People exposed to formaldehyde therefore can develop environmental sensitivity. The chemical easily penetrates lipid membranes. In the gut it increases the likelihood of developing leaky gut syndrome and irritable bowel. Penetration at the cellular level, especially the impact on mitochondrial function, is of concern. Mitochondria provide most of the energy of the cell, and disruption of mitochondrial structure and function is thought to be critical in the development of many of the chronic fatigue and chemical sensitivity syndromes.

PAHs (polycyclic aromatic hydrocarbons)

The carcinogenicity of PAHs has been known since the 1930s. These chemicals are found in cigarette smoke and air pollutants. They are the result of incomplete combustion of organic matter, such as in the tars from pitch and oil, and the combustion products of diesel. Charcoaled meats are the commonest food sources of PAH. The carcinogenicity of PAHs has been known since the 1930s.

Scrotal cancer in chimney sweeps in the 18th century was a result of these chemicals.

Research also indicates that they damage DNA. Because PAHs cling to the tiny particles of air pollution there is the suggestion that inhaling polluted air can cause genetic defects.[40]

IMMUNE SYSTEM DISORDERS

In the waiting room on any day, at least one patient will be feeling that their immune system is 'down' or 'weak' or malfunctioning in some way. Once they would have asked if they needed a tonic. Some of them still do.

The job of the immune system is to stand between the patient and ill-health. If it is not functioning well, what will happen?

Remember that the immune system developed to fight germs. Three types of maladaptive response can occur. Think about the war imagery in Chapter 3: Inflammation. When things go wrong, it may be due to an ill-equipped, understaffed army; or there may be problems with trigger-happy soldiers; or there may be death and misadventure through friendly fire. Translated into medical terms, this gives us immune deficiency, hypersensitivity (allergy), and autoimmune disorders.

There are three kinds of immune deficiency:

- *Acquired:* HIV-AIDS is one example; exposure to radiation or toxic chemicals is another.
- *Congenital:* These disorders may be benign, such as hereditary IgA deficiency; or life-threatening, as with widespread immune globulin deficiency where the sufferer must live in a 'bubble' to avoid all possibility of infection.
- *The result of overload:* This occurs where the immune system is functioning normally but a demand beyond its capacity has been made.

HIV is an example of deficiency at more than one level. The size of the viral dose seems to matter, so there is a (limited) capacity to fight back. Uniquely, HIV targets the immune system itself. The original insult of an overwhelmed immune system is then compounded by the fact that the immune system is systematically destroyed.

It is the other two responses — death by friendly fire and trigger-happy soldiers — which are the subjects of the rest of this chapter. Autoimmune disorders and hypersensitivity reactions are becoming increasingly common in the Western world. First we look at some factors that they have in common, and then discuss the two responses separately to uncover the basic science. However, it should be emphasised that they are highly interactive and share many common pathways and many control mechanisms, especially as provided by the prostaglandins (Chapter 5: EFAs).

The hygiene theory

The increase in childhood asthma and allergic illness has given rise to this theory, and it helps us to understand how immune disorders may occur.

With the fall of the Berlin Wall, it was realised that the genetically close populations of East and West Germany had very different asthma rates, and it was the economically deprived East Germans who fared better.

In Britain David Strachan, an epidemiologist at the London School of Hygiene and Tropical Medicine, is usually credited with formulating the hygiene theory. In 1989 he drew attention to his findings that children with a lot of older siblings were the least likely to develop eczema, hay fever and asthma — the group of illnesses usually referred to as 'atopic'.[41]

This finding was echoed around the world. Among Aboriginal Australians, poverty seemed to offer protection against asthma and allergy. Dirt, germs, even common parasitic worms apparently teach the immune system its job.[42] Sheltered by Western medicine from these benign assailants, a 'bored' immune system might practise on harmless antigens such as pollens and food particles. The list of practice targets may include the vaccine antigens, as this may be the closest thing to a real threat that the immune system has encountered (Chapter 2: Vaccination).

Crohn's disease, reactive arthritis, Type 1 diabetes, multiple sclerosis, lupus and coeliac disease are autoimmune disorders, and they too are on the rise. Some, such as Crohn's, were once rarities in children but are no longer. Both allergic and autoimmune disorders represent dysfunction of the immune system, and in particular, dysfunction of T-cell responses.

When a child contracts an infection in natural circumstances, the germ has to pass through one of the body's defence systems. This is typically the mucous membranes of the throat and respiratory tract, or of the gut. The invading germs are met by T-lymphocytes and other immune mechanisms.

In infancy the Th2 response predominates in producing antibodies, but in adults the Th1 system dominates. Maturation of the Th1 system is dependent on exposure to microbes. An Italian study showed that the incidence of atopy and respiratory allergy was inversely related to exposure to hepatitis A, *Helicobacter pylori*, and *Toxoplasma gondii*.[43] These two systems, Th1 and Th2, are known to have an antagonistic effect on each other. If Th1 does not mature, the organism is primed for atopic and allergic illness associated with an excessive Th2 response.

Autoimmune disorders are normally associated with an inappropriate expression of Th1. Certain viruses and bacteria can induce a shift toward the Th1 response. Both protection from germs on the one hand, and vaccination by injection on the other, are outside the range of experience of the human immune system.

When Junior is exposed to germs by vaccination, they do not run the gauntlet of the first-line defence mechanisms. Normally these first-line systems include skin, mucous membranes, and the immune cells located within and beneath them. Injected straight into the subcutaneous or muscle tissue, germs are essentially sending a signal that the normal defence barriers have broken down. Are we teaching the immune system to break the rules before it has even learned what the rules are? Having had little to practise on in the way of 'normal' germs, it may be honing its skills on an array of specific germs chosen by the medical profession and injected straight into the tissues. See Postscript 2008 at the end of Chapter 6.

No account of the rise in allergic and autoimmune diseases will be complete until we fully understand the impact of these factors on an immature immune system.

Breast-feeding

If breast milk is 'designed' for the baby, then by implication, all other milks are not. So formula-fed babies ingest a foreign protein for the immune system to recognise as 'non-self'. Moreover, breast milk contains a substance called *transforming growth factor beta* (TGF-beta), which among other functions facilitates oral tolerance (see below). Clearly this is not the only means by which tolerance develops, because many babies who are never exposed to this substance do not develop allergic and autoimmune problems. Notwithstanding, the consumption of breast milk is associated with a lowered incidence of asthma, eczema, food allergy, coeliac disease and other medical problems. Different disease names, similar pathways.

Hypersensitivity

Hypersensitivity reactions occur when the immune system is overactive and becomes trigger-happy. Asthma and allergy are examples. In this circumstance the immune response is out of all proportion to the damage the pathogen or foreign antigen might be expected to cause.

Hypersensitivity reactions are often further classified into Types 1–4. Type 1, which is the commonest clinical presentation, is mediated by IgE, one of the immune globulins produced by the B lymphocytes. IgE reactions are responsible for conditions such as asthma, eczema, hay fever and anaphylaxis. (Asthma is a complex spectrum of illness. Factors other than IgE are often involved.)

Contributing factors

Many factors affect the development of hypersensitivity reactions:

- *Genes:* In both autoimmune disease and hypersensitivity, genes are likely to be blamed (Chapter 3). The simple message is that it is not the genes we inherit, but what we do with those genes that determines the outcome.
- *Stress:* Physical and mental stress result in increased production of glucocorticoid steroids from the adrenals, and cortisol from the hypothalamus. These hormones often increase hypersensitivity reactions by increasing the production of inflammatory mediators.
- *Hormones:* Many female migraine patients notice the effects of pregnancy, menstruation and menopause

on their headaches. Thyroid disorders often present as allergic skin rashes.

- *Exposure in utero:* Highly allergenic foods such as egg and peanut via the maternal diet may increase the later risk of food allergy, although this thinking is constantly under challenge. Shortly we will see how the state of the gut flora in the mother during pregnancy has been shown to affect the development of asthma and eczema in the early years of the infant's life.
- *Breast-feeding:* The protection offered by breast-feeding is well established.
- *Vitamin and mineral status:* This has been discussed under the various vitamins and minerals (Chapters 4, 5). Just some of many examples include Vitamin B3 which inhibits mast cell degranulation, and therefore the release of inflammatory mediators like histamine. Selenium, as part of the enzyme glutathione peroxidase, modifies the effects of some of these mediators such as prostaglandins. Magnesium has a modifying effect on many messenger molecules at the site at which they attach to their respective receptors.
- *EFA status:* The modifying effect of EFAs in the immune system is discussed in Chapter 5.
- *The hygiene theory:* This is discussed above.

Autoimmune disorders

Autoimmune disorders, or friendly fire, occur when the system for recognising self from non-self breaks down and the body attacks itself. The archetypal autoimmune disorder is SLE, also known as systemic lupus erythematosis or 'lupus'. Coeliac disease is another contender for this crown. Other autoimmune disorders include rheumatoid arthritis, Sjögren's syndrome, Hashimoto's thyroiditis, and probably multiple sclerosis.

There is a definite connection between the presence of certain genes and the development of autoimmune disorders. This is particularly noticeable with certain variations of genes (such as HLA genes on chromosome 6). Although it may be necessary to possess such genes for autoimmune disease to develop, the presence of the genes alone is not sufficient to produce an autoimmune illness.

Contributing factors

Again, many factors affect the development of autoimmune disorders:

- *Bacterial, viral or other foreign antigens:* These can directly stimulate T-cells and B-cells and cause them to become overactive. Adenoviral gut infection is thought in this way to trigger the development of coeliac disease in susceptible individuals. An amino acid chain in gluten is responsible for the gut damage in coeliacs. Adenovirus type 12 shares a sequence of at least eight amino acids with gluten. In attacking viruses, the immune system may learn to attack food proteins which look like viruses.
- *Genes:* as above under Hypersensitivity.
- *Heavy metal poisoning:* Metals bind avidly to certain parts of proteins, including enzymes, co-enzymes and cell membranes. In this way they can alter function, permeability, Th1 and Th2 balance, and gene expression.
- *Synthetic chemicals:* Plastics, silicone implants and the gender-bending chemicals of industrial processes have all been shown to affect immune response, and have been causally linked to the development of autoimmune disorders (see Toxicity Disorders).
- *Medications:* A wide range of prescription drugs have been linked to the development of autoimmune disorders. They include the anti-psychotic medication chlorpromazine; the blood pressure pill Apresoline; isoniazid, used in the treatment of TB; and methyldopa, used for Parkinson's disease. Even the oral contraceptive is thought to adversely affect those at risk of lupus.
- *Trace element deficiency:* Zinc has established roles in both immunity and gene transcription. Selenium is important to the functions of the enzymes glutathione peroxidase, cyclo-oxygenase and lipoxygenase. These enzymes are all integral to immune pathways. Copper is a component in a wide range of immunological reactions, including the enzyme *superoxide dismutase*.

Copper bracelets have been used since ancient times for the treatment of arthritis. Deficiency in any of these nutrients will have an effect on immune regulation (Chapter 4).

- *Vitamin status:* Vitamin C is important to adrenal function. The role of the adrenal glands in modifying immune response is discussed presently. Vitamin E has been shown to activate T-lymphocytes, increase the release of interleukin-1beta, and induce the expression of genes associated with the immune response. The role of Vitamin B6 in the inflammatory response associated with raised homocysteine levels is discussed in Chapter 3. Once again, deficiency of such nutrients will disrupt normal control mechanisms in the immune system (Chapters 4 and 5).
- EFA status: Animal studies have demonstrated significant protective effects of omega-3 fatty acids in mice with a strong propensity for the development of lupus. Several human studies have supported a beneficial role of EPA and DHA in the treatment of rheumatoid arthritis (Chapter 7).44
- *Breast-feeding:* This gives proven protection against developing autoimmune diseases such as coeliac in later life. The health of the digestive tract in immune regulation is discussed in full in the next section.
- *Leaky gut:* For a doctor to confess, a few years ago, that they believed in the 'leaky gut' theory was to invite derision. All that is changing fast as is explained in the following section. Remaining cynics should do a simple net search on 'zonulin', the protein identified at the site of the leak. Zonulin research offers promise in the management of coeliac disease, type 1 diabetes and, possibly, even cholera.

Before we discuss gut disorders, a pre-emptive word is in order. Both coeliac disease and Type 1 diabetes are accepted autoimmune disorders. The interesting link is that the coexistence of both conditions in the one person is so well recognised that paediatric diabetic clinics in Australia now screen every patient for coeliac disease. What do we think is happening here? Alessio Fasano, a researcher from the University of Maryland, thinks he has an answer: damage to the gut caused by gluten allows the entry of other antigenic proteins into the circulation. Further antigen antibody reactions from these antigens attack targets such as the insulin-producing cells in the pancreas.[45]

Such antigens may include milk proteins (Chapter 2), as diabetes occurs more commonly in children who drink milk. Of course, gluten is not the only factor which can damage the gut mucosa, as we shall see, but it provides an ideal model for understanding 'leaky gut'.

The gut

Standing aloof in giant ignorance …

– Keats, 'On First Looking into Chapman's Homer'

Chapter 3 introduced the gut as a major part of the immune system, but this is not what I remember learning in my days in medical school. A doctor who has studied Ayurvedic medicine or traditional Chinese medicine, or gone to orthodox medical school in Germany, will not be surprised to consider that arthritis might have its foundation in the gut or that digestion is central to many health problems. In many cultures, this simple concept is a given.

No discussion of immune diseases can be complete without understanding how gastrointestinal factors might contribute.

Acid stomach and GORD

Drugs for gastro-oesophageal reflux disease, known as GORD, are one of the most commonly prescribed and expensive medications. That should tell us something about the way in which we eat, and how healthy is the state of the contemporary gastro-intestinal tract. The reality is the knee-jerk prescription of medications to stop us from producing stomach acid (proton pump inhibitors).

Indigestion is not always due to excess acid. Quite the contrary. Pain is nature's warning mechanism. If we get a stomach pain every time we eat, maybe this food does not agree with us. Maybe we should not be eating it, perhaps because of an allergy to foods like gluten or wheat or milk. One American researcher makes the case that we may be increasing food allergies by allowing allergenic foods through the gastro-intestinal tract with the aid of these drugs.[46] Not only do we mask one of nature's warning systems, we also reduce our ability to handle the problem food. When we insist on eating something that does not agree with us, our body deals with it by breaking it down into the smallest fragments—proteins into amino acids, food chemicals into more neutral forms. This is what the acid does for us.

It is well known that people with food allergies often don't produce enough acid. Maybe indeed, that is *why* they are allergic. If some of the factors to be listed shortly are operating, the net result may be the induction of food allergies.

And there is another point. During digestion the pyloric sphincter opens so the food can pass from the stomach into the duodenum. The signal that tells it to do this is the acid level in the stomach, measured as pH. The lower the pH, the more acidic, and the more likely the stomach will pass the food into the duodenum, where the acid will be neutralised. If there is not enough acid in the stomach, the food will sit there for longer, awaiting further acid to break it down. There may be a *lower* total amount of acid than the normal person has, but it feels worse because the food sits there for hours, waiting for *more* acid to arrive and get the whole thing moving.

The patient need not be worried about that, though, because we have another drug to hurry things up. A frightening list of side effects should not be cause for concern. We have outwitted Mother Nature again, and these 'prokinetic' agents have been submitted to clinical trials, after all.

In summary, your stomach may produce *more* acid in an attempt to digest a troublesome food. Or it may produce *less*, and this is why you are having trouble digesting it. We should be trying to find out why you aren't producing enough. In either of these cases, drugs to reduce acid secretion and accelerate transit time, although so frequently prescribed, are counter-productive. Acid does not hinder digestion, it helps it, which explains why so many cultures add acidic condiments to fatty foods—vinegar to chips, lemon to fried fish, sauerkraut to pork.

Contributing factors
Several factors affect acid production:

• *Chewing:* The signals to our stomachs to produce acid are manifold, and one of them is chewing. Those who bolt their food, or eat food that does not need to be chewed (junk food), do not give their stomachs time to prepare with adequate acid production (Chapter 8).

- *Stress:* Mother Nature knows that when we are running away from a tiger, it is no time to be thinking about food. At such times our leg muscles have priority, and blood supply should not be diverted to the stomach for digestion. When we eat while rushing, adrenalin suppresses acid secretion.

  It is better to defer a meal than to eat on the run.

- *Eating for the sake of it:* Modern lifestyles encourage us to take meals at scheduled or convenient times, rather than when we are hungry, or because we are told that it is 'healthy' to eat at particular times (Chapter 10). No-one should ever eat to *prevent* hunger. We should eat when we feel hungry, not before. The circadian hormones do not take kindly to food presented outside our natural hunger rhythms. Acid secretion has a distinct circadian cycle.

Irritable bowel syndrome (IBS)

Every day I see patients who have been diagnosed as having irritable bowel syndrome, or who feel that they are suffering from it. Following the simple principles in Appendix 3, most do very well. Interestingly, a recent study indicated that many cases of irritable bowel syndrome involved a food allergy which was best identified by looking for IgG food antibodies, as opposed to the IgE that is normally tested.[47] There are one or two laboratories in Australia where this test can be carried out. My own experience of it has been beneficial. The comments about acid secretion and optimal bowel florae apply to these patients.

The presence of abnormal bacteria in the gut has a significant impact on IBS. Gut bacteria, including the latest research, will be discussed in more detail shortly. Supplementation with probiotics can be a helpful. But there is a note of warning: a recent Dutch study showed that there were an excess number of deaths in a trial that used probiotic therapy in critically ill pancreatitis sufferers.[48] While this is a far cry from the average IBS patient, it warns us that good science needs to apply to natural therapies as much as to pharmaceuticals.

Coeliac disease

Coeliac disease has just been discussed as a candidate for 'archetypal autoimmune disease'. As we enter the 21st century, we realise that coeliac disease is not confined to the gut, and in fact it may not appear in the gut at all. When it does, the events visible at the mucosal surface may be no more than collateral damage to the maelstrom taking place in the lymphatic tissue below.[49] These events ramify throughout the entire immune system of the individual. Common associations include autoimmune disorders such as Type 1 diabetes, thyroid disease, lupus and scleroderma. We might assume that the linkage is the autoimmune predisposition, but I think the situation is more complex, involving extra factors like gut bacteria and the malabsorption of immune nutrients. Particularly curious is the association between Down syndrome, dementia, schizophrenia, epilepsy and cerebral ataxia, which might in part be explained by these other factors.

Among people of Northern European descent, 25 per cent have the genes for coeliac disease. Up to 1 per cent of Europeans are thought to go on to full expression of those genes. This number raises more questions than it answers. Why are there so many coeliacs? Is it simply that we are eating more wheat than before? Is it because wheat is bred for a high gluten content? Is it linked to issues such as the hygiene theory and reduced numbers of gut bacteria in the newborn of the Western world? Is it a reduction in breast-feeding, which we know is protective?

My feeling is that it will be a combination of all of these. One thing is certain; in unravelling coeliac disease we are going to find answers to many unsolved medical questions. As such, reference to coeliac disease appears throughout this book.

Inflammatory bowel disease (IBD)

The two commonest forms of inflammatory bowel disease are Crohn's disease and ulcerative colitis. A genetically determined predisposition is part of the story, but these conditions were uncommon in Asia until the adoption of the Western diet and lifestyle. Milk, gluten and sugar consumption have all been linked to these disorders, and Crohn's patients often also suffer from coeliac disease.

The hygiene theory described above has an interesting expression in relation to Crohn's disease. Several separate studies have shown that refractory cases of Crohn's disease can be treated by

252 THE GOOD BODY GUIDE

the deliberate infection of the gut with intestinal worms. The level of improvement was dramatic, exceeding that achieved by any pharmaceutical. Further support for the idea that the bowel might 'expect' a modest dose of worms comes from the fact that Third World countries which do not 'enjoy' all of the benefits of anti-worm (antihelminthic) treatments do not see much inflammatory bowel disease.[50]

The leaky gut—fact or fiction?
If the gut is part of the immune defence, anything that disrupts the integrity of the mucosal membrane that lines the gut weakens that defence. This situation is often referred to as a leaky gut, and was introduced in the discussion of autoimmune disorders.

The bowel's mucosal barrier is part of the immune system. Once the gut wall is damaged, its normal barrier function is compromised. Three types of problem can then supervene:

- It becomes easier for undesirable bacteria and viruses to establish themselves.
- Food particles can be absorbed in larger and less digested forms. The peptides from dairy and wheat ingestion are discussed in Chapters 2, 9 and 10.
- The passage of electrolytes back and forth across the membrane can be altered. Normally the gut mucosa controls what is absorbed from the intestines, and what is discarded into the intestines from the body. A damaged mucosa loses this discretionary ability, so that leakage occurs in both directions.

The gut is subject to many insults, and one of the earliest is often cow's milk. The gut mucosa of the newborn baby is 'designed' to be leaky, so that the large immune globulins in its mother's milk can gain access to the bloodstream. Nature did not 'expect' foreign proteins to be in the diet, especially not those as reactive as cow's milk. The exposure of the newborn's immune system to these complex molecules, even if only in one or two 'complementary' feeds in the nursery, may prime the immune system of that individual to react to dairy products throughout life. Other challenges to the gut mucosa include chlorine in the drinking water, preservatives and antibiotics in the food chain, therapeutic antibiotics, 'hygiene', and lack of friendly bacteria.

BSE (mad-cow disease), meningococcal meningitis and asthma can be seen as the result of the passage of challengers across membranes unable to deal with them. Thus all of these disorders could be seen as typifying leaky-gut or leaky-membrane phenomena. In the case of the meningococcal organism, the mucosal lining of the nasopharynx has been damaged by cigarette smoke. With BSE, the problem lies with the presentation of animal protein which the animal was never designed to process.

Gut flora

Chapter 3 looked at the normal function of the gut, and in particular its contribution to the immune system. We saw that the gut flora do a lot of work in protecting us. So how should we treat these little bugs?

Medical neglect and inappropriate intervention are at their worst here. Thirty years ago students were taught *nothing* about gut flora in medical school, apart from the mention that they existed and were thought to be harmless. Perhaps nothing was known, but if the vets of the day knew so much about ruminant flora, why was more research not under way in the medical schools? Where was the curiosity? Indeed, today's undergraduate curriculum indicates that there is still a long way to go.

Here is the whole sorry catalogue of what we do to our gut flora. We begin with Jean, a first-time mother.

Jean and Junior
When a baby is born it is covered in a white, cheesy substance. This provides an ideal medium in which to culture the bacteria it has picked up on its entry into the world. It is the nursery for this most important component of the baby's immune system. In our modern world, however, if the baby is born in the daytime, he is whipped away to be bathed in a soapy antiseptic (antibacterial) solution which removes the cheesy coating. Since Jean's baby was born at night he gets to lie in his mother's arms for few hours.

With the first breast-feed, Jean is shown how to wipe her nipples with a soapy sponge or an antiseptic wipe, ensuring that Junior ingests none of her (healthy) skin bacteria. After all, hygiene is everything with babies. Everything which comes near the baby will

254 THE GOOD BODY GUIDE

be sterilised, as you can readily see in the baby section of the nearest supermarket. Much of this avalanche of detergent ends up in the baby's gut. Detergents kill strong germs, as television advertisers regularly tell us; unfortunately they exterminate the friendly bugs in our gut as well. What chemicals Jean does not put there by rinsing, sterilising, and disinfecting, it can be assumed that the baby will. Baby's mouth is his own personal laboratory.

Back to the obstetric hospital. Jean may have had a forceps delivery (3.9 per cent in one major Australian hospital in 2003), a vacuum extraction (6.8 per cent), or a caesarean section (21 per cent). The hospital diet, while not likely to produce scurvy, isn't all that great either. Now she doesn't feel too well. The doctor thinks she has a urinary tract infection or a spot of early mastitis, and prescribes a 'safe' antibiotic, just to be sure. In the meantime, the nurses feel that Jean needs some sleep. So baby is abducted to the nursery, has another cleansing bath, and finds a bottle of cow's milk stuck in his mouth. (This is the first step in an unfolding immunological disaster.)

So what is happening in the baby's gut? The gut flora have only just moved in. They have not yet worked out which room to occupy, and they certainly haven't worked out how to arrange the furniture. Baby now has a stomach full of formula, and sated and asleep, is returned to his mother. Jean is just waking up, breasts full and ready to feed. Unconscious Junior could not be less interested. After all, it takes about 60 times more energy to drain a breast than a bottle. Baby has never filled his stomach so easily or so fully. And what about those bovine endorphins in the milk? No wonder he's out to it.

A couple of hours later, Jean's breasts are engorged. When Junior finally comes to, they're red and sore. There's talk of mastitis — she'll certainly need that antibiotic now. Junior may have to be bottle-fed. If he's lucky enough to keep breast-feeding, guess what will lace his dinner, playing havoc with his new gut flora?

Nonetheless, Junior survives, goes home, and has various encounters with the medical profession. Most are for things like nappy rash or routine vaccinations. Soon after he is weaned, he may start to develop some snuffles and coughs. Usually, these are not serious. The immune globulins he acquired through transplacental circulation are wearing off. The supply provided by breast milk has ended, and now he must develop his own immune system.

But Jean is a first-time mother and a little nervous. Unfortunately, the young doctor at the clinic is fresh out of teaching hospital. Normal babies are not his experience—he left the hospital with high praise for his management of babies with meningitis. He looks in Junior's ear and doesn't like what he sees. The eardrum is red. Junior doesn't like the examination and is crying vigorously. None of his teachers has told this doctor that when a normal baby cries its face goes bright red. So, he will soon learn, does the tympanic membrane. To put it another way, a red eardrum means almost nothing in a baby who is crying his lungs out.

The doctor is aware that antibiotics have little effect on the natural history of an ear infection, and that he'll need to treat 16 babies to benefit one (numbers needed to treat are discussed in Chapter 2), but there's always the more serious case to think of. Junior goes home on the first of many courses of antibiotics.

A recent study has indicated that mothers taking supplements of lactobacilli in pregnancy reduce the chance of their babies developing eczema and asthma.[51] Two things are thought to be at work. First, the good bacteria help to process the allergens in the mother's diet. Second, even more intriguingly, the lactobacilli may stimulate the production of anti-inflammatory substances such as transforming growth factor beta-2, thus 'calming' the developing immune system in the foetus. But why did the mothers 'need' these supplements in the first place? What are the consequences of dosing Junior with antibiotics at the first non-life-threatening infection he encounters?

Let's start with Jean. It is probable that in the past she has had an antibiotic. It is now thought that it can take months, or even years, to reconstitute normal gut flora after just one course of a common antibiotic. But even if she has diligently avoided the unnecessary use of antibiotics, she has lots of other opportunities for harming the gut flora. She may use a mouthwash. This is bactericidal; it says so on the label. Does the label also tell her the effect on the gut bacteria? She may like eating sweets. That will alter the flora in both her mouth and her gut, favouring the development of unhelpful yeasts. She may be on the contraceptive pill because her doctor feels she should give herself time to recover from the forceps or caesarean birth or mastitis before undertaking another pregnancy. The pill will drain a lot of her vitamin and mineral reserves,[52] contribute to her sugar cravings, and increase her risk of thrush.

What about Junior? The antibiotic he is on for his red ear is profoundly affecting the development of the colonies of friendly bacteria in his gut. Germs, normal everyday germs, are also under fire from the antibiotic. There's no point in attacking those; not enough of them are left. His immune system, in the form of the gut-associated lymphoid tissue, is casting around, looking for other antigens on which to hone its skills. What about food particles? Junior has just started on solids. How about those? Oral tolerance is not yet fully developed—there's still room for mischief.

The hygiene theory, discussed above, suggests that germs can be good for us. In laboratory experiments, the intestines of germ-free mice can display swelling and inflammation resembling that seen in inflammatory bowel disease. And we have seen how intestinal worms may be good too. When Junior comes home from kindergarten with his first dose of worms, he will be treated with worm poison (an antihelminthic). But humans survived for millennia without worm poisons, as did animals. Livestock in poor condition or kept in confined spaces can suffer from an intolerable burden of worms, but the rest seem to do just fine.[53]

If this sounds like pushing the natural approach too far, we might reflect on the individuals mentioned above, whose refractory Crohn's disease responded to roundworms. Perhaps bugs, parasites and their hosts have come to arrangements that we are barely able to conceive of.

John

What about Jean's husband, John—does he fare any better? Well, John has a sweet tooth, too. He's a junior solicitor in a big law firm and often misses lunch. He's found he can get by if he has a snack bar and some sweet black coffee from time to time during the day. He means to bring some fruit from home but often forgets. Still, the snacks must be okay because they're called 'muesli health bars'.

John rarely misses time from work, but he thinks he'd better see the dentist soon as a tooth is worrying him. Also his irritable bowel is playing up again. The doctor says there's not a lot you can do for irritable bowel, but he is going to order a test for helicobacter. This involves a radioactive drink, which the doctor has said is quite safe. If they find helicobacter, they will have to treat it with two different antibiotics and a proton pump inhibitor. The doctor says this will fix him: she hasn't yet explained that nearly 50 per cent of patients on this drastic treatment will have a recurrence within 12 months, or will go on to develop GORD. Better to deal with that one when they have to. As for discussing what that will do for Junior's chance at helicobacter exposure (see above, Hygiene Theory; also Chapter 8: Obesity), that is not even on the radar.

John doesn't have time for a big breakfast, but he does have toast — always wholemeal in deference to his bowel. His mother Vera keeps up a supply of her homemade marmalade, the good thick kind. No mould will grow on Vera's jam because it's full of sugar, which kills bugs (as food manufacturers know). After work John often goes for a beer, although he does this a bit less now that Junior has arrived. He only has one, but with the jam, the snack bars, the coffee and the beer, John has now consumed the sugar load in one day that might have served his hunter-gatherer forebears for a month.

What do his gut bugs think about this? They find it hard to combat the thrush which is building up, and sometimes they feel weakened by the effects of sugar on their own metabolism, but they are having some other problems too.

John likes to jog. When he comes back he is very thirsty and drinks a lot of water. What's more, his doctor has said that water will stop him from getting constipated and help with his irritable bowel. Jean would like to get a water filter, but John's father Stan, a council engineer, says there's nothing wrong with the town's water supply. Without chlorine, he says, we'd all be dead from cholera. After his run, John is sweaty and he likes to have a long hot shower. Under the shower John inhales and swallows the chlorine equivalent of drinking a couple of litres of unfiltered water.

Chlorine is toxic: why is it in our drinking water? It's only there in low doses, but those doses are enough to kill such pathogens as typhoid, cholera, giardia, cryptosporidia and *E. coli*. Chlorine is an indiscriminate killer; acidophilus and bifidus are fair game to any chlorine that enters the gut. Moreover, when chlorine reacts with organic matter at the treatment plant it creates a whole class of trihalomethanes and brominated by-products. These have been associated with a significant increase in the risk of bladder, bowel and lung cancer.[54] Are the extra cancers the direct result of the toxic effect of these substances, or an indirect effect on the bowel flora? As yet we don't know. In the meantime, John might do well to install the filter, despite what Stan thinks.

Preservatives

What other insults do we inflict on our gut flora? John's parents Vera and Stan are not doing too badly. They've always grown their own veggies and Vera likes to cook—hence the marmalade. But John and Jean are busy people, so they buy packaged and preserved foods, soft drinks, alcohol, sausages, hamburgers, snack foods, crisps, canned vegetables and fruits, dried fruit, instant soup, mashed potato. It's quite a list when you think of it. All these items tend to have one thing in common: sulphur-based preservatives. Sulphur dioxide, sulphites, bisulphites and metabisulphite can all be identified in lists of ingredients under the 'E' code as E220–E227.

Ever since she learned that Junior was on the way, Jean started to read labels. She has tried to avoid processed foods. But what about the salad bars and ready-to-go food sections of the supermarket? She has sometimes wondered why the greens in the prepared salads never seem to develop brown edges. When she makes a salad at home the leftovers don't look too good by the time of the next meal—but then, she does not add generous servings of metabisulphite to the salad dressing. And at the fish market, the fish always seem so fresh, the green prawns so green. Jean does not know about the man who had anaphylaxis after eating prawns and later at an allergy clinic showed no reaction to prawns but a severe reaction to metabisulphite.

How can we know what is in what? In Australia, packaged foods are subject to obligatory labelling laws. Open food bars are not.

Food that we prepare ourselves is somewhat safer (so long as we soak the fish). Appearance can help. A dried apricot or peach should be nearly black; if it's bright orange, it's full of sulphur. A strong smell of hydrogen sulphide (rotten egg gas) on the breath, especially after burping, is a sign of sulphur ingestion. If wine smells of sulphur when it warms up, then it's full of the stuff. If your asthma doesn't seem to respond to any medication, maybe you should check your sulphur intake.

There are two issues here. One is the health of the gut: collectively, GORD, inflammatory bowel disease, irritable bowel syndrome, peptic ulcers and gut cancers account for a large proportion of Western health problems. The other issue is that the gut provides a major chunk of our immune system.

Sulphate-reducing bacteria

In 1998 *New Scientist* reported that research from both the United States and Britain indicated that a high-sulphur diet has a remarkable impact on the composition of the gut flora.[55] Normally the gases produced by gut flora contain hydrogen, nitrogen, carbon dioxide and methane. The methane-producing bacteria, known as methanogens, represent the 'normal' or healthy state. (Excess methane production has environmental implications, discussed shortly.) Breath tests, however, were indicating that only about half of all North Americans and Northern Europeans appeared to be carrying methanogens in their gut.

At the same time, bacteria which feed on hydrogen and sulphur (known as sulphate-reducing bacteria) were increasingly identifiable. What these enterprising researchers then did was to look at the faeces of healthy people and compared them with the faeces of people suffering from ulcerative colitis. Among the colitis sufferers, 96 per cent hosted sulphate reducers; among the healthy people, only 50 per cent did. Cause and effect? People who host methanogens could be induced to host sulphate-reducing bacteria simply by being fed a high-sulphate diet.

Sulphate-reducing bacteria were first reported in the human gut in the late 1970s. They are named because of their ability to convert, or 'reduce', sulphate in the diet to sulphite, with hydrogen sulphide as the by-product. Not only known for its unpleasant smell, this gas rapidly converts to sulphuric acid in water. In mud flats, sulphate-reducing bacteria responsible for the characteristic smell produce sulphuric acid in a concentration sufficient to corrode metal pipes.

The effects of having metal-eroding sulphuric acid in our gut are worrying enough, but there are still more concerns. One of the sulphate-reducing bacteria is an organism that produces *beta-glucuronidase*. Excess numbers of beta glucuronidase bacteria are associated with an increased risk of hormone-dependent cancers. It works like this: when the liver wants to dispose of excess hormones such as oestrogen, it conjugates them to form glucuronide and sulphate compounds. These conjugates act as a glob of glue stuck to the oestrogen, which is then excreted in the bile. The hormone is prevented from being reabsorbed further down the gut by this glue glob. Unfortunately, the bad bacteria like nothing more than glue-globs for their lunch. They produce the beta-glucuronidase enzyme, which dissolves the bond between the glue and the hormone, and they settle in for a tasty meal. The hormone can then be reabsorbed from the intestine.

We should remember that the gut is no different to any other ecosystem. Much work remains to be done in the area of intestinal florae. It is encouraging to see that in Europe 64 research groups have combined to form the EU Human Gut Flora Project.

Genetically modified (GM) bacteria

The bacteria responsible for initiating tooth decay are called *Streptococcus mutans*. They secrete a sticky molecule known as glucan, which attaches to the teeth and provides a template on which these and other bacteria can grow. This reef of bacteria is known as plaque, and from it the bacteria convert sugar into the acid which is responsible for decay.

Sugar has been implicated in many other conditions — leaky gut, Crohn's disease and Type 2 diabetes, to mention just a few — so it might seem logical to reduce our consumption.

Certain foods have been demonstrated to have antibacterial activity against *Strep. mutans* (Chapter 7). One group of researchers, focusing on the symptom rather than the problem, are embarking on a program to genetically alter these bacteria so that they can no longer attach to the teeth.[56] (See also Chapter 7: Dental Health.) Apparently they seriously think that this is a helpful approach. But either *Strep. mutans* are a normal mouth commensal (bacteria which *belong* are usually called commensals) with a purpose, or they are not. If overgrowth is yet another manifestation of gut dysbiosis we should tackle the cause (Chapter 3). All the usual arguments against genetic engineering apply, but this research is going a step further.

These modified bacteria are designed to colonise mouths, and the mouths of babies at that. In short, just as we are beginning to learn how much we *don't* know about gut flora, we are proposing to modify them. Yet we know that transgenic crops out in the paddocks have jumped their lines of 'control'.[57] In fact, one American agricultural scientist who was asked about GM control said it all: 'I'm not an expert on confinement. Hardly anyone is.'[58]

Marker genes from GM foods were found in the colonic bacteria of human volunteers the first time they were looked for. These marker genes (for antibiotic resistance, as it happens) were isolated from the colostomy bags of those who had had bowel surgery. These transgenes had never been found in the faeces of people with intact bowels, leading to the assumption that transgenes do not survive the digestive process. Michael Antonio of King's College Medical School in London said: 'To my knowledge, they have demonstrated that you can get GM plant DNA in the gut bacteria. Everyone used to deny that this was possible.'[59]

The devastating 14th-century epidemic known as the Black Death is believed to have been caused by the organism *Yersinia pestis*. Researchers in the United States and Sweden have now confirmed that a single gene pilfered from another species transformed *Y. pestis*, a bacterium that caused a mild stomach upset, into one of the most feared diseases of all time that killed about one-third of the population. The gene in question codes for an enzyme that enabled *Y. pestis* to survive inside the gut of the flea. Having previously been a water-borne organism, it could now rely on flea bites for its transmission. As so often happens when an organism finds itself in a new environment, it also gained new virulence — HIV is another example.[60]

This is not to say that a modified mouth organism is about to start the next epidemic of bubonic plague or HIV-AIDS. It merely sounds a note of caution to those who take lightly the risks of genetic manipulation.

Some enterprising researchers in Belgium and The Netherlands propose to trial the release of genetically modified bacteria into the gut armed with proteins to target specific genetic defects. Their aims are worthy: the diseases involved include inflammatory bowel disease, insulin-dependent diabetes and other immune disorders. But as one geneticist commented, 'There is an awful lot that goes on in our guts that we're still totally in the dark about ... The prospect of genes for powerful immune system modulators breaking loose and spreading out of control is frightening indeed.'[61]

Another example of attacking the symptom rather than the problem is a novel Queensland proposal to reduce the greenhouse gas methane. Methane is the principal waste gas emitted by sheep, cows and humans; in contrast, kangaroos put out a brew dominated by carbon dioxide. Both methane and carbon dioxide are greenhouse gases, but in this context methane is the greater problem. The researchers propose recolonising the intestines of the domestic ruminants with the kangaroo bacteria. 'This is highly feasible, because the actual digestive process is the same ... It's the microbes that have evolved differently in kangaroos.'[62]

Of course kangaroos have their own distinctive gut flora. But the gut is designed not only to deal with the diet that the particular species has been consuming over millennia but also to meet its specific immune needs. The digestive mechanisms may be similar, but the *immunology* of the gut is species-specific. Failure to comprehend this most basic of facts was, in part, the basis of the BSE disaster.

Mother Nature is highly conservative. Amber from the Dominican Republic has been found to contain termites which are *20 million years old*, yet the bacteria in the termite gut bear a close resemblance to that in the gut of the termites' closest modern relative. If the goal is to reduce methane emission by domestic animals, the addition of fish oil to their diet can reduce it by as much as 80 per cent, probably because of the additional omega-3 fatty acids. The excess methane produced by domestic animals is a probable consequence of the change in their diets when they were domesticated. It could be remedied by cultivating crops closer to their original wild food. This would be healthier for the animals, and healthier for us.

Appendix 3 contains some recommendations for gut health.

POSTSCRIPT 2008: WHERE ARE WE NOW?

'If you don't understand the immunity, it sounds a bit like magic herbs, but it's straight immunology.'
—*John Stanford*

Since this chapter was first written, the rise in autoimmune and allergic disorders in the Western world has shown no sign of abating. Indeed, it has risen. Diabetes (autoimmune) is one of the fastest-growing diseases of childhood.[63] The urgency to find a solution cannot be overstated. It is my belief that this will not be found in a pill. New research gives hope to a more intelligent approach than the previous one. It involves bacteria and parasites in the gut, and infections in the body generally. It challenges our liberal use of antibiotics and anti-helminthics. In addition, the issue of epigenetics is changing much of our thinking, and will be discussed in Chapter 8.

The Modified Hygiene Theory

In the earlier part of this chapter, we saw that Th1 and Th2 have a braking effect on one another. But how do we account for the fact that both allergic *and* autoimmune diseases are increasing—and can be seen sometimes in the same person? Or that parasitic worms skew the immune reaction in the direction of Th2, but seem to also *protect against* a Th2 disorder?

A rethink has arisen as a result of work originating in the mid-1990s with Sakaguchi and his team at Kyoto University in Japan. Since then, there has been much research on molecules known as toll-like receptors (TLRs). The result is the 'modified hygiene theory'.

Distributed throughout our lungs, gut and in other tissues of our body, cells known as dendritic cells play a key role in the first-line defence system previously discussed. Receptors on these cells, the TLRs, act as go-betweens for 'foreign' matter and the lymphocytes in the lymph nodes. The conversation that takes place may determine whether the lymph node responds by producing Th1, Th2 or *regulatory* T cells that can switch off *both* Th1 and Th2.

The 'foreign matter' may include viruses, microbes, endotoxins, yeasts, parasites, worms and worm eggs. These things were once in the water that we drank from streams, on the animals we handled and in our day-to-day contact with the world in general.[64]

The implications of this research are profound.

Implications for cancer

To begin with, it is not just allergy and autoimmune disease we are discussing.

At a conference in London, UK, in April 2008, Californian researcher Patricia Buffler told the delegates that 14 studies involving 20,000 children indicated that those who attended day-care groups, experiencing a range of infections, were 30 per cent less likely to develop lymphoblastic leukaemia.[65]

It would seem that such kids also have a reduced risk in young adulthood of developing Hodgkin's lymphoma. Having several older siblings was also a protective factor.

Jessica Marshall the author of a *New Scientist* article ('Filthy Healthy', 12 January 2008) that tackles the cancer/germs debate, observes that the endotoxins on the cotton dust of textile workers seems to protect them from lung, breast, liver, stomach and pancreatic cancer. She notes that John and Cynthia Stanford at University College, London have been treating cancer patients with injections of a heat-killed Mycobacterium vaccine, cousin to the germ that causes tuberculosis. Fuelling the 'germs fight cancer' debate, she further observes that previous vaccination with either BCG or smallpox vaccine reduced the risk of developing melanoma by a factor of 2.5 to 4. The hypothesis is that one of the 'melanoma genes' is an old viral remnant, human endogenous retrovirus (HERV). The insertion of old viruses into the human genome was discussed in Chapter 3: Genetics. So, does infection with such diseases (or even the vaccine) fight off the retrovirus, taking out melanoma cells with it?

New applications

Research that explores how T cells react with the ecosystem fuels even more new thinking — and offers new surprises.

A study published in 2007 demonstrated that patients with MS who acquired intestinal parasitic infection experienced a beneficial modification of the progression of their disease.[66]

In Chapter 6: Inflammatory bowel disease, we saw that the use of round worms was beneficial in treating Crohn's disease. In that chapter, I asked if the rise in coeliac disease may be another manifestation of the hygiene theory. In 2008, we find a group of Australian researchers trialling hookworm infestation to modify the reaction to gluten in proven coeliacs.[67] The worm, Necator americanus, is a human parasite that does not usually cause illness. If this works, it will be highly significant. Until now, we have believed that once switched on, coeliac genes cannot be switched off again.

Depression
In Chapter 9: Mental Health, depression is discussed as the illness tipped by the World Health Organisation to become the second-leading cause of disease burden by 2020. One theory is that depression is an inflammatory disorder involving the release of cytokines. In Marshall's article, she observes that the people receiving mycobacterium vaccine treatment experienced improved cognitive function, vitality and pain tolerance. She also cites the work of Christopher Lowry from the University of Colorado, Boulder, who

found that serotonin levels were elevated in rats treated with this bacterium. Did these infections have a beneficial effect on our survival instincts?

Helicobacter and asthma

The stomach bacterium (described elsewhere in this book as 'much reviled' but, also, as 'possibly one of mankind's oldest friends') continues to attract attention. In the much-respected Archives of Internal Medicine (23 April 2007), a study of 7663 adults indicated that those infected with a virulent strain of Helicobacter pylori had a 40 per cent reduction in the likelihood of asthma before the age of 15, and protection against allergies that were due to pollens and moulds.[68]

Helicobacter and oesophageal cancer

Although gastric ulcers associated with Helicobacter pylori infection are known to lead to an increased risk of stomach cancer — infection with Helicobacter pylori has an inverse correlation with the prevalence of oesophageal cancer. This nasty disease is rapidly rising in the Western world.

Chronic Fatigue Syndrome (CFS)

Recognised as part of the immune system, gut bacteria are studied in the context of CFS. The presence of abnormal bacteria and the absence of normal bacteria are equally deleterious. Australian research in this area has been undertaken by the Collaborative Pain Research Unit at the University of Newcastle, by Henry Butt, Dunstan et al.

Autism and ASD (Autistic spectrum disorders)

This emotive field has spawned research beyond the scope of this book. In summary, the idea that toxic products arise from the gut when its bacteria are abnormal, enter the circulation and mess with a child's brain is entirely consistent with other theories of ASD discussed in Chapter 9.

The research

In Chapter 3: The gut's contribution to immunity, we saw that 95 per cent of gut bacteria are anaerobes. As such, the bacteria in question do not need oxygen to survive, and are often killed by it.

With routine faecal analysis, most of the anaerobes are dead on arrival at the lab. The Australian researcher Dr Henry Butt deals with this by a special collection method. In the US, Dr Alexander Bralley looks at the DNA of the dead bacteria. Such developments make specific therapy possible. Still other doctors sterilise the bowel, and recolonise it with the faeces and bacteria from healthy donors.

Doctor's dilemma
It is mid 2008 and I have just received data from the Australian government's Department of Health and Ageing advising me of a new vaccine, free to all children born after 1 May 2007.

Rotavirus, I am informed, is the most common cause of severe gastroenteritis in infants and young children. In Australia, it occasions 10,000 hospitalisations a year, while a further 137, 000 children visit an emergency department or a GP. On average, there is one death.

One death? The doctor in me laments that death. The scientist in me questions the virulence of the virus. In view of the foregoing, the immunologist in me asks if this new vaccine will deprive those vaccinated of the conversation between viruses and TLRs. And finally, the cynic in me asks how many of the children who become ill with rotavirus do so because of unnecessary antibiotics prescribed for minor illness in the past?

There is no clear answer here. In Chapter 2: Vaccination, I correctly acknowledged that vaccines save lives. But medico-legally, haunting questions remain. Marshall, in the article quoted above, acknowledged the ethical dilemma in trialling germs for combating cancer, since all trials require that 'best practice' options also be used. In the case of cancer, chemotherapy and radiotherapy are 'best practice'. But these treatments suppress the immune system, and may well stop the immune approach from working. Do I, as a trained medical doctor, advise against the rotavirus vaccine, because of the theoretical, but very persuasive, possibility of increased risk of autoimmune and allergic diseases, depression, or cancer? How many survivable illnesses must doctors vaccinate against as 'best practice'? How are we monitoring the outcomes as they become challenged by the new thinking that we have just explored?

Chapter Seven
SOME FIXED-NAME DISEASES

WHEN WE IDENTIFY A DISEASE by a name such as 'asthma' or 'hypertension', we risk the problem of semantic determinism. That is to say, the naming process itself presumes a cause. If we doctors were to apply the Burkitt approach instead, and tell patients to increase their stool size, what would happen? The addition of fibre, fruit and vegetables to the diet is the only effective way to increase stool size, and many diseases respond to such an intervention.

Once a fixed name has been given to a disease we tend to feel the name somehow *explains* the condition. Even today, there is no satisfactory explanation for the phenomenon of gravity, yet most of us are happy to accept that it is the reason we don't float off into space. The name is enough.

Most illnesses were named before we had any true understanding of causality. That the illness was a separate entity became embedded into the consciousness of lay people and doctors alike. Each disease was assumed to have a distinct cause, and consequently a specific treatment. Overlap between illnesses was a matter of curiosity. If such conditions co-existed frequently, then they became a 'syndrome'.

'Syndrome X' is a good example of this. This term is shorthand for saying 'junk food makes us sick all over'. Instead of this, we have a new disease. And to go with it, a whole new class of drugs.

For instance, I might send my patient Mary (Chapters 1, 4) to a psychiatrist for her depression, an asthma specialist for her asthma, and a gynaecologist for her heavy, painful periods. But what if these specialties no longer existed? If we were to reshuffle the pack of cards which constitutes the various medical disciplines, would we in the 21st century come up with the same nomenclature? Maybe we would have an essential-fatty-acid specialist who had been trained in the psychiatric, asthma and gynaecology wards to look at the manifestations of EFA deficiency. But this specialist would also need to know about magnesium, selenium and a whole host of other operatives, because all of these might be contributing to Mary's medical problems. Somehow the various disciplines would have to be approached as if in a grid. A deficiency in EFAs may contribute to each of 10 or 15 medical problems, but it will not be the sole cause of any of them.

Mary's treatment remains compartmentalised. As we tack through the illnesses which follow, let us observe how many different specialists Mary and her family might end up visiting just for the lack of a systematic approach.

ACNE

In Chapter 5 we met Mike. Acne was the problem that brought him into the doctor's surgery, but there were other issues. If we assume that acne was his main concern, then a script for antibiotics is a reasonable tactic. Mike will find his skin clears quickly, and he will be able to go to the school social next week. He will be out of the doctor's surgery after a brief consultation, which will suit him fine. (Remember he was reluctant to come in the first place.) And the doctor will be able to get on with the morning's list without the added complication of a challenging teenager.

In prescribing an antibiotic, we have accepted the notion of one problem, one treatment. But when we were first introduced to Mike, it was to look at ways in which something like an EFA deficiency could contribute to the other things troubling him — his parents were worried about depression, he has mild asthma, and he has problems in concentrating. Do we schedule a series of appointments to work through these one by one, or do we take a systematic approach?

To stress an important concept: just as one factor such as an EFA deficiency can cause multiple problems, any one problem can be caused by multiple different factors. The risk is that the network of seemingly unrelated symptoms will be treated by a network of genuinely unrelated solutions.

The conclusion which might be drawn from this is that problems like asthma, depression and acne are manifestations of the same deranged biochemical pathways. That they share in common deficiencies of nutrients such as EFAs, zinc and magnesium. That they cannot therefore be dealt with as separate entities, and should be seen as manifestations of system errors. If we look at *all* of the nutrients which might be used to help Mike's acne, the astute reader may detect the ways in which his other problems might benefit.

The physiology of skin

Many factors are involved in the maintenance of healthy skin. Skin is metabolically active, serving not only as a barrier to infections, chemicals and so on, but also as an organ for the excretion of waste products.

Skin, especially on the face and back, needs lubrication as protection against exposure to the elements. The discomfort associated with dry skin is well known. Tiny glands at the base of the hair follicles (sebaceous glands) produce a mixture of wax and oil to provide this protection, by secreting a fine film of these substances (sebum) onto the skin surface. If these oil glands become blocked by viscous sebum, then acne, or the inflammatory and disfiguring condition known as 'cystic acne', will follow.

Once the gland is blocked, a bacterium (called *Corynbacterium acnes*) flourishes. This bacterium produces enzymes which break down the sebum, but also release inflammatory cytokines. Steroid creams reduce the inflammatory process. Antibiotics attack the bacteria, and have immunosuppressive and anti-inflammatory functions. Unfortunately, one of the known side effects of steroids is the actual *production* of acne. The antibiotic effect will be discussed presently.

As we can see what goes on in our skin, it is probably no accident that it has become one of Mother Nature's prominent warning systems. Skin is one of the key responders to inflammatory mediators and cytokines. A rash is often the only notification we have, for example, of a food or drug allergy.

Food allergies, EFAs and sugar

Inflammation is a significant component of acne, and acne-like eruptions can occur as a result of ingesting allergenic foods. Chocolate and dairy products are both common culprits. The severe eruptions seen after the consumption of chocolate are well known to most sufferers. Migraine and acne seem to surge around Easter as chocolate becomes a staple. The contribution of milk and other food allergens is often less obvious because they are a part of so many daily diets.

The presence of EFAs in the diet exerts two important protective effects against the development of acne. First, they are a source of the anti-inflammatory prostaglandins (Chart 5.3). Second, by acting as dietary 'anti-freeze', they keep sebum in a fluid state. Fluid sebum does not clog up the sebaceous gland.

The consumption of sugary foods, over and above any allergenic effect, can precede an outbreak of acne. It has been proposed that the skin of people prone to acne actually exhibits insulin insensitivity (Chapter 8). Adults developing Type 2 diabetes may develop acne. Treatment with insulin can improve the acne, but this misses the point entirely. If acne is a marker for insulin resistance, it is also a warning for the development of this type of diabetes. A healthier diet and an increase in exercise are required.

Hormones

Cystic acne is often blamed on hormones. There is no doubt that acne is worse at times of hormonal change, notably adolescence. But a normal transition period such as puberty is not a disease and does not cause disfigurement. It is instructive to study some early 19th-century photographs of Australian Aboriginals who were still living a tribal existence. Their stage of pubertal development is in no doubt, as clothing is minimal. None of these photos indicate even the slightest evidence of acne. Protected by a diet rich in essential minerals and fatty acids, the adolescent skin is perfect. But for today's urban Aboriginals, the problem is as great as it is for their European equivalents.

Hormone 'imbalance' can occur in both sexes when the liver produces insufficient quantities of the protein sex-hormone-binding globulin (SHBG; see below, Reproductive Health).

Minerals and vitamins

Zinc is one of the best-known natural treatments for acne. It should not be given in isolation, because zinc by itself may reduce the uptake of selenium. Selenium also has been shown to benefit acne, presumably by means of its anti-inflammatory actions.

Zinc is particularly important for adolescent boys because the advent of puberty leads to an increased demand on zinc reserves. The metabolism of testosterone requires zinc. When there is a zinc deficiency, the 'nasty', or highly active, form of testosterone, dihydrotestosterone (DHT), is preferentially formed.

Chromium supplementation has also been found useful, perhaps because chromium depletion reduces insulin sensitivity.

One of the conventional treatments for severe acne is isoretinoin, a derivative of Vitamin A. But large doses of Vitamin A work just as well, as has been known for some decades.[1] Yet the synthetic retinoic acid has been favoured over the safer, natural product. We might ask how much Vitamin A is consumed by the average Western adolescent. If potato is the main vegetable consumed, and apples the main fruit, the range narrows. Sardines were a convenient source of both EFAs and Vitamin A.

Finally, Vitamins C and E, in various trials, have been shown effective in the treatment of acne.

Gut bacteria

Abnormal gut bacteria often flourish in the presence of a sugary diet. Apart from the contribution of sugar itself to acne, products of abnormal bacterial fermentation enhance the inflammatory process. Recycled hormones from the activity of undesirable bacteria, such as those producing beta glucuronidase, contribute to the hormonal imbalance already discussed.

Which brings us to the currently popular antibiotic treatment of acne. There is no doubt that this treatment works. But at what cost? We know that such treatment is injurious to the normal flora of the gut. In a healthy gut well-chewed and well-digested food is far less likely to induce an inflammatory or allergic response. With every antibiotic we swallow, we increase the risk not only of all the disorders associated with disturbed gut flora, but also of the very response we are trying to avoid — excess inflammation. Recent studies have indicated that antibiotic use is associated with increased asthma risk, and the author of one study has directly attributed responsibility to the alteration of gut flora.[2] Will Mike thank us for that?

The risk is of the self-fulfilling promise: take the medication and you'll need the medication. The quick fix becomes the self-perpetuating 'drug deficiency disorder'.

THE ARTHRITIS FAMILY: SICK JOINTS

The arthritic family of diseases fits into a broader group of disorders known as musculoskeletal disorders. This term embraces all the maladies that can afflict the bones, the joints between bones, the tendons that connect muscles to bones, and the ligaments that connect bone to bone. It can also include the nerves that supply those structures, and even the skin overlying the joint.

The word arthritis, strictly speaking, means 'inflammation of the joint'. Any aspect of the joint can be involved: the synovium (the 'lining' of the joint), the synovial fluid, the articular cartilage, the meniscus or its capsule, the adjacent bone.

Despite its name, not all forms of arthritis involve inflammation. The common name was used before the underlying pathology was understood. As medical science progressed, arthritis became divided into two groups, inflammatory and non-inflammatory. However, even this separation is seen to be somewhat artificial. Osteoarthritis, long thought to have no inflammatory component, not only responds to anti-inflammatory medication but is now thought to have a greater or lesser degree of inflammation most of the time.

Better terms for arthritis therefore are:

- arthropathy, meaning sick joint (collectively, the arthropathies)
- the arthritides.

There are many conditions in the arthritis family. They include rheumatoid arthritis, osteoarthritis, reactive arthritis, tuberculous arthritis, pyogenic arthritis, gonococcal arthritis, psoriatic arthritis, gouty arthritis. There are other forms associated with specific conditions, most notably those associated with inflammatory bowel disorders.

The classification of arthropathies is confusing. They can be classified on the basis of the underlying cause, or they can be classified by age. Thus arthritis in children is often called *juvenile arthritis*, because it is an uncommon disorder in children. At the other end of the age spectrum, we are not surprised to see arthropathies, and we often then refer to the arthritis as 'degenerative'.

Arthritis can also be classified according to the location, the number and the distribution of the joints involved. Certain medical conditions seem to target particular joints. Ankylosing spondylitis favours the sacroiliac joints and the remainder of the spine. It is often referred to as a 'spondylo-arthropathy'. The terms 'monoarthropathy' and 'polyarthropathy' describe the location of the arthritis. Monoarthropathies can be seen in conditions such as gout, and curiously, can be a marker for coeliac disease. Only one or two joints are afflicted. Monoarthropathies can also be seen at sites of trauma, often years after the original injury. Polyarthritis refers to the arthropathies which are usually not confined to one or two joints. Rheumatoid arthritis is a classic example of a polyarthropathy and is often symmetrical.

Sometimes tiny joints such as the little ossicles in the inner ear can be affected, thus causing hearing impairment. Other forms, such as osteoarthritis, target large joints, such as knees and hips, and are less likely to be symmetrical.

Sometimes arthritis is acute and self-limiting. Sometimes urgent medical intervention makes the difference between cure, and permanent and severe damage to the joint. This is particularly true in the case of infective arthritis. Surgical drainage and the use of appropriate antibiotics can prevent destruction of the joint, or the complete loss of joint function. 'Slipped epiphyses' occur in young people when the growing end of the bone is physically detached. Surgical intervention here prevents long-term problems of growth and arthritis.

It is not hard to understand all the possibilities that go through the mind of a doctor when a patient complains of 'arthritis'. Let us say that I have two arthritis patients this morning. Mrs Green has not long been through menopause, and ever since then she has been gaining weight. She feels that her left knee, and the joints at the base of her thumbs, are growing stiff. She is almost certainly going to have osteoarthritis. David is more of a worry. He is in his late 30s and has had a couple of severe attacks of confirmed rheumatoid arthritis. He takes anti-inflammatory medication, and mostly his disease is under control. Today he has come in with an acutely swollen, sore right knee.

Rheumatoid arthritis and osteoarthritis are two of the most common arthropathies in our society. I will see more patients with these problems before the day is over. There are protocols for managing both conditions. In most cases, the aim of treatment is to arrest the underlying problem, known as 'disease modulation', and to supply pain relief, or both.

The drug approach

In the past, available treatments centred mostly on aspirin-like medications and paracetamol. Some conditions such as gout were treated with a variety of disease-specific medications. In the 1950s, steroids were added to this range.

A few decades ago, Mrs Green was most likely to be prescribed paracetamol, and David would be prescribed an anti-inflammatory. His regime might start with an aspirin-like medication, steroids when things were bad, and possibly paracetamol to attenuate pain relief. Nowadays, there is a whole range of drugs to choose from. In the December 2004 edition of *MIMS* (the catalogue of available drugs which sits on every doctor's desk in Australia), there were no less than 14 pages of entries for drugs normally used for the arthritis family (and this excludes entries for narcotic analgesics, steroids, and the drugs specific to gout). It is true that most of these medications are variants on aspirin or paracetamol, still the mainstay of arthritis treatment. COX-2 inhibitors will make up most of the remainder.

Disease modulation

Steroids and the aspirin family reduce inflammation, and pain relief is a welcome side effect of this. These anti-inflammatories are divided into those which are steroid-based, 'steroidals', and those which are not. The latter are known therefore as 'non-steroidal anti-inflammatories' or NSAIDs. Early in the history of the use of steroids for this and other medical conditions, it became apparent that they had serious side effects. Thus, NSAIDs were used as first-line treatment, with steroids added for acute flares. As time passed, some other drugs were introduced for the more severe forms of the inflammatory arthropathies. These drugs acted directly on the immune system to make it less trigger-happy. Some of these have been useful agents, but also have side effects.

A new class of drug, based on the aspirin family, was introduced in the late 1990s. In many ways these drugs seemed to be a great improvement on the parent drug. These new medications, which belong to a class known as COX-2 inhibitors (Chapter 2), will be discussed shortly.

Pain relief

Traditionally, paracetamol was believed to have little effect on inflammation. It provides pain relief by altering the cerebral interpretation of pain signals. Other drugs have a similar function, but some of these are limited by their addictive potential. Paracetamol is not addictive, but it has serious side effects, including fatal liver toxicity in over-dosage. About 10 per cent of people are thought to lack an enzyme which is necessary to convert paracetamol into its active form. As a result, they experience little, if any, benefit from this drug.

Treating symptoms

There are several disturbing features about treating a condition by providing relief of the symptoms without dealing with the cause. Neither anti-inflammatories nor pain relievers can be said to target underlying pathology.

Pain and/or inflammation remain the key problems in arthritis. It is true that joint inflammation, unchecked, may lead to joint destruction, and must therefore be treated. The question remains: why has this patient succumbed to an inflammatory process? Although inflammation becomes a problem in its own right, it is, nonetheless, a symptom. As an immunological process, inflammation has always been one of our short-term defence mechanisms. If it persisted, it was because the threat to the organism persisted.

Throughout this book, the role of inflammation in the disease process is discussed. This is because nearly all health problems in the Western world are problems of oxidative stress and/or inflammation. So if we take the medication-based approach to arthritis, we are again falling into the trap of treating the symptom as though it were the disease.

Sometimes the anti-inflammatories used to reduce the joint inflammation may have other beneficial effects. For instance, we believe that small doses of aspirin may reduce the risk of bowel cancer. But often, the reverse is true. Steroids can increase the risk of depression and of cardiovascular disease. Aspirin can cause gastrointestinal bleeding, stroke, asthma.

By looking at the fixed name 'arthritis', we risk neglecting the actual disease process. Few people on arthritis medication are being treated for arthritis alone. Put in epidemiological terms, co-morbidity in arthritis is high. We might argue that because arthritis is a disease most commonly found in the older age group, we would expect other problems on the basis of probability alone. But if these 'other problems' are the result of chronic inflammation, then an integrated approach to the problem is warranted.

Pain is also nature's warning signal. Pain relief can actually allow the patient to use the joint and perpetuate the injury.

Side effects

Most medications have side effects, and arthritis drugs are no exception. About 10 per cent of people are sensitive to aspirin. In these people, the use of aspirin and NSAIDs can cause an immunological 'cascade' that can lead to asthma, haematological disorders, gastric ulcers and even death.

Chart 5.3 highlights other problems with the anti-inflammatories. Aspirin and steroids non-selectively interrupt all three prostaglandins pathways. Although these medications may assist in reducing inflammation, and therefore pain, they are also interrupting other pathways. The implication of this is twofold.

Remember that inflammation is not always a foe. Its primary purpose is to *protect* us. It is one of the means by which we fight germs. Second, the interruption of the PG-1 and PG-3 pathways reduces the natural anti-inflammatory defence. For example, there's a problem with eating fish to fuel the PG-3 pathway if you take aspirin at the same time (see Chapter 5).

In short, aspirin and the NSAIDs reduce the formation of inflammatory PG-2—that is *why* they are used. But at the same time, they also reduce the conversion of DGLA to PG-l, and the conversion of eicosapentaenoic acid into PG-3. The arthritic pain is reduced by aspirin, but the loss of the protective benefits of the PG-1 and PG-3 pathways is the price we pay.

Another side effect is this. Both steroids and aspirin increase gut permeability (leaky gut), even to the point of bleeding. The relevance of this side effect should become clear presently.

The 'breakthrough' drugs

The COX-2 inhibitors were introduced in Chapter 2 as an example of dubious safety in clinical trials. They were originally marketed for their selective interruption of the conversion of arachidonic acid by the enzyme cyclo-oxygenase-2 into PG-2 (Chart 5.3). They are not tolerated by aspirin-sensitive people. The main advantage was that they did not act on the PG-1 and PG-3 pathways.

But serious side effects cause us to question this. We saw that heart failure was a risk for elderly people on these drugs. The combination of COX-2s with antihypertensives was even more dangerous.[3] Yet in a survey of 3500 people from 400 general practices, between 5 and 8 per cent of all people on COX-2 inhibitors were also taking an ACE inhibitor *and* a diuretic for hypertension. Up to one-third of all people on the COX-2s were taking at least one of these anti-hypertensives. Combining *either* medication with COX-2s is regarded as risky. Combining *both* was described as a triple whammy. Renal failure is the possible outcome.

The manufacturers advise against such combinations in the small print. Offsetting this, in huge print, these drugs are portrayed as the ideal medication for most arthritis sufferers. Advertisements for these drugs showed elderly people leaping into the air—but the angle of the feet to the legs makes it is clear that the photographs were taken with the feet firmly planted on the ground.

Arthritis is most common in the elderly, and there are few people in this age group of whose kidney function I could be confident. Or, to put it another way, I would be *extremely* confident that there would be some renal compromise in all but a few. Hypertension and poor renal function are common in later life.

Despite the hype about these drugs, they come with a long list of contra-indications, precautions, adverse reactions and interactions. I wrack my memory to think of just one of my elderly patients to whom I can safely say these warnings might not apply. The very pathways which lead to the arthritis are the pathways leading to the asthma, the cardiovascular disease, the hypertension, and all the other conditions requiring steroids, anticoagulants and diuretics. All of these had been listed as risky problems when using drugs like Celebrex.

Another approach

Let us look at the arthropathies in general terms. Even rheumatoid arthritis and osteoarthritis, in many ways representative of the two extremes in arthritis, can usefully be discussed in generalities.

Rheumatoid arthritis is a classic inflammatory condition: heat, swelling, pain. Osteoarthritis, by contrast, has always been considered the result of wear and tear. But is the problem wear and tear, or is it the inability of the body to repair the damage?

If multiple conditions are co-morbid with arthritis, and these occur often enough to warrant special warnings, why aren't we looking for common underlying causes? After all, how many medical problems are there which are *not* due to wear and tear or chronic inflammation? The same building blocks which repair worn and torn bones and joints are also the materials with which we defend ourselves against all degenerative and inflammatory processes.

To put it another way, the inflammatory arthritis *is* the asthma, *is* the cardiovascular disease, *is* the depression. The particular way in which our biology reacts to the deprivations or toxic insults it faces is largely a matter of the weaker links in our genetic chain. Look at Chart 5.3 again. If the Western diet favours a predominance of PG-2 over PG-1 and PG-3, of course we will succumb to the conditions as listed.

Far from blaming our genes for our disease, we would do better to look at those deprivations and insults, and correct them. Indeed, we can probably thank the inherent robustness of our genes that we don't actually get the entire list of diseases possible as indicated by deficiencies of EFAs and other nutrients.

Some things to consider in rheumatoid arthritis

There is a strong genetic component in rheumatoid arthritis. This is also true of psoriatic arthritis and the arthritis which accompanies Crohn's and other inflammatory bowel disorders. However, we have seen that Crohn's was once relatively rare in Japan (Chapter 2). With the adoption of the Western diet the incidence of these disorders has grown out of all proportion. The gene pool has changed little in that time.

It has been proposed that foods including gluten-based cereals, dairy products, sugar and fructose can provoke immune-based inflammatory arthropathies. A patient who is hospitalised and fed only fluids through a drip often experiences complete remission in rheumatoid arthritis. This is strong supporting evidence that dietary influences can trigger the inflammatory response, and this highlights the reasons for avoiding drugs which increase gut permeability.

Other food groups have also been implicated as suspects. It has been observed that in the skeletal remains of peoples from cultures prior to the agricultural revolution, the classic rheumatoid deformity is not seen.[4]

The immunological role of 'good' or 'friendly' gut bacteria deserves full attention in these patients. In differentiating 'food as friend' and 'food as foe', these bugs are an unexplored resource in the management of rheumatoid arthritis. A reduction in both hydrochloric acid (Chapter 6) and hydrolytic enzymes has been observed in patients with active inflammatory arthropathies. Acid helps break down food particles into sizes which are less immunogenic. Is this why some people swear by apple cider vinegar for their arthritis?

There is an age-old adage about sitting down to eat. Our digestive processes (and acid production) are inhibited by stress. Does David rush his food in order to get to the office on time? Does this account for his flare-ups? They are always worse when he is under pressure. Such observations may seem either mundane or irrelevant. They are anything but. Inflammatory arthritis is one of the commonest correlates of inflammatory bowel disease. (We have to ask whether the anti-inflammatory drugs might help to perpetuate the arthritis, given that gut damage is one of their known side effects.)

Plant-derived hydrolytic enzymes can be found in the circulation and have been shown to break down immune proteins, believed to be directly responsible for joint inflammation.[5] These enzymes include bromelain and papain. A diet rich in fruit and vegetables abounds in such 'pharmaceuticals'. Vegetarian and vegan diets have both been shown to benefit inflammatory arthritis. The Western diet is notoriously low in fruit and vegetables. The more we cook these foods, the more we destroy those enzymes. As such, the rise in the inflammatory arthritides should hardly come as a surprise.

Bacteria, viruses, and even moulds and fungi have been associated with the development of inflammatory arthropathies. This highlights the fact that molecules other than food particles can act as antigens. People whose joints ache in damp weather may well be responding to a rise in mould levels. There have also been reports of spectacular cures of rheumatoid arthritis when antibiotics are prescribed. This is by no means universal because the factor which precipitates the immune event will vary from person to person, and there may be several factors involved.

Fish oil and its omega-3 EFAs is one of nature's most potent anti-inflammatories. 'Persuasive studies have now emerged which indicate that the activity of COX-2, which is associated with inflammatory reactions, can be suppressed by diets supplemented with fish oil.'[6] A diet rich in fish would be a better choice than Celebrex.

In his *Textbook of Nutritional Medicine*, Werbach cites many well-referenced studies indicating that the minerals copper, zinc, boron, selenium, molybdenum, iron, and Vitamins C, D, E, B5 and folic acid may all exert benefit in rheumatoid arthritis.[7] The mode of action relates to enzyme function. Both zinc and copper are essential to the superoxide dismutase (SOD) enzyme. Another form of this enzyme requires manganese. Glutathione peroxidase needs selenium. Some of these enzymes have been discussed in the context of quenching free radicals (Chapters 3 and 6) and the reduction in the formation of inflammatory prostaglandins and leukotrienes.

So the separation of arthritis from cancer, or any of the other degenerative disorders, might seem increasingly arbitrary. Indeed, this is one of my key themes.

Some things to consider in osteoarthritis
Osteoarthritis is often divided into two kinds:

- *Primary:* generalised and often affects multiple joints. This kind appears to have a strong genetic predisposition.
- *Secondary:* often seen at the site of old injury. Having 'osteoarthritis genes' certainly appears to increase the risk of this complication when there is a history of trauma or deformity.

Osteoarthritis is also associated with food allergies and sensitivity. Sensitivity to the nightshade family (*Solanaceae*) — potatoes, capsicum, peppers, eggplant and tobacco — has been highlighted.[8] The alkaloids in these vegetables are thought either to inhibit collagen repair or to provoke an inflammatory degradation of the joint. Gluten, dairy, soy and other foods have also been implicated.

'Leaky gut' is thought to have an impact on osteoarthritis like the effect seen in rheumatoid arthritis. In both experimental and clinical studies, the use of aspirin and NSAIDs inhibited cartilage synthesis and accelerated cartilage destruction.[9] These concerns have been reinforced by the findings that in young people Celebrex relieved pain but delayed healing (Chapter 2). Whether these effects are the result of the 'leaky gut' or an independent chemical process is unclear.

Oestradiol, the most potent of the female hormones, appears to accelerate osteoarthritis. It is not surprising than osteoarthritis is far more prevalent in women than men. The oestrogen-blocking drug Tamoxifen appears to slow cartilage degradation. Before we initiate a knee-jerk prescription for Tamoxifen, we should remember that nature has supplied many oestrogen buffers in the plant world. These are discussed in Chapters 6 and 10; they include the legumes, asparagus, fennel, celery, nuts, parsley and apples. It is not hard to recognise a few 'traditional' arthritis remedies in this list.

Although under challenge in 2008, glucosamine has been seen as a natural remedy success story. I suspect that it will be the dose and delivery method that will explain the discrepancies in studies of commercial preparations, but this remains to be seen. What we do know is that glucosamine is an extract from the cartilaginous material of animals and shellfish. What did our ancestors do before glucosamine was available in pill form? They chewed on the wings of the birds they caught; they ate shrimps, small insects, locusts, small fish — shells, bones and all. Grandma boiled the chicken carcase for soup, ate sardines with their little bones, and did not throw away the bones from the canned salmon.

The inflammatory aspect of osteoarthritis is responsive to EFAs in the same manner as any other inflammatory process.

Vitamin C has a critical role to play in the cross-linkage of molecules vital to the stability and repair of articular cartilage. Defining characteristics of scurvy include joint pains and effusions. The reduction of fruit and vegetables in the modern diet, and the high risk of Vitamin C deficiency in the diets of elderly people living alone, all contribute to cartilage degradation. As an anti-oxidant, Vitamin E is vital in stabilising the membranes lining cartilaginous surfaces. Vitamin A and all the B-group vitamins, especially B3, B5 and B6, have all been shown to have a role in the maintenance and repair of cartilage (Chapter 5).

Of the minerals, zinc, selenium, copper, boron, and molybdenum are all required in the maintenance of cartilage and bone. These roles are sometimes structural; sometimes the minerals act indirectly via their influence on hormonal pathways, and sometimes as anti-oxidants. German doctors have used boron in the treatment of osteoarthritis for over 30 years.

The lessons

To avoid the arthropathies we should avoid refined carbohydrates and excess animal fats, and eat nutrient-dense foods. A diet rich in fruits, berries, vegetables, nuts and fish is ideal. Elimination diets are worth a trial, especially eliminating the *Solanaceae* (nightshade family), dairy products and gluten.

ASTHMA

It is important to discuss asthma as a disease because of its prevalence, but we must avoid the trap of fixed-name disease. Asthma is an inflammatory disease, and so it appears under the discussion of inflammation and essential fatty acids (Chapters 5 and 6). It has links to autoimmune and genetic disorders, and it has associations with magnesium and selenium status. The emergence of gut bugs as important players in the asthma story shows that the disease cannot be seen simply as a disorder of the respiratory system. Thus, like most fixed-name conditions, asthma is best understood when seen in the context of the health of the entire organism.

Two or three generations ago in Australia one in 20 people would at some time in their lives be diagnosed with asthma. Typically, this diagnosis was made in early childhood, and at least one parent had a similar history. Many asthmatic children were expected to, and often did, grow out of the condition as they approached their teens. Many of these children did not go to a doctor with their condition at all. Mild wheezing was often seen as a temporary event that followed infantile eczema, a related condition. Severe asthma attacks were treated with an injection of adrenalin by the family doctor.

About 30 or 40 years ago, all this began to change. Drugs which had actions similar to adrenalin were put into pills, syrups and inhalers. Small doses of sedatives or antihistamines were sometimes mixed in with these. Over time, steroids were seen as a valuable adjunct in the more severe cases.

The age profile also began to change. People who developed asthma in young adulthood were often experiencing a return of the asthma that they had grown out of, and these cases seemed to be increasing in number. More cases of adult-onset asthma began to appear. This term refers to those people who have their first-ever asthma attack in adulthood. Thirty years ago adult-onset asthma was regarded as unusual, and potentially very serious.

By 2006, the disease pattern had changed beyond all recognition. At some stage of their life, one in four to five of all Australians can expect to have an asthma diagnosis and to be prescribed asthma medication. Doctors are no longer surprised when asthma turns up for the first time in a family lacking an asthma history.

Adults having an attack for the first time in their fifties draw little comment. Young people who have their first attack as they move out of home or go to university are far from unusual. While patients and their families may be surprised that the illness appears to have come from nowhere, the doctor no longer expects family history to help explain or confirm the diagnosis. What has happened in the last 30 years for such drastic changes to occur?

A few facts are established. Allergists and respiratory physicians agree that this change in numbers is not just a matter of better diagnosis, nor of greater access to medical care. Also agreed is that these trends are largely confined to the Western world. As developing nations adopt Western customs, the asthma statistics rise.

Another point of consensus is that asthma has a complex aetiology. Few centres nowadays try to find 'the cause' of asthma, as if one villain could be identified. Just a few years ago, it was not uncommon to blame the asthma epidemic on one 'bad guy', which often became the subject of the research endeavours of a particular university. Thus, pollens after rain, dust mites trapped in hermetically sealed homes, cockroaches, all had their moment of glory as *the* cause of asthma. Nowadays it is much more common to acknowledge that multiple factors contribute, probably because the public is tired of conflicting advice.

The experts had told us that everything depended on hygiene — dust mite hygiene, to be precise. Parents spent half of their waking hours vacuuming and the other half washing and sunning the sheets. If there was no improvement in Junior's asthma, the weekends might be spent looking at houses that were further from, or nearer to, the coast, depending on the theory of the day. Carpets were ripped up and replaced with polished floorboards. Then it was household pets and garden plants—the weekends were spent digging up grevilleas, wattles and rye grass, and new homes had to be found for Mogsy, Flopsy and Rover. Crying children farewelled their four-legged friends, their dismay ending in another asthma attack.

The advice about medication kept changing, too. Studies showed that you should treat asthma with bronchodilators, but only during an attack. (Bronchodilators are the adrenalin-like drugs such as Ventolin and Bricanyl.) Severe asthmatics should have steroids added. Then other studies showed that it was better to *prevent* attacks, with drugs such as steroids and cromoglycates. Some parents were a bit uneasy about medicating kids *in case* they got sick, and so education programs were designed to reassure them. Further studies seemed to show that children on continuous steroids were stunted in growth, and were not much better off than under previous regimes. The pendulum swung back to treating attacks, and only using continuous prevention in chronic severe asthma.

Then, of course, there was the mode of delivery. Administration straight into the lungs allowed smaller doses than pills and syrups. Turbuhalers were better than puffers. Nebulisers were better than turbuhalers. Spacers were best for younger children. The whole thing began to look like an IQ test. I remember one elderly GP approaching me with a spacer in his hand, guiltily asking me what he was meant to do with it. He was ashamed that he didn't know. This man had delivered babies single-handed in remote areas and had operated on farmers while they were trapped under their tractors, but now he felt inadequate.

Parents who found it difficult to keep up might be comforted to know that doctors were also confused. In hospital emergency departments it was no better. 'Never give oxygen to an asthmatic' gave way to 'oxygen is the first line of treatment in severe asthma'. 'Steroids are a last resort' became 'steroids are the lynch-pin' in emergency management and even maintenance.

Meanwhile, public concern grew. Everyone heard stories of a child dying of asthma on a school camp. Despite the plethora of medications and regimes, the problem seemed to be getting worse. Various kinds of asthma were described: allergic asthma, exercise-induced asthma, 'intrinsic' asthma (asthma for which there is no clear precipitant).

Every school had a chart on the wall reminding teachers of the danger signals for severe asthma. Schools equipped themselves with nebulisers. At the same time a growing number of children were being diagnosed with severe food allergies, most commonly to foods such as peanuts and eggs. Should culprit foods be banned from school canteens, or should affected children learn to protect themselves?

The pathology of asthma

There are two key features in the pathology of asthma: chronic inflammation of the airways and bronchospasm. Let us look first at inflammation.

- Inflammatory mediators are an important aspect of the asthmatic response (Chapter 5). These include the leukotrienes (Chart 5.3).
- The immune system was 'designed' to protect us from pathogens. In order to do this, the immune system must distinguish between 'self' and 'non-self'.
- It is essential to life that the immune system develops a tolerance to certain 'non-self' items, such as foods, inhaled matter, sperm, and (in females) a foetus.
- An adaptive immune system will not make its response to the 'non-self' threat worse than the threat itself.
- A braking effect on the inflammatory response is provided by anti-inflammatory prostaglandins, notably PG-3, derived from omega-3 fatty acids.
- Children who eat fish once or more per week were shown in an Australian study to have half the morbidity and mortality from asthma of those who ate less or none (Chapter 5).
- Selenium and other nutrients act as anti-inflammatories via their roles in redox enzymes. Diets deplete in these minerals and vitamins increase the chance of 'asthma genes' being expressed.

- Asthma may result from a hypersensitivity reaction in the immune system. Some people have a genetic predisposition to hypersensitivity reactions.
- One of the means by which such genetic predisposition is expressed is through a relative deficiency in enzymes such as delta-5 and delta-6 desaturase. These enzyme variants are far too prevalent to be regarded as true defects. As such, illness arising from them should raise the question of what we are doing to render benign genetic variants harmful. The impact of excessive hygiene and early vaccination are discussed presently.

Bronchospasm is the other cardinal feature in the pathology of asthma.

- An asthma attack occurs when the protective ability of our airways to build up the head of pressure needed to expel a foreign agent (pollen, dust) cannot easily be reversed.
- The diameter of the airway is controlled by tiny smooth muscles in the wall of the bronchioles. If these muscles are continually in spasm, muscle thickening, or 'hypertrophy', will occur. Smooth-muscle hypertrophy is a key finding in the pathology of the chronic asthmatic.
- The ability of the muscle to relax depends, among other things, on the magnesium status of the individual. The effect on peak flow readings (a simple monitoring tool used by asthmatics) in response to magnesium supplementation has been discussed in Chapter 4.

Hygiene and the immune system

As asthma rates increased, treatment regimes proliferated. Parents began to challenge the received wisdom—'The doctor doesn't seem to be able to do anything, so I took him to a naturopath.' The medical profession also began to ask questions.

Pollens and dust mites have been on the planet longer than people; dogs and cats have been with us for thousands of years. And, anyway, kids with one pet had less asthma than kids with none. (But kids with *two* pets seemed to have *more*. Don't expect this to be easy!) Should we be looking at the immune system itself, rather than just the things that set it off? Sure, dust, pollen and animal danders were all allergens. But why were so many kids becoming allergic to them?

As we have seen, it soon became apparent that first-born children were the most affected. In many ways, this was counter-intuitive. First-borns got undivided parental attention. Their mothers were younger and often healthier, and had more time to breastfeed without toddlers underfoot. They had more time to keep the house clean, vacuum the floors, sterilise everything that came near Junior. There were no older siblings to bring home nasty germs. The hygiene theory (Chapter 6) seemed to offer some explanation.

Breast-feeding
The protective effect of breast-feeding on asthma and eczema development has been discussed in Chapter 6.

Pollution
Pollution was once thought to have little to do with asthma. But a decade or so ago, a public health doctor in Sydney called George Rubin plotted hospital asthma admissions against the official pollution count for any one day, and found an indisputable correlation. His work was repeated in other parts of the world with similar findings. 'Pollutant' can mean anything that we come in contact with which can have an adverse effect. Most of these are particles that we either inhale or ingest.

Inhalants
An 11-year-old boy I treated had used his mother's hair mousse for the first time (in itself, an interesting comment on our culture). Within half an hour he was clinically hypoxic, a situation that frightens even the most experienced doctor. He had never had an asthma attack before. Fortunately, he responded rapidly to bronchodilators.

Another inhalant is pollen. Many pollens associated with the allergic response are from hybrid plants—that is, plants modified by human intervention. Grevillea Robyn Gordon, developed for attractive flowers and hardiness, is currently one of the main allergens in Australian gardens and poppys and peonys are among the worst culprits in the Northern Hemisphere. Of inhaled pollutants, though, the particles from car exhausts are the worst.

Food

The various kinds of food additives were discussed in Chapter 6. Of particular concern for asthmatics are the sulphite preservatives, signified by the numbers E220–E227. There have been an alarming number of incidents where people have developed severe, and sometimes fatal, attacks of asthma after consuming cask wine. Wine, especially cheap wine, has a high sulphite content. In warm weather the sulphites become gaseous, and are inhaled as much as swallowed.

Pesticides, fungicides and other toxins are unintentional additives which can increase the chemical burden on the immune system. Preservatives of any kind affect the gut bacteria and lower the threshold for asthmatic episodes.

If the notion of a 'bored' immune system has any validity, it is not surprising that common foods are becoming increasingly the cause of allergic reactions, including asthma. In the past the advice has always been that, unless there is a classic IgE allergy (skin rash, anaphylaxis, etc.), food plays little role in asthma. It was customary to say that 'less than 5 per cent of asthmatics have to worry about what they eat'. But the immune system can respond with IgG and IgA reactions (Chapters 3 and 6) to cause food sensitivities, and there are also the reactions caused by foods containing natural glutamates, salicylates and amines. Fortunately there is a growing awareness of these factors. Peanuts and eggs are well known IgE allergens. Usually, the reaction to eating them is rapid and therefore obvious. Oranges, chocolate, yeast extracts (such as Vegemite), gluten and dairy foods have all been implicated as triggers for asthma. Perhaps these foods would have once caused mild eczema, but a trigger-happy immune system turns them into villains.

And foods themselves have changed. Genetic modification, or even selective breeding, ensures that these are not the same foods as great-great-grandma was eating. The public is usually not aware as to whether GM products are included in their staple foods.

Genetics

In Chapter 5 I noted that Herb, Mike's grandfather, probably had 'asthma genes'. Asthma is almost certainly a multi-gene phenomenon, and the effect of a 'sluggish' set of delta-6 desaturase enzymes was discussed in Chapter 3. It may even be that sluggish delta-6 enzymes are one of the major genetic determinants of asthma.

Delta-6 desaturase requires a list of co-factors before it can be activated (Charts 5.3, 5.4). Also, it is sensitive to toxic stimuli. It seems to be less efficient in certain individuals, including the elderly, and those with diabetes and allergic and immune disorders.

If this is one of the genetic factors that disposes people to allergies, perhaps we should regard eczema, asthma and autoimmune disease as part of a spectrum of delta-6-deficiency syndrome. The result of all this will be a greater difficulty in producing PG-3 from dietary precursors. This is not a problem, provided that the intake of fish, nuts, leafy green vegetables and other sources of omega-3 fatty acids is high. But we know that people are eating less of these, and that selenium, zinc and magnesium intake is at an all-time low. In such a climate, we can only *expect* a rising asthma rate, not to mention a whole raft of co-morbid conditions. Mike is almost a *representative* teenager.

A child with a learning impairment is much more likely to have a history of eczema or asthma than population averages would lead one to expect. The EFAs have been successfully used in the treatment of all of these conditions. As such, it is no coincidence that one treatment modality solves several problems.

The modern child with asthma and learning difficulties or depression is *not* carrying lethal genes. *But the modern diet, with its reduction of omega-3 fatty acids, magnesium, selenium and zinc, has unmasked the problems inherent in an otherwise harmless delta-6 inefficiency.*

The medical dilemma

If vaccination or the use of antibiotics is contributing to the epidemic of asthma and allergies, then it should be held to account. Vaccination may have to be started later. Extreme caution may be needed in the prescription of antibiotics to pregnant women and young children. An American study shows that children given antibiotics in the first six months of life were *2.6 times* more likely to develop allergic asthma than those who were not; for broad-spectrum antibiotics this figure became an alarming *ninefold* increase. There were also increases in other allergic responses to grasses and animals.

One might argue that kids with twitchy lungs are more likely to get the respiratory problems that signal the need for antibiotics in the first place. However, the increase held true for children receiving antibiotics for non-respiratory illnesses, such as kidney infections.[10]

What has been the medical response to these various issues to date? So entrenched is the idea of universal vaccination that it is impossible to run a controlled trial. Data is only available on biased samples of children: those whose parents fail to vaccinate through poverty or neglect, or are conscientious objectors. Mothers are still castigated if they delay or withhold vaccination from infants. Doctors sympathetic to them run the risk of censure, as we saw with the challenge to MMR vaccines (Chapter 2).

Despite some improvement, doctors still prescribe non-essential antibiotics to pregnant women and to small babies. Increasing numbers of births by caesarean section add another vexatious dimension. Although the obstetric outcome might be as good as in vaginal birth, caesareans are associated with higher antibiotic usage and greater failure in establishing breast-feeding.

It is easy to attack doctors for the direction that their research takes. But as long as industry provides the majority of asthma research funding, research will find the nebuliser or drug or carpet shampoo that is 'necessary' to treat asthma.

What you can do

Asthma can kill. People do not develop asthma because they have a Ventolin deficiency, but in acute asthma Ventolin, steroids and related drugs save lives. Moreover, acute withdrawal from any medication is potentially very dangerous. The assessment and overall management of asthma belongs in the hands of competent medical practitioners. The ideas I have raised about vaccination and the use of antibiotics should be openly debated. The following suggestions are aimed at improving health, not at treating established disease.

Exposure *in utero* to highly allergenic foods such as eggs and peanuts via the maternal diet may increase the risk of later development of the relevant food allergy, but it has not been proved. Certain food taboos have been recorded among Australian Aboriginals on the consumption of 'strong foods' in pregnancy. This intriguing list includes honey, nuts, eggs and fish. The derivation of such a taboo is certainly food for thought.

Asthmatics may be able to improve or control their condition by being careful about what they eat.

- The diet should be high in fresh fruit and vegetables. These are the best source of anti-oxidants, and they contain many substances whose contribution to good health has yet to be established. Organically grown produce is best because it is likely to have higher levels of nutrients and fewer chemicals.
- Unless allergy to seafood has been established, a diet in which fish is eaten once or more per week reduces the severity of asthma, as we have seen. In cases of true fish allergy capsules of flaxseed oil should be used, because there is a small risk that fish oil capsules may be contaminated by fish protein — the factor responsible for allergy.
- Avoidance of food colourings, salicylates, amines, chocolate, oranges, peanuts, dairy and gluten can often bring spectacular results. In Western countries the asthma incidence has been observed to parallel the consumption of dairy foods, so dairy elimination is certainly worth a trial.
- Elimination diets can be trialled. This is best done with the supervision of a doctor or dietician with expertise in this area. An inadequately performed elimination diet is worse than useless.

Exercise and sunshine can also be useful. Sunshine provides Vitamin D, the benefits of which are being increasingly recognised. Swimming, preferably not in chlorinated pools and definitely not in cold water, seems to be one of the most beneficial of all forms of exercise for asthmatics.

Moderate exposure to germs and pets might also assist asthmatics, although it would be a brave doctor who told a parent to deliberately expose their child to germs. But somewhere between 'sterile' and 'filthy', there is 'hygiene'—guided, one might hope, by good sense.

We have also seen that the simple administration of normal gut flora to pregnant women reduces the incidence of eczema and asthma in babies at risk (Chapter 6).

Vitamin and mineral status in the hypersensitive individual was also discussed in Chapter 6, including the inhibition of mast cell degranulation by Vitamin B3, thus reducing the release of inflammatory mediators. Selenium, as part of the enzyme glutathione peroxidase, modifies the effects of some of these mediators such as prostaglandins. Magnesium has a modifying effect on many messenger molecules at the site at which they attach to their respective receptors.

Asthmatics should avoid continuous low-level stress. Physical and mental stress result in increased production of corticosteroids from the adrenals and cortisol from the hypothalamus. These hormones often intensify hypersensitivity reactions by increasing the production of inflammatory mediators. Hormonal change can take the form of worsening (though sometimes improving) asthma during menstruation, pregnancy, menopause, adolescence, or when thyroid disorders are present.

CANCER

This section is not a comprehensive discussion of either the prevention or the treatment of cancer. It focuses on a few salient aspects of this most feared of diseases in order to help those keen to undertake preventive measures, as well as those already dealing with a cancer diagnosis. In Chapter 2 I discussed many of the issues surrounding the subject.

Certain carcinogens, such as cigarette smoke, are associated with specific cancers, such as lung and bladder cancer. These are the easy ones because we understand cause and effect. However, the identification and avoidance of other possible carcinogens, while harder, is still a realistic goal.

It helps to view a cancer cell not as something that is out to get us, but as an undifferentiated cell that has lost its direction. Cell differentiation is the key to normal cell growth; it is the process by which a new cell develops and matures. If something interferes with that process, the cell becomes autonomous and begins to read bits of the genetic code which you would rather it did not. For instance, the instruction 'reproduce yourself at all costs' is an appropriate part of the code when a wound is in need of healing. Cancer cells are in effect healing wounds which are no longer there.

In Chapter 3 I discussed the free radical as an unruly child. It is not inherently 'bad', and it can be an effective member of society so long as the normal controls operate. The process leading to cancer is similar. It normally begins as the result of direct DNA damage, either from oxidative stress or from an unresolved inflammatory response. Many cancers begin in visible inflammation, such as the membranes lining a smoker's lung. If the stress goes on for too long (as with continued smoking), and the anti-oxidant and anti-inflammatory reserves are exhausted, then the stress exceeds the ability of the cell to cope.

The scene I'm trying to set is this. An inflammatory process activates a cell, which starts to act beyond its mandate. The cell is 'confused' and damaged, and in its attempts to heal, or to differentiate, it exaggerates the weaknesses in its DNA. Some of these weaknesses will be inherited, some brought about by environmental stress. To avoid cancer, we need to reduce the stressors on the cell, and to increase our lines of defence.

Defences

The value of vitamins, minerals, EFAs and others is discussed throughout this book. Zinc is an important factor in translating the genetic code; magnesium is important as a messenger molecule and hormone modifier; selenium has been detailed at length (Chapter 4). Falling soil levels of zinc, magnesium and selenium, and of vitamins in our diets, all play a part in the rising cancer rates.

The question of what people eat is sensitive. A morbidly obese journalist recently lashed out in the Australian press at the suggestion that some controls be exerted over the national eating behaviour. No doubt he will happily take a priority hospital bed when his own eating behaviour adds to the burden of the national health budget. Estimates vary, but figures ranging from 30 to 90 per cent have been given for the numbers of cancers arising from what does and does not go into our mouths. In this most critical area, we have a large measure of control.

We can take care to eat the cancer-fighting foods — the brassicas (cabbage family), the yellow vegetables for carotenoids, and the red fruits and vegetables for bioflavonoids and anthocyanins. In August

2007, Monica Giusti, from the University of Ohio, demonstrated the benefits of anthocyanin pigments for rats with colon cancer. In the same year, University of Pittsburgh researchers showed that anthocyanins killed cells from all tested lines of human leukaemias and lymphomas. An Australian biochemist, Dr Greg Jardine, conducted similar studies, through the University of Sydney, with prostate cancer.[11] These pigments are found in foods such as purple grapes, beetroot, chokeberry, purple corn, eggplants, red cabbage and bilberries.

More cancer fighters can be found within the mushroom family—in particular, in Asian mushrooms like shiitake and maitake. Professor Tom Borody, from Sydney, asks: 'How much evidence do we need?' He says, 'Cancer patients [have been prescribed mushroom extract] in Japan for decades and we in Australia, have been oblivious to it. And perhaps many would feel more comfortable keeping it that way'.

Cancer-fighting foods also include fish, herbs, nuts and seeds, and also the hormonal buffer foods, that is, those containing phyto-sterols (Chapters 6 and 10).

We can avoid nutrient-depleted foods and toxic foods, which include fats heated to high temperatures, especially if they are reheated, and fats with high levels of trans fatty acids (many of the margarines). We can avoid foods with artificial colourings, flavourings, preservatives and sweeteners (Chapter 6).

Other important defences against malignant degeneration of cells include the functions of intestinal bacteria, as hormone buffers, toxin destroyers, and producers of short-chain fatty acids. Chapter 3 discussed the effects of preservatives, antibiotics, chlorine and other substances on normal gut flora, and Appendix 3 gives recommendations for gut health. Because gut bacteria constitute a frontline defence against toxins, anything that alters the composition of that flora contributes to the development of the toxin-related cancers.

Butyric acid, the by product of lactobacillic fermentation, has a direct relationship to the prevention of bowel cancer. The relationship to the development of breast, pancreatic and prostate cancer is harder to establish, but there is speculation that butyrate will prove to have a similarly important role in preventing these cancers as well. (See also Chapter 3: A done deal; Chapter 3: Epigenetic inheritance.)

Various studies have purported to show that certain personality types predispose to cancer survival. One commonly held belief is that a response of helplessness is associated with a lowered survival rate. By contrast, those who either go into denial, *or* come out fighting, fare best. It is assumed that denial is actually a passive way of saying 'I won't accept this diagnosis and I am going to live my life despite it.'

Other studies claim that attitude has little to do with outcome. In the meantime, those who respond with anger should direct it towards unacceptable commercial practices and the governments which condone them. A Western mother who was told that her child had a one-in-seven lifetime risk of contracting HIV would be devastated. And yet these figures are associated with only *one kind* of cancer (of the breast).

Some common cancers

Breast cancer

Breast cancer, including screening and chemoprevention, was discussed in Chapter 2, and some helpful books are listed in the reading list.

The recent explosion of breast cancer cases has nothing to do with an increase in the BRCA1 and 2 genes, and everything to do with an environment that allows breast cancer to develop. Multiple epidemiological studies have confirmed that breast-cancer risk moves with individuals. People moving from an area of low risk to an area of high risk adopt the risk of their new milieu. This is not genetic.

There is an accepted correlation between breast cancer and a diet high in animal fat. This may reflect the fat-solubility of environmental carcinogens, particularly pesticides and industrial chemicals. Epstein points out scathingly that university departments of nutrition are the last place to go on this subject, as many of them 'have no expertise in toxicology and carcinogenesis', and 'many of them are recipients of major support from the food industry.'[12] If it is true that breast cancer is 'a rich woman's disease', many features other than the consumption of dairy products might be involved. However, dairy intake may be a significant factor, and should be considered. Various studies have linked milk consumption to breast, ovarian and prostate cancers.[13] Proposed mechanisms include:

- IGF-1 in milk acting as a growth factor (Chapter 2)
- pesticides

- high calcium levels blocking the action of Vitamin D
- an inflammatory response evoked by the A1 casein protein (Chapter 2).

The drugs designed to prevent breast cancer (SERMS) have a molecular structure that resembles oestrogen and progesterone. Their function is to sit on, and therefore block, the appropriate receptor sites of cells. The comparison is with the key which enters a lock but will not turn. This has been discussed in Chapter 6. If environmental chemicals exert their carcinogenic effects through hormone imitation, we can see why the Asian diet is protective, as these foods are rich in phyto-sterols, and seem to serve a similar function to the SERMS. There is a good case for arguing that such a diet is just as protective as, and infinitely safer than, the use of SERMS.

Optimal treatment includes establishing the extent of the disease, surgical removal of the primary, assessment of lymph node involvement, and the whole discussion of what to do next. There is the question of whether to remove *all* the lymph glands if only some are involved, and there is the question of whether to perform a biopsy on a gland known as the 'sentinel node' before removing *any* axillary glands.

If the disease is thought to be confined to the breast, a choice must be made between lumpectomy and mastectomy. Many women prefer not to lose their breast. However, the removal of the lump is usually followed up with local radiotherapy. When the chest wall has been irradiated it is a much worse candidate for breast reconstruction should a later lesion develop necessitating mastectomy. Radiotherapy can result in lung damage, and an increased risk of coronary artery disease through radiation damage to those arteries. Though it goes against the current thinking, I see mastectomy as the better option.

Lung cancer
This cancer still kills more people than any other cancer. It most nearly conforms to the paradigm of single-cause disease, and in this regard it is more the exception than the rule. Exposure to cigarette smoke is the commonest cause of lung cancer. Exposure to asbestos causes another, rarer lung cancer, mesothelioma.

Since the link to smoking became accepted, many men have given up smoking and a fall has resulted in the number of men dying from this disease. Social change has seen an unfortunate rise in female deaths. The risks and costs involved in a chest X-ray every two years are still thought in some places to justify the benefit of earlier diagnosis.

Bowel cancer

Currently, in Western countries, bowel cancer kills someone every two hours, whereas breast cancer kills someone every five hours. Most forms of bowel cancer bleed from time to time. The bleeding is often dismissed by the patient or the doctor as piles, but this is a risky assumption.

Patients with familial polyps or a strong family history of bowel cancer are often investigated on a regular basis with a colonoscopy. While not all polyps become malignant, almost all bowel cancers begin as polyps. Although colonoscopy is invasive, the cost-benefit analysis supports it so that polyps can be removed, and cancers can be detected before they spread.

An effective screening process looks for microscopic traces of blood in an apparently normal stool. This is totally non-invasive and is far more effective than mammography in detecting cancer, yet there is no national screening program.

It might be noted that in the American Cancer Trial (Chapter 4), the single greatest indicator of bowel polyps was a low level of selenium in plasma.[14]

Ovarian cancer

This is a rare cancer. It is significant because it is on the increase, it often strikes very young women, and it has an association with breast cancer and the BRCA genes. Often it has already spread at the time of diagnosis. Fewer, and later, pregnancies are thought to explain part but not all of the increase in incidence.

It has a poor prognosis: approximately 35 per cent of women diagnosed after spread will be alive five years after the diagnosis. Caught early, the survival rates approximate 90 per cent.

Until now, the main diagnostic tool has been a blood test for the levels of a protein called CA125, pelvic examination, and pelvic ultrasonography. These are only minimally invasive, although the best ultrasounds, done transvaginally, are a little more so. Ultrasound is not cheap, but it is a justifiable cost if there is any suspicion of ovarian disease. As a mass screening procedure, it may not meet the criterion of cost-effectiveness unless the incidence of ovarian cancer continues to rise. Recent reports have appeared of a more sophisticated blood test based on techniques known as the 'fingerprinting' of a blood protein.[15] Further research should be awaited with interest.

A recent study has shown that drinking more than two glasses of milk a day significantly increases the risk of developing this deadly cancer.[16] When we add up the cappuccinos, the yoghurt and the cheese, this amount is not hard to reach.

Even after diagnosis, there is something else that we can do. A study showed that adding selenium to the treatment regime seemed to prevent ovarian tumours from becoming resistant to chemotherapy.[17]

Prostate cancer

Testing for prostate cancer is more contentious than for the previously listed cancers. The blood test has an error rate of about 20 per cent in both directions. Confirmation is difficult, as normal ultrasounds and scanning procedures can miss small clusters of malignant cells. So, too, can biopsy, which is both invasive and unpleasant. A person with a positive blood test faces the dilemma of living with the anxiety of cancer, or undergoing treatment which may not even be necessary.

It is often said that men are more likely to die with prostatic cancer than of it. Prostate cancer can be very slow-growing, taking decades before it spreads or becomes aggressive. Often the patient will die of some other age-related condition before the prostate cancer causes him significant ill health.

Surgery often leaves the man with urinary incontinence and impotence. Other treatments such as radiotherapy, chemotherapy and hormones all have side effects.

Urologists and epidemiologists around the world are divided on the issue of routine screening. Those who strongly favour the testing are no doubt influenced by the aggressive form of the disease, especially in young men. In the past, both Britain and Australia have rejected routine screening as a policy, though it is often carried out at the discretion of individual doctors. Recent cost-benefit analyses seem to be steering opinion in the direction of screening. In the United States, especially where patient pressure is strong, it is already done widely.

The American Cancer Trial found that selenium supplements significantly reduced the risk of prostate cancer after only a few years of usage. This may be because selenium can provoke cancer cells into 'committing suicide' or programmed cell death.

We saw under Breast Cancer above that a high intake of dairy products has been linked to an increased risk of prostate cancer, and we know that soy-consuming nations like Japan have a much lower incidence than Western cultures. Diets rich in fruits and vegetables—particularly lycopene, the anti-oxidant found in tomatoes—appear to confer significant protection.

REPRODUCTIVE HEALTH

Many topics can be discussed under this heading. For women, they include menstrual difficulties, polycystic ovary syndrome, endometriosis, pregnancy and menopausal issues. For men, there can be erectile difficulty, ejaculation disorders and prostatic problems. For both sexes there are fertility problems and the whole spectrum of reproductive cancers. Problems in any of these areas could be said to represent various fixed-name diseases.

Mother Nature wanted us to have a healthy reproductive system so that the species will reproduce itself. The sexual act is normally painless, and indeed, highly pleasurable. It is part of an intimate bonding process. This contributes to an optimal environment for the rearing of the young.

Any of the problems listed above can be seen as a warning that something is wrong. The role of nutrition in other areas of sexual health is discussed directly or indirectly throughout this book. Erectile difficulty, for example, is as much a cardiovascular problem as anything. Libido disorders have more to do with overall health and well-being than hormone levels. If those levels are abnormal, it is more instructive to find out why than to attempt to adjust them synthetically. In Chapter 4: Iodine and bromine, we saw the influence that iodine deficiency alone may have on fibrocystic breast disease, breast cancer, PCOS, ovarian cancer and insulin resistance. Little under this heading, therefore, is likely to respond to the approach typical of fixed-name disease.

Fertility

Infertility (male or female), and polycystic ovaries are two of the commonest reproductive problems seen in general practice. Infertility can arise as a result of many factors including previous infections or toxic exposure. In this context we should remember not only the effects of chemicals like the gender-benders (Chapter 6), but also other chemicals such as nicotine, which are known to damage sperm.

Polycystic ovaries are one 'cause' of infertility, and a look at the factors leading to their development gives insight into fertility issues in general. The ovarian cysts are not the cause of the infertility. Cysts form when the environment is not optimal for pregnancy. If the hormonal environment is wrong, or the developing egg is not receiving enough of the zinc, selenium, magnesium, EFAs, and whatever else is necessary for normal maturation, it is doomed, and so the body does not waste precious resources on developing it.

Similarly with sperm. Many men whose sperm is abnormal in number, shape or motility achieve significant improvement in sperm quality after interventions such as giving up smoking and taking vitamin and mineral supplements. But improved sperm quality is not the end point. The ability to impregnate their partner with a viable foetus is. Doctors practising from these basic starting points can all tell stories of ' miracle babies'.

Polycystic ovary syndrome (PCOS) and infertility

Gudrun and Hans have been married for about three years, and for the last 18 months have been trying to become pregnant. About six months ago, Gudrun, who is 28, was diagnosed as having polycystic ovaries. A similar diagnosis was made in her early 20s, when she sought help for irregular, long menstrual cycles and excess facial hair. At that time, she was put on the oral contraceptive, and the cycles became predictable again.

Gudrun has always tended to be overweight. She has not minded this too much, as many of the women in her family look the same. She admits to a sweet tooth, and although she has tried a succession of diets she regains any weight she has lost. I shall return to Gudrun and Hans shortly, but first let us look at some aspects of the sex hormones.

The balance of hormones in the human body, male or female, is finely orchestrated. Men need testosterone, along with a small amount of oestrogen. It may be oestrogen which is responsible for men's libido, in a manner analogous to the action of testosterone in women. Women need oestrogen and progesterone, along with a small amount of testosterone. Too much testosterone causes unwanted hair and other undesirable symptoms.

This is where the liver comes in, by producing a substance known as *sex-hormone-binding globulin*—SHBG. In Chapter 6: Sulphate reducing bacteria, we saw one way in which the liver keeps hormones in balance—by disposing of excess. Here is another. SHBG acts as a different type of 'glue' to which excess hormones can attach as they travel around in the bloodstream. This helps maintain hormone balance and ensure that free hormone acts only when and where needed. The production of SHBG requires first that there is adequate soluble fibre in the diet. Included in this category are soy, flaxseeds, lentils, legumes, asparagus, nuts, seeds and certain tuberiferous vegetables like yams and sweet potatoes.

Gut bacteria then ferment these foods and produce short-chain fatty acids or SCFAs, as discussed in Chapter 3. Of particular interest here is the SCFA known as propionic acid, because this stimulates the liver to produce SHBG. Any study purporting to prove that isoflavones (from soy, etc.) have no effect on female hormone or prostatic disorders is meaningless unless gut florae have been taken into account.

A woman who is hirsute (hairy) may have a serum level of testosterone that is in the normal range for females, but an abnormally high level of 'free testosterone'. That is to say, she is not producing excess testosterone, but she does not have enough SHBG to act as a buffer. Low levels of SHBG are a common finding in women with polycystic ovaries.

Although SHBG will bind to most of the sex steroids, it has a particular affinity for oestrogen. This is possibly because oestrogen, of all the hormones, has one of the widest fluctuations. Both high and low levels of SHBG may be a cause for concern.

- A high level can indicate pregnancy, but it may indicate excessive oestrogen exposure. Levels rise when a woman is on the oral contraceptive pill or, more worryingly, exposed to environmental oestrogens or oestrogen-producing tumours. It is not the high level of SHBG

itself which is the problem, but what it may stand for.
- Low levels are a different kind of worry, because the buffering effect on hormones is lost. This is usually easy to fix by dietary intervention.

A parallel strand to this story is hyperinsulinism. People with PCOS often show signs of insulin resistance, and many of the drug treatments are based on increasing sensitivity to insulin. Thinking critically, we should ask what features of the diet produce high levels of insulin *and* low levels of SHBG.

A diet with high levels of refined carbohydrates is deplete in the foods just listed, and also predisposes to insulin resistance. In other words, the diet which leads to hyperinsulinism is also the diet which is lacking certain protective elements. It is important to understand this concept, because many people will point to cultures in which a moderate degree of obesity is the norm (Pacific Islander for example), and protest that obesity is a healthy state. In the Western culture, however, it is the means by which that obesity is attained, as much as the obesity itself, which is the problem.

Polycystic ovaries are a symptom, not a disease. When Gudrun sought help five or six years ago, the response was to impose regularity on her cycles. Irregular cycles are a feature of PCOS, so let's fix the irregularity! The cysts represent immature egg follicles, let's stop her from ovulating!

Under normal circumstances, a single follicle in the ovary develops each month. It looks like a small cyst. When the egg is ripe, the follicle bursts open and releases the egg. This opened follicle then re-forms as a little gland called the *corpus luteum*, which produces progesterone. If pregnancy occurs, the corpus luteum will supply progesterone for the first three months, after which the foetus takes over and maintains the progesterone level.

The cysts in polycystic ovaries do not mature, for reasons which we will discuss presently, and therefore progesterone levels remain low. Without progesterone to mature the uterine lining, there is a build-up of friable material, and periods, when they finally arrive, can be heavy, and unpredictable.

As Gudrun's concern at the time of her first presentation was heavy irregular periods and facial hair, a discussion on weight loss may or may not have taken place. If she had been referred to one of the obesity/endocrine clinics, she would have been put on a strict diet, and might have been given an anti-diabetic drug known as Metformin. The reason for this is that insulin resistance is playing a part in the formation of the cysts in her ovaries. High levels of insulin act as a growth hormone and stimulate the production of multiple follicles, an undesirable anabolic effect of insulin (Chapter 8).

The rationale for Gudrun's treatment is both easy and difficult. On the one hand it is easy because she has a metabolic disorder that is producing symptoms, whether irregular cycles at age 21 or infertility at age 28, and you have medications which can help her. On the other hand, you have a young woman, *still in her 20s*, being educated to think that a diet and lifestyle that can result not only in infertility, but hypertension and diabetes, are best treated by taking the oral contraceptive pill, using Metformin, or going to a fertility clinic.

The better clinics do not take this either-or approach. It is important for Gudrun to realise that the source of her condition threatens not only her fertility but the well-being of her future baby as well. And she may have more control over the situation than she realises.

Charts 3.5 and 3.6 show that the hormones derived from cholesterol are structurally similar and can be converted into each other. Indeed, this interconversion is one of the fine-tuning tools used by the endocrine system. These reactions are mostly controlled by enzymes. The enzyme that converts testosterone to oestrogen is an aromatase, and is inhibited by insulin. So if Gudrun is eating too many sweet things, her elevated insulin levels may favour testosterone production over oestrogen. Hence the facial hair. This is another of the ways in which insulin can act as a growth hormone. Oestrogen lays down fat; testosterone helps to build up muscle tissue.

In evolutionary terms, the increased musculature of the male enhances his hunting, fighting and protective roles, so he gets the testosterone. Oestrogen increases fat reserves, which the female needs for pregnancy and lactation. Fat cells themselves can make oestrogen, increasing the levels available. Of course, nature did not 'plan' for the type of obesity produced by the junk food diet of the modern world.

So Gudrun may have three problems: high levels of insulin, stimulating multiple follicles; oestrogen 'dominance' over progesterone from an excess of fat cells; and progesterone deficiency because these multiple follicles cannot mature and produce progesterone. All three of these hormone profiles are common in PCOS.

If excess insulin results in high testosterone levels in a woman, she may develop a masculine build and male distribution of body hair, and have fertility problems. Importantly, the growth hormone action of insulin in producing multiple follicles mean that the follicles are the symptom, not the disease.

These follicles are destined to go nowhere. One reason is that the change in the ratio of oestrogen to testosterone is not conducive to pregnancy. The crucial reason, though, is that the diet that leads to excess insulin not only lacks SHBG precursors, as we saw above, but is also low in micronutrients. A normal follicle, with its egg contained inside, needs key nutrients in order to develop and mature. Unsurprisingly, these include vitamins, minerals such as selenium, zinc and magnesium, and the essential fatty acids. In Chapter 4 we saw that even the most primitive life forms, prokaryotes and eukaryotes, have selenium-dependent enzyme systems. Yet these vital elements are missing from Gudrun's bad diet (not to mention the fertility clinic's treatment).

Perhaps this explains something else. There is a higher incidence of foetal abnormality in babies conceived by the various IVF methods. Researchers have tried to find which, of the many possible, environmental effects could be causing this. They have overlooked the fact that the fertility problems might have arisen in the first place because of nutrient and micronutrient deficiency (a deficiency which may subsequently cause foetal defects).

We can understand why obese women develop PCOS, but PCOS also occurs in women of normal or even slim build. Perhaps we can better understand this if we stand back for a moment. PCO refers to a condition whereby a woman may have polycystic ovaries but not the pathology associated with PCOS. She may even still be ovulating. It is conjectured that up to 25 per cent of women may have PCO, and that this may even have had an adaptive benefit for hunter-gatherers.

Depending on the build of these women (fat or thin), and the availability of food, PCO may have helped some women turn ovulation off in circumstances where pregnancy was best avoided (such as during long treks). Alternatively, it may have helped other women to avail themselves of appropriate circumstances in which to switch ovulation on. The appearance of PCOS in the Western world may be another example whereby the diet and lifestyle of the 21st century render otherwise adaptive genes 'deleterious'.

The trekking woman does not have high levels of insulin; but her city cousin, even if she is not overweight, is still living on a refined carbohydrate diet. She is blissfully unaware what muesli bars and other sugary snacks are doing to her insulin levels. High insulin levels paradoxically mimic the very effects of infertility produced in nature as a protective device. Despite all these 'energy bars', it is likely that the diet of the city cousin will be deplete in essential micronutrients. To keep slim, she may work out at the gym. This reduces her body fat, and thus her oestrogen levels. With high exercise levels and the lack of nutrients to mature the follicles, her endocrine system has interpreted the situation as a desert trek. She develops PCOS, and everybody is mystified.

This account helps us to understand many of the other causes of infertility, including male infertility. Healthy conception requires a healthy egg, a healthy sperm, and a normal hormonal environment. From this standpoint it should be apparent that, while excess insulin is typically accompanied by obesity, it is still possible for thin people to suffer from insulin resistance and PCOS when they consume the wrong diet.

The healthy pregnancy

Pregnancy should be a time of good health and pleasurable anticipation. Many women say that they have never felt so well as when they are pregnant. This is not hard to understand, as the levels of oestrogen and progesterone give them, in effect, a steroid 'high'. Remember how closely these hormones resemble other steroids. Often women experience a reduction in asthma, skin and other problems, because of this steroidal effect. For reasons that may be similar, many women with migraine lose their headaches.

For other women however, pregnancy may be blighted by morning sickness, back strain, fatigue and dental problems. Whatever the underlying causes, these problems are always made worse by stress. The modern nuclear family differs from the tribe, where help was always at hand.

Although answers to these health problems are far from clear, there are some clues. Nausea in pregnancy is thought to act as a warning of toxic foods. Sensitivity is heightened to any chemical, mould or toxin that could harm the developing foetus. The use of zinc, chromium and Vitamin B6 has been helpful to some. Does pregnancy highlight the toxins and deficiencies of the modern diet?

We have seen in Chapter 4 how magnesium deficiencies might affect the ease of labour and the development of pre-eclampsia. Magnesium, as well as calcium, is important for the baby's bones. Mother may be short-changed as the baby gets preferential access to the supply. *Her* bones and joints start to ache, and paracetamol is not the solution. All of the nutrients which we have discussed in earlier chapters are required by the foetus, and it may get first option.

Most women will put up with an uncomfortable pregnancy: their goal is a healthy baby and their worst fear is a birth defect. Nowadays, many tests along the way put some fears to rest (although sometimes they raise others).

Recurrent miscarriages can be due to antibody formation, and this is often treated successfully with aspirin. But aspirin, as discussed in Chapter 10, is a form of salicylic acid, a common ingredient in fruit and vegetables. The tendency to form these antibodies can be genetic; it is called the 'phospholipid' or 'cardiolipin' syndrome. Is this just another example of the modern diet unmasking harmless genes as 'bad'?

Sometimes miscarriages occur because the foetus is non-viable. The inability of such a foetus to maintain its progesterone supply (as described above) explains why so many miscarriages occur at three months.

The risk of spina bifida may be increased when the diet is deficient in folic acid, or when the mother has two copies of the gene for the less effective form of the enzyme methylenetetrahydrof olate reductase (that is, she is homozygous for this gene). This risk increase could be a direct result of raised homocysteine (Chapter 8). However, as folic acid (as folate) is involved in multiple pathways, there are various means by which a deficiency could exert its deleterious effects. The consumption of alcohol uses up the body's stores of folic acid. Some of the effects of the foetal alcohol syndrome are thought to be due to the acute deficiency of folic acid. *Some* of the severe problems seen in spina bifida and foetal alcohol syndrome may be the extreme examples of acute folic acid deficiency in the developing foetus.

Simple folic acid supplements (along with Vitamin B12, which is also involved in homocysteine metabolism) are effective in reducing blood levels of homocysteine. Folic acid has been held responsible for the dramatic reduction by about two-thirds of babies born with spina bifida in supplemented mothers. Folic acid has been given to alcoholic pregnant women as part of an attempt to reduce the effects of the foetal alcohol syndrome, notably on Native American reserves, but as this is usually part of an overall nutritional program it is difficult to unravel the individual effects.

In the future other cause-and-effect nutrient trials may identify the problems of nutrient-deplete diets and ensure better pregnancy outcomes.

Dysmenorrhoea and endometriosis

Dysmenorrhoea is the medical term for painful periods. Pain can be experienced prior to the onset of bleeding but is most common during the period itself. The basis of this is not difficult to understand.

The uterus is shaped like an upside-down pear. The bulk of the uterus is muscle tissue, with the thickest part at the top. This enables contractions to start at the top of the uterus and travel downwards in a co-ordinated manner to expel the uterine contents, whether a baby or the monthly blood loss. Several factors are important for muscle contraction and relaxation. The role of magnesium as a smooth muscle relaxant has been discussed (Chapter 4). Prostaglandins (from the EFAs) are important in the co-ordination of muscle contraction (Chapter 5). They accumulate in the uterus at the time of childbirth, and are thought to help initiate the contractions which lead to the expulsion of the foetus. They are also necessary for the smooth, and ideally painless, loss of the endometrial lining during menstruation. Many of the drugs used to treat dysmenorrhoea act by blocking the actions of the PG-2 series (Chart 5.3).

Remember Mary in Chapters 2 and 4, who had mild mood swings and mild asthma as well as painful periods? Magnesium and EFAs play a role in mood and asthma. Can we realistically think of her dysmenorrhoea as separate?

If Mary is unlucky, her pain may become so severe that someone will give her a laparoscopy to see if she has endometriosis. 'Endometriosis' is a condition in which the type of tissue that lines the uterus has somehow made its way into the abdominal cavity or peritoneum. The term for this is 'ectopic' tissue, meaning something which is in the wrong place. When the uterine lining bleeds, so does this tissue. This causes severe pain. There is nowhere for the blood to go, and the way the body deals with this is to create scar tissue known as 'adhesions'. Adhesions can glue organs together and stop their normal action of gliding over each other with movement. They are tethered together and the result is very painful.

There are two theories on how the tissue gets there. One is that it forms when the woman is an embryo. The other theory is that it occurs as a result of retrograde bleeding. The uterine lining, instead of being neatly expelled downwards, travels back up the fallopian tubes and enters the abdominal cavity. As part of the patient's own tissue, it readily 'takes', rather like a graft. We can imagine how this might happen. When a uterus contracts in a co-ordinated manner, top to bottom, the contents are expelled. When it goes into spasm, its liquid contents can be sent in all directions. If the contents is a baby, the nett effect of spasm is to hold on to the baby (delayed labour) rather than to deliver it.

Prostatic disorders

Prostatic disorders occasion much medical intervention in the Western world, and it is not hard to understand the distress they cause. The fixed names applied to the most common of these are prostatism, benign prostatic hypertrophy (BPH), and prostate cancer. The incidence of all of these appears to be on the rise. By contrast, the Japanese have a lower incidence of these disorders, with the risk increasing in those who migrate to Western cultures.

Some factors seem to be common to all three conditions, notably increased levels of circulating 'free testosterone'. In this unbound form, testosterone is available to be taken up by prostatic cells.

Prostatism and BPH
In the male, the urethra traverses the prostate gland. Any inflammation in either the urethra or the prostate gland will cause discomfort, and possibly swelling. When infection is present, antibiotics may be used. Often the basic pathology is as much to do with inflammation as infection *per se*.

Any enlargement of the prostate obstructs urinary flow. As a result, urination becomes difficult, urinary retention and secondary infection can occur, and the patient may have to make multiple trips to pass ever-decreasing quantities of urine.

Surgery is sometimes recommended. One approach is simply to bore a larger hole. Another is the removal of the prostate, which can have the unfortunate side effects of impotence or retrograde ejaculation. Men often show a distinct lack of enthusiasm for such procedures. Let us look at some other treatments.

In the male, the concentration of zinc in the prostate is higher than in any other organ in the body. When people are deficient in iodine, the thyroid gland enlarges as if to trap more of whatever iodine might be available. The comparison with BPH is unavoidable. Among its other actions, zinc acts to inhibit the activity of the enzyme 5-alpha-reductase. This is the same enzyme targeted by the drugs used to treat BPH. Men with BPH often gain symptomatic relief from the addition of zinc supplements (Chapter 4).

As the prostate gland clearly has a requirement for selenium, the same rationale applies as for zinc. Selenium was also discussed in the context of prostate cancer.

As we saw in Chapter 5, EFAs produce the molecules called prostaglandins. They are so named because they were first isolated from prostatic secretions. A deficiency of EFAs may go a long way towards explaining prostatic disease. When testosterone enters the prostate cell, it converts to dihydro-testosterone and stimulates the release of prostaglandins. These in turn inhibit the further binding of testosterone to the cell. Furthermore, BPH is characterised by inflammatory symptoms, and we already know that EFAs are important in reducing inflammation.

The low risk of prostate disease in soy-consuming cultures such as China and Japan has been attributed to the action of genistein and other isoflavones derived from plants. As phyto-sterols they stimulate the liver to produce SHBG, keeping free testosterone levels in the safe range.

Sexual health

It is accepted that a healthy sex life benefits a wide range of physical and mental conditions. One of the main concerns for males can be erectile dysfunction, or ED. The entry of this term into common parlance was rapidly followed by the term 'female sexual dysfunction' or FSD. Curiously, the debut of these disorders was soon after the release of Viagra. It did not take long before Viagra was mooted for treating FSD. A good account of this story appears in *Selling Sickness*.[18]

As erectile dysfunction is more often than not the result of a medical or vascular problem, and as the side effects of Viagra can be quite alarming, we might ask if there are more benign interventions than Viagra. Preventing and treating diabetes is a major start. A recent report indicated that there might be others. Let us take a step back for a moment.

A common problem of ageing is faecal and urinary incontinence. For women, problems often begin with childbirth and may worsen around menopause; but men are not spared either. There are suggestions, however, that cultures which use squat toilets and individuals who practise pelvic-floor exercises have much reduced rates of incontinence. A small three-month trial indicated that such intervention might be as effective as Viagra in the management of erectile dysfunction.[19]

Menopause

Menopause is a normal phase of the human condition. It is unusual in mammals: most go on reproducing into old age.

Various reasons are put forward to explain why humans differ. One of the most intuitively appealing is that human society is so complex that the raising of children falls not only to the parents, but also requires the wisdom and skills of other generations. In evolutionary terms, human groups that include grandmothers survive better than groups that have no grandmothers. Freed of the burden of their own young, grandmothers are able to help out with the care of their grandchildren. There is the interesting possibility that the insomnia which besets middle-aged women is programmed into them to do the night shift with sick or restless grandchildren.

Many older patients remark that menopause was not a problem for them or their mothers and grandmothers. The Japanese, we know, do not have a word for the event. Among the list of possible culprits for menopausal associated disorders are these:

- *diet:* low intake of omega-3 fatty acids, magnesium, selenium, boron and zinc, and of phyto-sterol-rich foods such as beans, lentils, root vegetables, nuts, seeds and wholegrain cereals

- *gender-bending chemicals:* environmental and also cosmetics such as nail polish and deodorants
- lack of physical exercise
- medications, many of which impact the endocrine system
- reduction in the number of pregnancies and the duration of breast-feeding (most modern women, myself included, would rather not think about this one)
- disturbed diurnal rhythms: a function of artificial lighting and travel to other time zones.

Somehow, menopause has become so medicalised in recent years that the terminology begins to imply that it is a medical condition requiring treatment. HRT was discussed in Chapter 2.

The treatment of menopause has two distinct phases. One is the treatment of the symptoms surrounding the menopausal period, and the second is the long-term management of the effects of the alleged hormonal 'deficiency'.

Normal menopause
It would be odd if half the species could expect 20 or more years of post-menopausal life without appropriate defences against memory loss, arthritis, osteoporosis, and the other effects of the alleged hormonal deficiency. It would also be odd if the libido of the male remains intact while local problems in the female genital tract render sexual relations either difficult or impossible.

It seems more likely that the transition from fertility to the non-fertile state was once seamless and the symptoms minimal. What were the factors that kept women from the ill effects so common today?

Oestrogen
The body does not produce one oestrogen; it produces many oestrogenic molecules (Chart 3.6). Predominant among these are oestrone, oestradiol and oestriol, known as E1, E2 and E3 respectively.

While all of these are produced throughout life, oestradiol and oestriol are the main hormones of the fertile years. Oestrone provides women with oestrogen in the post-menopausal years.

Many HRT preparations try to mimic the normal situation by

using oestrone. Some use oestriol, because it is a weaker oestrogen and, therefore, deemed safer. In an earlier edition of this book, I discussed the rationale of various preparations, based on assumptions about which oestrogen does what. My current thinking is that we are not all that certain of the specific functions of each oestrogen, and our neat calculations overlook the following:

- oestrogen sensitive tissues — such as breast — can convert oestrone to oestradiol
- the assumption that oestriol is benign just because it is weak is unproven
- supplemental oestrogen, at any stage of life, raises a woman's SHBG level. As we have seen, SHBG can combine with other hormones, and as such, can remove testosterone from the circulation
- testosterone is both antiproliferative and apoptotic which, in plain-speak, means that it can kill (breast) cancer cells. (This alone is a powerful argument against HRT, and does not look too good for the oral contraceptive, either).

In 2006, the World Health Organisation declared that exogenous hormones — whether as HRT or the oral contraceptive — should be labelled as human carcinogens.[20] In short, I believe that the use of HRT signals a failure to understand the biochemistry and physiology of menopause, and the use of the oral contraceptive for trivial reasons, such as the regulation of periods or to treat acne, is very questionable indeed.

Progesterone
John Lee is an American physician with an unusual view on HRT. He argues that menopausal women are suffering not from a deficiency of oestrogen, but from an excess relative to the amount of progesterone in their bodies.

As menopause approaches, the hypothalamic-pituitary axis (the link between the structure at the base of the brain called the hypothalamus and the pituitary gland, which is suspended from it) continues to stimulate the ovary to produce oestrogen just as it has always done. The ageing ovary is slow to respond, but when it does there is a burst of oestrogen, often quite high. In the fertile woman the formation of the corpus luteum after ovulation triggers a cyclical rise in progesterone, but without ovulation, progesterone remains low. The oestrogen highs, combined with chronic low levels of progesterone, are thought to contribute to the menopausal symptoms.

Although high levels of oestrogen are part of the normal menopausal process, modern industrial chemicals ensure that the menopausal woman of today is floating in a 'sea of oestrogens'. We have already seen that many commercial chemicals degrade to oestrogen-like molecules. Notable among these are the pesticides and plastics whose ability to mimic hormones has given rise to the term gender-bender (Chapter 6).

Progesterone and oestrogen look very similar (see Chart 3.5). An environmental contaminant which could mimic one of these hormones could easily mimic the other. But hormones become active only when they find a receptor site which matches their structure. In chemical terms, oestrogen receptor sites are regarded as 'promiscuous', while progesterone receptor sites tend to be 'monogamous'. Thus environmental contaminants are far more likely to mimic the functions of oestrogen than progesterone. Lee argues that if *imbalance* is the problem, HRT logically should constitute replacement with progesterone.

This idea has appeal, as many of the undesirable aspects of HRT come from the oestrogen component. Moreover, many of the progesterone formulas can easily be delivered as the bioidentical molecule, that is, a progesterone molecule identical to that made by the human body.

If Lee is correct, why does conventional HRT control the symptoms of menopause? Perhaps it does not work by *replacing* oestrogen. As we have seen, just because a substance has beneficial effects, it does not imply that the patient had a deficiency of that substance, even if it is a natural part of the biochemistry. The high doses of oestrogen may act by 'flooding' the system, like the over-enthusiastic use of the choke in an automobile when we are attempting to start a cold engine. Just as the engine can stall in this circumstance, the HRT can turn off the pituitary stimulus to the ovary.

Lee's ideas are interesting but difficult to test. Environmental contaminants may well be sitting on oestrogen receptor sites and creating havoc. They may be mimicking the real thing and promoting cancers. They may be blocking the real thing and preventing it from doing its job. But our commonest measurement tool is the absolute blood level of the wrong oestrogen (E2) and we have no easy measure of activity at the receptor site because of the 'second messenger' functions of minerals like magnesium (see below and Chapter 4). Lee's idea that a bioidentical progesterone is preferable to a synthetic oestrogen-progestogen has merit, but is yet unproven.

Other options

Nature provides plenty of examples of how things were managed before HRT. Asian countries have their share of industrial pollutants — in some places, due to the unscrupulous dumping policies of the First World, more than their share — but menopause appears to cause few problems. What seems to differ markedly are the dietary factors.

- EFAs are anti-inflammatory. Many of the illnesses associated with menopause are inflammatory disorders. Mood swings, depression and memory loss may or may not be inflammatory conditions, but EFAs play a role in the central nervous system (Chapter 5), and the consumption of a diet high in the EFAs should certainly be part of the treatment regime of the menopausal woman.
- Vitamins and minerals all play an important role in the menopausal woman (Chapters 4 and 5). Selenium is possibly one of her best defences against the gynaecological cancers - breast, ovarian and uterine. Magnesium is essential to allow hormones to attach to their receptor sites to exert their effects. Rather than topping up with synthetic hormones, maybe we should be helping our existing hormones to get their message through. Magnesium is also important in the biochemistry of neurotransmitters and other mood molecules and for the maintenance of healthy bones. Boron is also believed to have roles in bone maintenance, memory and the production by the woman's own body of the hormones we are so concerned to 'replace'.

Many of the foods Grandma ate afforded the kind of protection we expect from the Asian diet. Sardines and the selenium they contain helped her avoid cancer, arthritis, and heart disease. Sardines also have Vitamins A and D. The calcium and magnesium in the little bones (now sometimes removed) were all the calcium tablets Grandma ever needed. The cartilaginous material in the joints of those bones supplied her with the glucosamine her grand-daughters now buy in capsules.

Baked beans were Grandma's source of the phyto-sterols, an inexpensive, low-fat source of good quality protein. Westerners who cannot adapt to soy products need look no further than baked beans. They provide the substrate on which the healthy gut flora feed and use to produce their cancer-protective short-chain fatty acids. Nourished in this way, the good bacteria keep harmful ones, like the producers of beta glucuronidase, under control, thus preventing the recycling of potent hormones back into the circulation. Unlike meat as a source of protein, legumes like soy and baked beans do not increase the loss of calcium to the body, thus offering another protection against osteoporosis.

DENTAL HEALTH

Dental health has an intimate relationship with overall health. The person with no teeth is usually confined to eating soft foods and therefore has a limited diet. Even those who can afford good dentures find that eating foods such as apples can be difficult. Some stop eating nuts, because they stick under the plate, and so on. Chronic gum infection — periodontal disease — almost doubles the risk of heart attack and almost triples the risk of stroke.

Here we will discuss three topics concerning teeth that show the characteristics of fixed-name diseases: dental decay, periodontal disease and orthodontics.

Dental decay

Teeth decay when the tooth loses so much calcium from its enamel that it cannot remineralise. The main minerals are the various salts of calcium phosphate, principally as hydroxyapatite and hydroxyfluoroapatite crystals. The greatest risk factor for demineralisation is theWestern diet because of its refined carbohydrates, especially sugar.

Under ideal circumstances, a thin layer of *pellicle* coats the tooth. This is made up largely of salivary elements, but also contains some enzymes derived from normal mouth bacteria.

Saliva

Normally saliva is an ideal buffer solution. It contains bicarbonate-carbonic acid, phosphate, protein, ammonia and urea. It demonstrates one of nature's finely tuned balances. A small amount of acid in the mouth activates digestive enzymes and helps in the defence against fungi and undesirable bugs. A large amount rots the teeth. However, the development of plaque prevents the protective elements such as bicarbonate from reaching the tooth surface.

Saliva flow seems to be one of the best defences against tooth decay. This has been borne out in trials of sugarless chewing gum.

If saliva flow offers protective benefit, we should be asking what promotes the production of saliva? For starters, nothing makes the mouth water like the smell of good food when we are truly hungry. The other great promoter of salivation is vigorous chewing. Because we eat by the clock true hunger is rare, and little of the food consumed by Westerners really needs chewing. The most energetic mastication nowadays is most likely to be the consumption of stick-jaw toffees and candies. The complex carbohydrates our ancestors chewed on not only produced good saliva flow, but also cleaned the teeth and inhibited the development of acid forming bacteria.

Bacteria

Bacteria colonise the mouth from a baby's earliest days. Certain components in maternal milk act as antibacterials. These are thought to assist in establishing desirable bacteria, and prevent undesirable bacteria from colonising. By the age of two or three a child has the bacterial strains which will be with it for life.

The enzymes in the surface pellicle help to maintain the teeth. Problems arise when dietary sugars encourage the bacteria to form excess amounts of a sticky substance called *glucan*. A small amount of glucan is thought to provide a foothold for desirable bacteria such as *veillonella* on tooth surfaces, where they tend to neutralise acid. Once a large amount of glucan is present however, other bacteria, and the acid they produce, become trapped, forming the substance we know as plaque. The damage done by the acid from these bacteria is a result not only of the amount of sugar in the diet, but also of the *frequency* of ingestion. 'Plaque attack' occurs each time we eat foods containing refined carbohydrate.

Over 200 species of bacteria have been identified in the mouths of humans, and the largest mass live on the teeth. At least 92 different strains taken from the tongue have been genetically sequenced. In one study in Boston, Massachusetts, people with halitosis were shown to be lacking in three kinds of bacteria common to the mouths of people with sweet-smelling breath.[21] Presumably when the 'good guys' are missing, the 'bad guys' will predominate. The parallels with bacteria in the rest of the gut are obvious.

Fluoride

Fluoride has been a mainstay of the preventive dentistry. The compulsory fluoridation of town water supplies has been controversial because fluoride in excess poses definite health risks. There is also a matter of principle involved for those who object to enforced medication.

There is little doubt that fluoride helps to reduce tooth decay (although some of those objecting to its use would contest even that statement). It increases resistance of enamel to acid attack, promotes remineralisation, and inhibits the bacterial enzymes which result in the formation of acid. But that protection comes at a cost.

High fluoride intake, occurring when children eat fluoridated toothpaste or otherwise ingest a toxic dose, can cause a condition known as 'dental fluorosis'. This has a mottling effect on the teeth, and is said to be of cosmetic concern only. Acute fluoride poisoning is rare, but can be fatal. It produces salivation, sweating, vomiting, headache, low blood pressure, and possibly cardiac arrhythmias. Chronic toxicity has been associated with allergies, birth defects, cancer and genetic mutations.

These matters are highly controversial, with a small but determined sector challenging the assurances of the various experts. Their concerns are understandable. There is a narrow range between the effective dose of fluoride and a toxic dose. The doses from all combined sources used in the prevention of dental decay represent pharmacological amounts, not physiological. The fact that a substance has a pharmacological benefit does not necessarily mean the substance is essential.

Fluoride is found in very low amounts in maternal milk, a time of rapid tooth development. This suggests that its incorporation into teeth may not be a significant part of the natural process, or at least that only a tiny amount is needed.

In 1990 the American National Toxicology program reported a clear linkage between fluoride and the nasty bone cancer osteosarcoma.[22] Striking primarily adolescents and young adults, this cancer has a high fatality rate and is increasing.

Fillings
In the past one of the main materials used in the filling of tooth cavities was mercury. Although mercury, even in tiny amounts, is highly toxic, there are still those who defend its use, or argue that it is more dangerous to remove amalgam fillings than to leave them in place. Mercury can be removed with safety by a skilled practitioner, and this course of action is worth considering.

Prevention
Despite improvements in the various treatments for tooth decay, prevention is the hallmark of good dental care. This should be primarily a dietary approach for several reasons.

Cost benefits alone would make this worthwhile. Many people spend more on their teeth than they do on the rest of their personal health. Dental care for those most in need is often hard to find. More importantly, the diet which produces dental caries is the same one which contributes to all the other diseases of Western civilisation. This goes far beyond the association between periodontal disease and cardiovascular risk, encompassing diabetes, obesity and many other conditions. Bad teeth are more than a dental problem: they are a symptom.

Perhaps it is not excessive to suggest that all sweets and snack foods carry the same level of warning as a cigarette packet. Diabetes, for example, is not only a fast-growing health problem, but also the second most common cause of blindness in our community (see below, Ophthalmology). Putting fluoride in the water may reduce tooth decay; it doesn't prevent blindness.

The *frequency* of food ingestion has been mentioned. In our society constant snacking is the norm. It is depressing to count the supermarket rows dedicated to sweet drinks, biscuits, lollies and 'snak paks'. Our society grows obese, blows out its health budget and rots its teeth, just for a snack. These snack foods break two rules of good dental health. We eat far more sugar than we should, and we eat it in multiple sittings, thus increasing the opportunities for plaque attack.

The *order* in which food is eaten is also worthy of comment. The Western habit of concluding a meal with a sweet also contributes to dental decay. Foods such as nuts and cheese (see below) offer better protection when they are consumed at the conclusion of the meal.

Many whole foods, such as apples and carrots, contain the sorts of sugars which contribute to dental decay. However, they seem to pose a lesser problem when eaten whole, raw, and as part of a mixed natural diet. So often nowadays they are consumed as juices, or in some other processed form.

What is new?

Along with all the other foreign antigens we thrust on the developing immune systems of babies, there is now talk of *vaccinating* them against the bacteria which cause tooth decay. The effects that this might have on the health of the baby may be imagined. One researcher did admit that 'certain risks' were associated with the prospect.[23]

A second line of research is tackling *Streptococcus mutans*, as discussed in Chapter 6.[24] The plan to *genetically engineer* it so that it does not produce acid, and to introduce the resulting mutants into the mouths of babies before other colonies (finely honed since the early days of *Homo sapiens*) have had a chance to take hold, is a worry. The particular characteristic of these bugs, other than failing to produce acid, is to be *aggressive colonisers*. It appears that they achieve this by producing an antibiotic which destroys all the other bacteria in their immediate vicinity! The researchers do not discuss what might happen should the mutant *mutans* make their way down into the gut and begin a friendly gene-exchange with the gut bugs.[25] How early in life do the scientists propose to commence this process? Before cell differentiation of the immune cells in the gut? Before a potential coeliac has their first exposure to gluten? And just as certain genes increase the risk of coeliac disease, the chromosome 6 class I gene HLA-B27 predisposes to the development of ankylosing spondyltitis and Crohn's disease. Food allergens and organisms such as klebsiella have been implicated. How do we know that this mutant mouth organism may not set off a similar immune process?

Then there is the proposal to create preventive chewing gum. It will be impregnated with casein, or even calf saliva. The casein provides bioactive peptides to bind calcium and phosphate in a form readily available for absorption onto the tooth enamel. The calf saliva provides antibodies and antibiotics against bacteria.

All of these strategies may offer something. However, one could also argue that we should show more respect for the bacterial milieu of a healthy gut, *as it might have evolved in the natural environment*, rather than to introduce mutant strains, antibiotics and foreign antibodies into that environment.

Nature's way

Change of diet is an obvious approach, but there are some other defences as well. The contribution made by the ingestion of calcium, phosphate and fluoride was dealt with in Chapter 4. Other elements such as copper and boron have been thought to contribute in various ways.

In rat experiments the addition of copper to sugar reduced almost to zero the capacity of the sugar to create dental caries.[26] Copper has antibacterial properties, and in these experiments it reduced acid production by the unhealthy bacteria in the dental plaques. Boron is beginning to be appreciated as an important element in human health (Chapter 4) and it has been suggested that boron intake may have a beneficial impact on dental decay. Boron forms a weak acid which may exert antibacterial effects in the mouth. The modern diet is low in copper and boron. Foods rich in copper include nuts, apples and molasses. Foods rich in boron include pears, apples and honey. Molasses even contains traces of fluoride, an irony which does not need expansion. When molasses is refined to produce sugar, those protective agents are lost.

Various studies have shown that some essential fatty acids can inhibit the growth of *Strep. mutans*. Similarly, the effect of certain amino acids is to increase the alkalinity within dental plaque, thus reducing acid-caused decay.[27] Foods such as cheese and nuts may be protective not only because of their mineral content, but also because of their fat and protein content. The virtues of the Stone Age diet, in which carbohydrates had a relatively minor role, may show that our teeth manage a diet high in fat and protein far better than a carbohydrate-based diet. Of course, 'high fat' does not refer to the heated, processed fats that make up so much of the content of the junk food diet.

Certain foods do not contain any of the substances which promote dental decay, some actively suppress the acid-forming bacteria. They are widely distributed across the food spectrum. For example, seaweed, algae and certain fruits and vegetables contain natural sorbitol, which is poorly fermented by oral bacteria. *Strep. mutans* is capable of fermenting it, but produces little acid from it. We can be sure that such foods will not contribute to tooth decay and they may actually increase resistance to decay.

The shiitake mushroom, widely consumed in Asian countries, has some remarkable properties. Both in the laboratory and in real life, shiitake has been shown to protect against caries.[28] The consumption of shiitake appears to increase the amount of non-adherent plaque, and reduce the amount of adherent plaque, with a resultant decrease in caries formation. With the delightful economy of nature, shiitake mushrooms also lower blood sugar.

Fruits, vegetables (and coconut shells and birch trees) all contain a substance called xylitol, which stimulates salivary flow, enhances remineralisation of enamel, and reduces the numbers of *Strep. mutans*. Many sweet things in their natural state have inbuilt decay protection. In nature, bitter often denotes 'poison' but sweet indicates 'edible'. So it is natural that we are attracted to sweet things, but it should not be at the expense of our teeth.

The mineral content of molasses and honey has already been mentioned. Honey has other attributes. Its medicinal properties are discussed in relation to *Helicobacter pylori* in Chapter 10. The possibility that it may be effective against both halitosis and tooth decay is currently under research.

Chocoholics will be delighted to know that their favourite treat may also hold anti-decay properties. Researchers at Osaka University in Japan have found that cocoa beans and cocoa bean husks inhibit the ability of *Strep. mutans* to produce glucan. The active ingredients are also found in other plants, chewed by Africans and other forest dwellers.[29] Of course, sugar-laden chocolate probably negates the benefit. Good quality sugar-free chocolate is not difficult to obtain.

Periodontal disease

The same conditions which produce dental decay also lay the foundation for periodontal disease. In young people, tooth loss is mostly the result of decay. In the elderly, gum disease is the more common cause.

The relationship between periodontal disease and cardiovascular disease continues to attract attention. There has been a move to treat gum disease as a way of preventing heart attacks. The idea is that infection may trigger the rupture of a coronary clot, either as result of bacteria entering the bloodstream or from an immune response to the bacteria. Chronic infection results in the release of inflammatory mediators and cytokines, and these, so the theory goes, may be the last straw in precipitating a vascular event.

However, the same junk food diet produces both conditions. While treating the gum disease is important in its own right, focusing on the last straw in cardiac disease seems to be a case of the tail wagging the dog.

Orthodontistry

It is hard to find someone these days who has *not* worn braces or had some other corrective process. People have their teeth straightened to get the perfect smile. But a lot of orthodontistry is undertaken because of complications from the disposition of the teeth within the mouth. The list is long: sinusitis, snoring, migraine and other headaches, increased wear and decay, and temporo-mandibular joint disorders. Malocclusions and crowding of teeth are often to blame for these.

The 'adenoid face' is well-known in medicine. A high arched palate and dental crowding are associated with infected tonsils and adenoids, chronic sinusitis, and even asthma. Unerupted molars cause abscesses and even osteomyelitis of the jaw. Surgeons and dentists remove tonsils and adenoids, drill sinuses, fit braces, remove wisdom teeth, change 'bites' and perform various other feats, all for valid health reasons.

The number and placing of teeth in our heads seem not to have kept pace with the evolution of the jaw; the size of the jaw seems to be receding. A book called *Nutrition and Physical Degeneration* challenges this.[30] Originally published in 1945, it is the story of a dentist, Weston Price, who had a keen interest in anthropology. He travelled the world, painstakingly collecting photographs of the peoples who consumed the 'primitive' diet. Their teeth and jaw alignment were perfect and every last one had the perfect smile. More remarkable were the photos showing generational variance within the members of the same family or tribal group. Those born after the introduction of the Western diet had obvious decay, which might be expected with the rapid change of diet. Far more remarkably though, they demonstrated the crowding of teeth and narrowing of the dental arch that are so common in the Western world.

This is only one book of photos, subject to all the usual criticisms of field surveys. But it is hard to look at these photos and be unimpressed. Evolution of genes for facial structure cannot occur so rapidly. Diet does not change other features such as skin colour or eye shape. In short, all the characteristics which we accept as needing correction, and which are often present at birth, should probably be seen as *congenital and developmental malformations*.

The most likely culprits when deformity is present are either toxic exposure in one or both parents, or dietary deficiencies in the pregnant mother. Price's photographs were taken long before pollution was widespread. (Alcohol and nicotine may be exceptions. The foetal alcohol syndrome produces a characteristic facial appearance. And I remember seeing a quiz some years ago in which doctors had correctly identified from photographs babies whose mothers had smoked in pregnancy, although many of the doctors believed that they would not be able to tell.) Weston Price claimed that nutritional inadequacy in the maternal diet started to alter the facial features. This effect was then exaggerated by the child's diet: softer food, less chewing, and so on. Indeed, the transition to the Western diet may have induced facial changes so extreme that they could reasonably be classified as birth defects were we not so inured to their effects.

There is good medical rationale for this consideration. Folic acid deficiency, in tandem with some genetic inputs, can produce spina bifida. Hare lip and cleft palate have multiple causes, including a genetic contribution; maternal nutrition is thought to play a part. Even foetal alcohol syndrome may be caused not only by the mother's alcohol intake, but also by her inadequate nutrition.

I said that the implications of his studies are enormous. If diet can have a visible physical impact on facial structure to the extent that it over-rides the genetic template, we should be asking what contribution a nutritionally impoverished diet during pregnancy is having on many other childhood diseases and syndromes.

OPHTHALMOLOGY

If you ask the average person what matters most to them about their health, they usually reply with something that relates to their mental capacity, their vision or their mobility. The ability to think and plan, to see and to get around are the basis of independent living. Even hearing, unless the person is a musician, is often rated after these three.

Less-than-perfect vision can have many causes, such as accidents, infection and Vitamin A deficiencies; the latter are the scourge of the developing world. But in the Western world, the commonest cause of visual impairment in the young is refractive error. For older age groups, blindness, either partial or complete, is usually the result of diabetes or of age-related macular degeneration (ARMD).

Diabetes is discussed in Chapter 8. Until recently, it was thought that little could be done to prevent the development or progression of refractive error or ARMD. Both now seem, in part at least, to be affected by the lifestyle and diet of modern civilisations.

Refractive errors

Refractive errors include *myopia* (short sight) *hypermetropia* (long sight) and a related condition of advancing age, *presbyopia*. Myopia increases with age and thus is the clinically more significant condition.

Refractive errors are common in the Western world, and increasingly being recognised in the developing world. They are believed to be increasing, and are responsible for considerable inconvenience at the very least. In the developed world it is estimated that 30 per cent of people of European descent are affected by some degree of myopia.[31] Mother Nature certainly seems to have been careless here.

In the developing world, refractive errors account for increased morbidity and even death. It has been estimated that up to 100 million people worldwide who would benefit from spectacles do not have them. Moreover, it is thought that 12 per cent of blindness and 55 per cent of visual impairment results from refractive errors. 'In Africa, half of the children in blind institutes aren't actually blind. They just need glasses.'[32] It is thought that early last century fewer than 1 per cent of Inuit and Pacific Islanders were myopic. In places that figure is now as high as 50 per cent.[33]

The problem in both long and short sight is a mismatch between the shape of the lens at the front of the eye and the length of the eyeball.

- *Long sight:* The lens is too flat for the 'shortness' of the eyeball, and the focal point is located behind the retina. These people see well at a distance but require a positive lens in front of the eye to focus on near objects. As the eye grows, the problem often corrects itself.
- *Short sight:* The eye is too long for the 'roundness' (convexity) of the lens, and the focal point falls in front of the retina. A negative lens extends the focus back to the retina. People with this defect can see well at close range, but everything beyond a few metres is a blur.

I have employed the terms 'too flat' and 'too long', but these are subjective. There is in fact no 'right' length for an eyeball, or 'right' bulge for a lens: all that is required is that the two match up. However, this is a precise requirement, measured in fractions of millimetres.

It has been assumed that the inheritance of good or poor refraction involved a gene for the matching process. There is no doubt that genes do play some role in this function, although it is difficult to imagine how the gene actually codes for the required precision.

In the modern world, the problem is relatively minor because spectacles to correct errors are easily available. But without spectacles significant refractive errors are almost incompatible with life. If you cannot see the snake, you will tread on it; if you cannot see the tiger in the jungle, you will become dinner. And if you cannot see the food plants at your feet, you may starve.

One would expect that people with such refractive-error genes would simply breed themselves out. One does not see wild animals stumbling about in the jungle, bumping into things and falling off cliffs, or lining up at the vet clinic for a change of spectacles. Nature, as Darwin observed, is a ruthless culler. (Aquatic animals are short-sighted on land, in order to accommodate the refraction of light in water. Seals sitting on rocks 'squint', using the resulting pinhole effect to filter out the diffracted rays.)

It is hard to explain by genetic means why, in some cultures, so much of the population is now legally blind. In Asia, and increasingly throughout the Western world, obtaining a driver's licence, or even going about the business of daily living, frequently requires some kind of visual aid.

Myopia

It used to be argued that the high percentage of myopic individuals in countries such as China was due to their long history as the world's oldest civilisations. Urbanised cultures can support their visually disabled citizens. There are few snakes and tigers in cities, where nature's tendency to cull is somewhat thwarted.

Myopic people even had a mild selective advantage in such environments. They seem to enjoy close work, even if it is for lack of other options. Scholars are often portrayed as short-sighted in the extreme. Myopia confers a degree of magnification for vision at close range. Myopic people doing needlework or reading fine print usually remove their spectacles. (From my own experience, I can attest to the advantages of myopia when suturing lacerations. Mask on, remove spectacles, face into the wound, microsurgery, no problem!) When decreased flexibility of the lens gives rise to presbyopia in the mid-40s age group, short-sighted people can still read or sew without requiring long arms. Although laser surgery has made it possible to correct refractive errors, many myopics are not prepared to sacrifice the close-range benefits.

It is attractive to argue that, in this manner, civilisation allows 'bad' genes to persist. However, despite an obvious genetic basis to myopia, its prevalence leads to speculation about the interplay between our genes and the environment. There are at least two lines of enquiry.

Discussions about vision suggest that in Asian cultures which valued art, pottery and written text, the gene for close work was perpetuated. In parallel with this was the observation that short-sighted people seemed to be 'brainy'. Were the genes for artistic skill or braininess co-inherited with myopic genes? If you can't see very well, it takes intelligence and cunning to survive. Only myopics with high intelligence lived to reproduce themselves. Less intelligent ones did not. For some time this was the received wisdom. (Various studies to determine an association between intelligence, or giftedness, and myopia have produced widely varying results.)

Another line of thinking said that people who can't see beyond their own nose will naturally develop their abilities, whatever they might be, for occupations which can be conducted at close range.

Recently, a whole new concept has emerged, which might accommodate all of these theories. It seems that when the *rate* of deterioration in myopic children was observed, rather than finding a more or less consistent deterioration as the child grew, the refractive error would remain constant for a while, then drop a 'step', stabilise for a while, then drop again. Remarkably, and all the more so for being unexpected, the periods of deterioration coincided with *school terms*, and stabilisation occurred during *vacation*. School is bad for your eyes!

Far from the genes being 'fixed' in the match they provide between eye length and lens shape, it appears that they *take their cues* from what the eye itself is doing. The eyeball continues to grow until the child stops growing. The lens however, maintains a degree of adjustability throughout life as muscles in the eye act on a relatively flexible lens. This function is known as 'accommodation'. For people with refractive errors, the range of accommodation available to them, while as great as people with normal vision, is insufficient to overcome the mismatch.

The conclusion has been that because children on vacation spend more time out of doors, they accommodate to distant vision and *cue* the growing eyeball to see at a distance, not simply at close range. Today's children start school earlier, learn to read at a younger age, have more expectations placed on them by ambitious parents, and consequently express myopic genes more frequently.

There are several corollaries. Children in less privileged cultures tend to read less. Highly successful parents (possibly genetically favoured for academic traits) encourage their children to read. People who have good distance vision excel at sports, spend more time out of doors, neglect intellectual pursuits, and so on. And with increased urbanisation, there is less open space in which to play. Many parents believe that the outside world is dangerous and keep their children indoors. The advent of television and computers as entertainment simply completes this cycle.

The theory that eyes are cued by the environment receives some support from the people known as the Mokens (living in South-East Asia, especially Thailand) who can see underwater twice as well as European holidaymakers. The Moken live by fishing and diving, and researchers wondered whether selective advantage had resulted in an evolutionary effect in this group. In fact, Moken vision above water was similar to that of the holidaymakers. But underwater, where refraction of light results in relative long sight, the Moken children's eyes accommodated by narrowing the pupils. To *narrow* pupils in this environment is counterintuitive; the normal response to dimness is dilation. But when the dimness was brought about by being under water, the eye took the cue and acted appropriately. These children had also learned (or at least, their eyes had learned) to improve their vision by maximising the convexity of their lenses. This is a natural response to being underwater. What impressed the researchers, however, was the extraordinary adeptness with which these children did this.[34] There is much anecdotal support for the idea that Aboriginal children, and those from other 'primitive' cultures, have superior visual adaptation.

Another theory might explain myopic increases in both the West and the developing world. One research team has suggested that the increase in refined carbohydrates in the diet may be playing a role because it results in a higher output of insulin. This in turn acts as a growth hormone (Chapters 7 and 8) and produces biochemical effects which may interfere with the delicate matching process described above. Experiments are under way to test this hypothesis.[35]

Age-related macular degeneration

Macular degeneration is the leading cause of blindness in the developed world. (The second most common is diabetes. In the developing world, river blindness, trachoma, cataract and Vitamin A deficiency remain the major causes.) The *macula* is that part of the retina which is responsible for central vision. When we look at an object we focus it onto the macula of each eye. Without reception by the nerve endings in the macula, we are unable to read. Peripheral vision, what we see out of 'the corner of our eyes', may be quite unaffected by macular degeneration.

There are two common forms of macular degeneration, often called 'wet' and 'dry'.

- The wet form accounts for about 5–20 per cent of all ARMD. An excessive growth of blood vessels in the area obstructs vision. Diabetic retinopathy is similar. In both

cases the offending blood vessels are treated by laser surgery.
- The dry form is responsible for 80–95 per cent of ARMD. Cellular debris accumulates in the layer known as 'retinal pigmented epithelium', giving a patterned appearance to the retina known as 'Drusen'.

The main risk factors for macular degeneration include increasing age, smoking, high blood pressure and atherosclerosis. Thus, many of the risk factors for cardiovascular disease are relevant (Chapter 8).

Eyes can give direct information on the health of arteries, and even nerves, which in other parts of the body we can only obtain by secondary means. When we introduce a treatment in ophthalmology, we can *see* whether this has stabilised the condition, improved it, or had no effect.

It has been established that the introduction of anti-oxidant supplements — notably zinc, selenium, Vitamins A, C, E, and the bioflavonoids — can stabilise or *even reverse* macular degeneration.[36] The other players in this story are the essential fatty acids. People who eat fish (fresh or frozen) once a week have half as much risk of macular degeneration as those who consume it less than once a month.[37] Suppose this effect was 'cure' instead of 'prevent'. Imagine the headline: 'Doctors cure half of those suffering the Western world's commonest form of blindness'.

This statistic applies to omega-3 fatty acids alone. Add in the anti-oxidants just mentioned. Would the effect be additive? Geometric even? If we were talking about a drug of similar profile, whether for treatment or prevention, the *failure* to employ it could be seen as medical negligence. We are talking about blindness after all, not ingrown toenails. Of course, the supplements should not be used by themselves in preventing or treating this condition. Many nutrients exist in fruits and vegetables, the benefits of which we are only beginning to appreciate. In particular, a group of carotenes which do *not* get converted to Vitamin A appear to be important here, including lutein, zeaxanthin and lycopene, found in brightly coloured fruits, berries and vegetables.

Essential fatty acids, vitamins and trace minerals do not just prevent macular degeneration, as this book has been at pains to demonstrate. When we think in terms of a fixed-name disease, we fail to see illness as a 'systems fault'.

For further reading on the various influences on myopia, see Rachel Nowak's interview with Brien Holden and the article by Matt Ridley.[38]

Chapter Eight

Two Leading Causes of Death: Obesity and Cardiovascular Disease

ALTHOUGH THE PREVALENCE OF THESE TWO CONDITIONS earns them a chapter of their own, obesity and cardiovascular disease are further examples of conditions normally treated by the fixed-name approach.

OBESITY

By the early 1990s the coexistence of conditions such as diabetes, hypertension, raised cholesterol, polycystic ovaries and obesity became increasingly hard to ignore. Stuck for a name, doctors began to label this condition 'syndrome X'. The use of the letter X, symbol of the unknown, is ironic when the causes are all too obvious. The solutions are equally obvious: the Burkitt approach of doubling the size of the patient's stool would probably be all that was required. Yet doctors join ranks with the pharmaceutical companies to promote the idea that the answers lie in a pill.

Syndrome X is now also known as 'metabolic syndrome'. This term acknowledges the existence of the complex and interacting pathways which, in this condition, have become deranged.

The health problems may stem from bad eating habits and

inadequate exercise, but once the problems are labelled a syndrome the patient becomes a victim, removed from responsibility. If we can demonstrate that there is a genetic predisposition to this syndrome (which we, the medical profession, have been at pains to do), then the syndrome is hereditary. And if we can produce a drug, or drugs, to treat this condition, the patient has a hereditary condition which can only be treated by the wizardry of modern medicine. The patient's choices and lifestyle obviously have nothing to do with it. Similarly, asthma has become a Ventolin-deficiency disorder and depression a Prozac-deficiency disorder.

When diet and lifestyle are so destructive that a whole raft of medical conditions ensue, *each* of them an independent risk factor for increased morbidity and death, the time has come to challenge the drug model of health care. We have allowed commercial interests to outstrip public well-being. Products advertised on television as comestibles are things which you would be ashamed to feed the family dog. The voice-over declares, 'Naughty but nice!' But these products are lethal and should carry a government health warning. In the 21st century no one would allow an advertisement for cigarettes as 'Naughty but nice'.

There is no way to overstate the importance of the obesity epidemic. Most of the medical conditions which kill or incapacitate at a premature age occur more frequently in the overweight and the frankly obese. These problems include cancer, cardiovascular disease, diabetes, arthritis and depression. Also in this list are hormonal disorders, ranging from thyroid malfunction to polycystic ovaries, and including menopausal, menstrual, prostatic and fertility problems.

This is not simply a matter of obesity making some medical problems worse, as when excess weight aggravates arthritic joints. The point is that the diet that leads to obesity sets up biochemical pathways which *directly cause* the development of these illnesses.

If we view obesity as a biochemical condition, the accumulation of fat is a side effect. The cosmetic factor may be what bothers the patient, but the medical problems are far greater. Fat is not inert. It is highly metabolically active; once it is on 'overload', fat begins to contribute to the problems which beset the patient. Engineers call this a positive feedback loop. Many medical conditions fit this paradigm, and obesity is an archetype.

The statistics relating to obesity are familiar and depressing: 66.3 per cent of Americans over twenty years old are overweight or obese and approximately $132 billion annually is spent on the direct health costs of obesity in the US. 67 per cent of Australian men and 57 per cent of Australian women are overweight or obese. An estimated 20 per cent of Australian children fall into one of these categories. In the UK the figures for adults are remarkably similar as for Australia but for children, the amount of overweight or obese children rises to 30%. The indirect costs are inestimable. If the epidemic is not checked, the future of health in these and other developed nations is unthinkable.

Many children already have early arteriosclerosis, hypertension and insulin resistance. Some are even being diagnosed with Type 2 diabetes, a clinical syndrome *never* in the past seen in childhood.

Metabolic syndrome

Metabolic syndrome or syndrome X is not diabetes, but it is one of the commonest pathways by which diabetes will develop. Each component is a health risk in its own right. The goals in treatment are to reduce these risks, and to prevent progression to established diabetes. The features which characterise metabolic syndrome are:

- raised blood fats (triglycerides, with or without raised cholesterol)
- insulin resistance (with or without raised blood sugar)
- hypertension.

The cells of the muscles, liver and fat stores are the place to start when trying to understand the metabolic syndrome. Under fasting circumstances, the body's needs for energy are met in the form of liver and muscle glycogen, and by fats (triglycerides) from the liver. Triglycerides, which are important players in the metabolic syndrome story, are discussed presently.

If food has been properly digested in the gut, the proteins are broken down into amino acids, carbohydrates into their component sugars, and fats into fatty acids. Proteins and carbohydrates are absorbed into the general circulation. Fats, by contrast, are fast-tracked to the liver.

Sugar
There are many different kinds of carbohydrates. For the purpose of this chapter, we are discussing refined carbohydrates, such as sugar,

and the breakdown of refined flours into sugars. Sugar can be found in many forms:

- *Glucose:* the basic form of sugar used by the body for energy. Other dietary sugars can be used for different purposes, but many will be converted into glucose for energy. Glucose is also used for the manufacture of important molecules known as glycoproteins, glycolipids and proteoglycans.
- *Sucrose:* the most common form of sugar, as in table sugar. It is a *disaccharide*, made up of two sugar molecules joined together. One molecule is glucose, and the other is fructose.
- *Fructose:* thought to have particular influence in the development of diabetes. Its name shows that it was isolated from fruit, but fruit in fact has quite low fructose content. (Honey, too, is relatively low in fructose, and unless consumed in large quantities these foods are unlikely to be a problem).
- *Lactose:* the sugar found in milk. It is another disaccharide made up of a glucose and a galactose molecule.
- *Maltose:* the other main dietary disaccharide. It consists of two glucose molecules joined together.
- *Glycogen:* not a dietary sugar as such. It is a branched-chain polymer of glucose, formed by a series of enzymes for the purpose of energy storage. The polymer may contain as many as 100,000 units of glucose. The liver can store up to 10 per cent of its weight as glycogen. Skeletal muscles can store only 1 per cent of their mass but because of the absolute mass of muscles in the body they account for approximately two-thirds of total glycogen stores.

Insulin

Insulin plays a critical role in dealing with sugar. It is a hormone-like substance which is produced by the 'beta' cells of the pancreas.

As soon as food starts to enter the circulation, insulin is released. One of the roles of insulin is to facilitate the transport of sugar into all bodily cells to provide their immediate energy supply. Excess sugar is stored in muscle, liver and fat cells, either as glycogen for current energy needs, or as fat for long-term energy storage.

As well as handling sugar, insulin is also responsible for the entry into cells of amino acids from protein, and fatty acids from fats. This explains why a diabetic cannot avoid the need for insulin simply by avoiding dietary sugars.

Amino acids are used for various purposes in the repair and maintenance of tissues (Chapter 3). They are remodelled into new proteins of many types, including enzymes, muscle cells and skin cells. When there is an excess of dietary protein, the amino acids are converted and stored as fat.

After a meal, fatty acids — either from the meal, or previously released into the circulation from the liver — enter muscle and fat cells, also under the influence of insulin. Insulin gives the message that glucose is in abundant supply and should be used as the preferred fuel. It is telling the body that fats and protein can be diverted for the other purposes just outlined. As such, insulin is an *anabolic* hormone, referring to that state when tissues such as muscle are promoted and developed. As an anabolic hormone, insulin stimulates other growth factors, including a hormone known as insulin-like growth factor 1 (IGF-1; Chapter 7). The relevance of these actions to the development of the metabolic syndrome will become apparent shortly.

The state that contrasts to anabolic is *catabolic*, in which tissues are broken down for energy supplies. In times of deprivation or ill-health, survival takes precedence over a fine set of biceps.

As a logical extension of the post-prandial process, insulin also acts to inhibit any release of fat from the liver. After a meal the release of stored energy is unnecessary: the organism is now fuelled by the food it has just ingested.

Insulin resistance

What has been described so far represents the normal state. Insulin rises and falls throughout the day with the intake of food. What happens, however, when the organism is constantly snacking, especially if those snacks are made up of sugary foods and drinks? In this circumstance, the periods in which there is a fall in circulating insulin become shorter. Insulin, as a messenger molecule, conveys the message that there has been a change in the status quo. When a messenger repeats its message incessantly, the recipients tend to become deaf to the message.

Thus the pancreas, honed by evolution to deal with a diet of whole foods eaten at spaced intervals, is presented with high sugar loads at frequent intervals. What does it do? It simply responds to the carbohydrate load in kind, pumping out extra insulin.

At first, the increased levels of insulin achieve the desired effect. Blood sugar levels do not exceed normal, though insulin levels may soar. Eventually however, the cells become 'deaf', and relatively greater amounts of insulin are required to achieve the same effect. This is known as 'insulin resistance'.

After a while, the pancreas simply cannot keep up the supply necessary to remove excess glucose from the circulation. Blood sugar levels start to creep up, whether the person is overweight or not. (Usually, though not always, they are.) Moreover, as liver cells become insulin-resistant, insulin is unable to inhibit the liver from releasing its fats.

Now there is a double problem. Not only are bodily cells failing to pack away recently ingested sugars from a meal, but the liver is spilling out the dangerous fats in the form of VLDL molecules (Chapter 5: Vitamin E; and below, Cardiovascular Disease). These sticky sugars and fatty substances are easily deposited at sites of inflammation. The reasons for this were discussed in Chapter 5: Vitamin E, where the biological purpose of 'bad cholesterol' was explained. The endothelial membranes lining arteries become prime targets. And to make matters worse, the fats are sources of free radicals, adding to the inflammatory damage already present.

Excess levels of glucose cause other problems. As discussed earlier, glucose forms compounds with other molecules, including proteins. Under normal circumstances this is an important function. These compounds are of structural significance in cells and connective tissues as diverse as brain, nerves and joints. Excess sugar, however, can disrupt the maintenance of these glycoprotein compounds. The stiffening of arterial walls and joints, the damage to kidneys, nerves and retina, and the clouding of the lens protein to produce cataract — these are problems for the diabetic which, in part at least, are thought to be due to excessive sugar-protein reactions.[1]

Complicating this picture even further is fructose. As mentioned, it is one of the two sugars making up table sugar. After a meal, fructose — like fat and unlike glucose — is selectively shunted towards the liver. This may be because the liver uses it as one of the building blocks of triglycerides. Whatever the reason, fructose appears to be instrumental in causing the liver to spill triglycerides into the circulation. Fructose is discussed further below, Diets Based on the Glycaemic Index.

Glucose tolerance

As the increased levels of insulin fail to keep the blood sugar in the normal range, the person is said to have 'reduced glucose tolerance'. At this point the patient may still not meet the formal requirements to be diagnosed as diabetic, but they are on the way. Diet and exercise are the key interventions, and in common with treating insulin resistance, should be used preferentially. Certain medications can be used either to boost the production of insulin or to increase insulin sensitivity, but their use signals failure to correct the metabolic fault.

The medical problems

Diabetes

The medical problems associated with diabetes are protean, and in particular occur as a result of cardiovascular disease. The effects are those of compromised blood supply to the end organs, whether kidneys, eyes or nerves. It should be stressed that one of the main aims in treating obesity and metabolic syndrome is to avoid the progression to diabetes and all its complications.

Hypertension

There are various means by which obesity is associated with high blood pressure or hypertension. Lack of exercise alone, either as a cause or a result of the obesity, is an independent risk factor for hypertension.

Raised blood sugar and insulin directly contribute to hypertension in several ways. The process of 'stiffening', or hardening up the arteries by the excess formation of glycoproteins, has just been discussed. As arteries stiffen, resistance increases, and blood pressure automatically rises. With this comes an increased risk of 'blow-out' lesions, one of the causes of stroke, aneurysm and blindness.

Kidney damage, brought about by a similar mechanism, promotes a hypertensive response. Furthermore, as a consequence of the anabolic state induced by insulin, the kidneys retain sodium, contributing to hypertension. Insulin also increases the tone of the sympathetic nervous system, which puts further pressure on the kidneys.

To round off this picture, the stimulation of IGF-1 causes hypertrophy (thickening) of the smooth muscles which regulate the diameter of blood vessels. Thickening and hardening of the arteries is another of the undesirable anabolic effects of insulin. This also favours a hypertensive outcome.

From a lay person's point of view these details may seem insignificant, but they show how these different aspects of the metabolic syndrome feed into each other and contribute to the alarming list of diabetic complications.

Aproximately one in four adults have been diagnosed with hypertension in the US, one in five in the UK and more than one in ten in Australia. In Aboriginal populations this is closer to twenty five per cent. Other factors contribute to these statistics and will be discussed under Cardiovascular Disease; excess insulin brought about by a junk food diet is a significant player in the hypertension story.

Polycystic ovary syndrome (PCOS) and infertility
The definition of the metabolic syndrome does not include these problems, but they are common medical complications of it. They are listed here for completeness, but have been dealt with in Chapter 7.

Dyslipidaemia and fatty liver
One of the criteria for the metabolic syndrome is a raised level of fat in the blood, usually as triglycerides. Cholesterol may or may not be raised as well. The term dyslipidaemia refers to elevation of any of the blood fats, with the probable exception of elevated 'good' cholesterol.

As the Western diet is usually replete with the 'bad' fats, and as dietary sugar is readily turned into these fats, it is likely that such fat will accumulate in both the fat storage cells and the liver. Some of the mechanisms for this effect have already been discussed. The body, already battling an excess fat and sugar load, finds itself in a positive feedback loop. The rise in insulin has been interpreted as it would have been throughout evolutionary history—that is to say, in the presence of all of this abundance, we should store the surplus for future use.

Unfortunately, then, some of the direct effects of insulin are to promote 'unfavourable' lipid pathways. This includes the conversion of protective HDL into the 'bad' fats such as VLDLs. Of course, these pathways are 'unfavourable' only when they are not followed by the expected fast.

Cancer
A 2003 study confirmed what had long been suspected: that decreased glucose tolerance alone was a significant risk factor for death from colon and other cancers.[2] The high levels of circulating insulin seem to act as a growth factor in the development of cancer cells. This is another aspect of the anabolic effect of insulin.

Chapters 2 and 10 discuss the role of dairy and gluten in the Western diet. One of the problems with these foods is their opiate-like activity. Opiates, whatever their source, can deregulate the activity of natural killer (NK) cells. These cells are one of our most important defences against cancer. Once again, the diet which contributes to one problem—addictive eating leading to excess insulin and diabetes—also contributes to other related problems.

A genetic disorder?

The 'thrifty gene'
One of the first steps in turning obesity into a genetic problem was to find a gene or genes that predispose certain individuals to weight retention. In primitive cultures food deprivation was common, so the ability to store energy as fat in times of plenty had a clear adaptive benefit. Like most biological variables, the ability to do this is carried in the genes.

Depending on our genetic makeup, some of us burn calories quickly and are said to have a high basal metabolic rate, or BMR. By contrast, those with the thrifty genes burn calories less easily. For the same caloric intake, they gain more weight. These people are said to have low BMR

But the body is adapted to changes in food supply. To prevent unnecessary weight fluctuation therefore, it *resets* the BMR as intake fluctuates, at least for a modest period of time. Thus dieters may reduce their food intake drastically, and yet see no weight loss for some weeks. As a protective mechanism, the body treats the current weight, *whatever it may be*, as the ideal weight. When food intake drops over days or weeks, the BMR also drops to conserve energy. If intake rises, the BMR also rises. Everyone has this capacity. It is the flexibility of the process, and the rapidity of the response, which is determined by the 'thrifty genes'.

On a shorter time scale — hours during the day, for example — the metabolic rate rises and falls. Exercise and eating both raise the metabolic rate, as does shivering when we are cold. People with thrifty genes may have to exercise more than others to raise their metabolic rate, but it will happen. And conversely exercise, rather than breakfast, may be the sensible way to start the metabolism in the morning. (This is discussed below under The Biochemistry of Breakfast.)

These interactive processes increase the energy supply when we need it, and save it in lean times and when we are resting. They provide energy to perform a task when we have eaten and make us hungry when we are cold. The ingestion of food gives us both immediate warmth and reserves for a possible winter shortage. Most people notice their appetite change with the seasons and know that they 'warm up' once they have eaten and that listlessness disappears after a meal.

Nature's signalling systems are a source of wonder: we interfere with them at our peril. Yet that is the effect of the proposed treatments of obesity. Nature's signals, it is argued, evolved when privation was a constant threat and obesity can be tackled by changing some of these signals. But is this true? Surely in human history there were times of plenty and many Gardens of Eden.

Since the first edition of this book, there have been challenges to any simplistic view of the 'thrifty gene'. New thinking relates to epigenetics (see Chapter 3: Epigenetic Inheritance). As foreshadowed in that chapter, a junk food diet may switch genes on or off permanently. The idea is scarier than simply passing on unfortunate genes. Effectively, we may be creating them by re-wiring normally silenced genes. We know that both Type 1 and Type 2 diabetes have increased. The increase in Type 1 has been linked to the hygiene theory, Vitamin D deficiency, viruses, and gluten and dairy consumption. The Western diet shoulders blame for the rise in Type 2. But now there is discussion of 'double diabetes' and Type '1.5'. With other increases in autoimmune and allergic disorders, epigenetics looks set to take centre stage. In regard to these emerging forms of diabetes, fructose, particularly as high-fructose corn syrup (used in many processed foods) is part of the debate.[3]

The addictive gene

Many overweight people experience genuine hunger despite recent and adequate food intake. Others, however, feel no hunger but eat because they have difficulty in controlling the desire to eat. Such people are thought to have 'addictive personalities'. Alcohol addiction is known to run in families, and there is a general acceptance that some individuals are disposed genetically to develop addictive behaviours of all kinds.

A key suspect for this gene is one which results in a reduced number of brain receptors for dopamine. Certain foods, such as fat-sugar combinations, chocolate, cheese and meat, appear to trigger the release of opiates in the brain, providing some compensation for the reduction in receptor numbers.[4]

Some other genetic factors

Thrifty genes were originally thought to be involved with production of a hormone called leptin (see The neurohumoral loop, below). A whole range of appetite-control hormones has now been uncovered, and doubtless more will follow. It is almost inevitable that variants in the production of these hormones will be found, and each promises to provide another 'genetic cause' for obesity and the metabolic syndrome.

Metabolic syndrome is often associated with the elevation of cholesterol, and almost always with an increase in triglycerides. Predisposition to these elevations is known to be under the control of several genes (see below, Cardiovascular Disease). These genes do not give us raised blood fats and premature cardiovascular disease (with the exception of a few rare homozygous states). They simply increase our vulnerability to the Western diet and lifestyle. Genetic predisposition to both diabetes and hypertension is well known.

No less than 70 genes have been implicated in the obesity epidemic. Far from supporting the concept that it is all genetic, this highlights the difficulty of attributing the condition to genes. If obesity is an unhealthy state, why would there be so many genes for it? Once again, it is not what genes we have which make us sick: it is what we do with those genes which counts.

Appetite control

Many of the approaches to the treatment of obesity will be based on an understanding of why people eat, why they overeat, and why they seem to favour the more 'fattening' foods.

We eat because of hunger, and the pleasure associated with relieving it. Through conditioning we learn to associate the act of eating with pleasure. As a result we may eat for pleasure, even when not hungry.

In societies where there is no certainty about the next meal, a tendency to overeat could be protective. However, a complex control system should be able to adjust to extremes of both kinds. We would therefore assume that there are signals for satiety, just as there are signals for deficit.

Modern research into obesity concerns itself with the cerebral mechanisms of hunger and satiety. If we can understand the signals to which the brain is responding, we might use this knowledge in order to reduce appetite, and thus food intake. Few believe that food intake is simply a matter of responding to hunger signals. But the temptation to overeat is harder to resist when satiety signals are weak. These signals therefore have been under intense scrutiny in recent times.

The neurohumoral loop

One of the first pieces of obesity research to attract public attention was to do with *leptin*, a hormone which is isolated from fat. As fat increases, more leptin is produced. Leptin, it seemed, was responsible for putting the brakes on appetite. By administering leptin, it was hoped, appetite would decline. Unfortunately, this did not happen. Overweight people already seemed to have a lot of leptin, and extra made no difference. It was as if the satiety centre had become deaf to the message of the hormone, just as overstimulated insulin receptors lead to insulin resistance.

This research increased understanding of appetite control. Leptin acts on two kinds of neurones: one which stimulates appetite, and one which shuts it down. Leptin up-regulates the inhibitory circuits, and down-regulates the stimulatory. These circuits are located in the hypothalamus. The hypothalamus is a very old part of the brain that has to do with hunger, thirst, sleep and sex, among other things.

The chemical messengers in this system are neuropeptides, or neurotransmitters. In the 'eat' circuit, the neuropeptides bear forgettable names such as *neuropeptide Y* (NPY), and *agouti-related peptide* (AgRP). In the 'don't eat' circuit, there is a neuropeptide called *melanocyte stimulating hormone* (alpha-MSH).

Enter stage left, *grehlin* and *PYY3–36*, hormones released from the stomach and intestines respectively. Grehlin makes its appearance when you are fasting, and PYY3–36 is there to signal satiety. So now there are several players telling the brain whether we should be searching for food, or whether we should be setting about some other activity.

These neuropeptides are not dedicated to hunger and satiety. Such substances rarely have a single function, and are to be found throughout the brain. In fact, 'appetite' has a cast which includes scores of hormones, neuropeptides and neurotransmitters. There are physical messengers as well. When we are hungry, the sight and smell of food is pleasing. Our gastric juices flow audibly. If we are full, exposure to food is a matter for indifference, or even nausea. Nerves such as the olfactory and the vagus (two of the cranial nerves) transmit information to the conscious and unconscious brain, which interprets and acts on the information. Together these systems are referred to as the 'neurohumoral loop'.

Dopamine and friends

Dopamine, serotonin, GABA and adrenalin are some of the other players in this scenario. Serotonin is related to depression, and alteration of appetite is a major characteristic of depression. Adrenalin mobilises stored energy and suppresses appetite: hunger would be a distraction during a flight-or-fight response.

Another influence on appetite is *dopamine*. Under normal circumstances dopamine suppresses appetite. Dopamine production is deeply connected to the pleasure circuits in the brain. Its presence signals feelings of contentment, satisfaction, sexual pleasure, reward and general well-being. Perhaps those who continue to eat after an adequate intake do so to prolong the release of dopamine, despite the satiety message.

Indeed, most of the substances of addiction exert their addictive effects either by stimulating neurones to release (and deplete) their stores of dopamine, or by mimicking the action of dopamine at the receptor sites. When certain activities, or the use of certain substances, begin to dominate life, one might be said to be addicted. The so-called runners' high refers to the 'addictive' aspects of the normal pleasure associated with healthy exercise. Excess exercise can be likened to the use of food to give pleasure at a level beyond that required to sustain life.

There has been controversy as to whether the word addictive can be properly used of activities such as eating. This was highlighted in two lawsuits: one was known as the 'cupcake trial' and the other was a mass action by several obese people who blamed their condition on the manufacturers of fast food. Few will be unaware of the latter, which is still before the courts. And when a former police officer shot dead the mayor and one other in San Francisco, he was found guilty of 'involuntary manslaughter' on the grounds that a large number of sugar-laden Twinkie cupcakes had produced hyperglycaemia and a loss of impulse control.[5] One might say 'Only in America ...', but for how long?

From a biochemical point of view, these lawsuits raise some interesting issues. Are the addictive properties of junk food any less reprehensible than those of nicotine, if they share the same biochemical pathways and cause the same amount of disease in the community?

There is one group of obese patients who do not seem to eat much junk food. In Chapter 2 we saw that healthy foods may contain opiates, and milk and wheat seem to be main culprits. A diet free of dairy and wheat (or gluten) often results in significant weight loss with no caloric or other restrictions in place.

Interconnections

As scientific endeavour unravels the workings of hormones, neurotransmitters and other chemical messengers, it becomes apparent that all of these complex systems are highly interconnected. People will report a loss (or sometimes an increase) of appetite when they are under stress, getting the flu, pregnant and so on. But none of these circumstances are new to the human species. Why do we have an unprecedented epidemic of obesity and its related ills?

Perhaps it has to do with a confusion of signals. If we drink a lot of water or eat an entire head of lettuce, our stomach stretches and we feel bloated, but this only reduces our hunger in the short term. A chocolate bar may meet or exceed our caloric needs, but still leave us hungry because the stomach still feels empty. The ideal meal is neither a bowl of lettuce nor a chocolate bar, but one which provides clear signals such as 'stretch' and 'energy value'.

At this stage of research, we can conclude that the neurohumoral loop is responding to a variety of cues. Foods which are slowly digested, such as fat and fibrous food, seem to promote the satiety signals. One researcher in this field has suggested that the modern refined-carbohydrate diet gives the poorest of signals in producing appropriate appetite-control messages.[6]

Appetite leads us to make food choices that can have far-reaching effects. As in a game of chess, the movement of one piece on the board changes the entire dynamic. To play the game successfully, we have to watch the whole board. In arguing about the semantics of addiction and proposing drug treatments, perhaps we are just playing with the pawns. What is missing in our culture, either at a social or a biochemical level, which prevents us from producing enough dopamine? Dopamine-production is one of the job specifications of the normal healthy brain. All of our endeavours, at some level, should make us feel good, or relieve uncomfortable feelings. The basic pathways for dopamine production are outlined in Chart 3.3.

If our diets attained some sort of ideal proportion, if we began to exercise properly, would we be able to enjoy social drugs, pleasant behaviours and good food at an appropriate level for survival and recreation, regardless of our 'addictive' genes? Or perhaps are we suffering from some brain damage as a result of exposure to toxic chemicals such as PCBs, lead and mercury, and we are actually self-medicating with food, alcohol and drugs?

Primitive cultures, animal experiments and general observation indicate that the nutrient-deplete Western diet should shoulder a fair proportion of the blame.

Nutrients

Animal experiments have shown that it is easier to induce alcoholism in rats fed on junk food than in those on a good diet.

Zinc
At low levels, zinc deprivation seems to direct the search for food, especially tasty food. In Chapter 3 we saw that when rats were fed a low-zinc diet the deprived animals became obese in comparison with their lean litter-mates. The role of zinc in appetite control has been noted by several observers. In his book, Bryce-Smith comments: 'We feel that there is a large amount of evidence that anorexia (nervosa) has a nutritional basis and that zinc is the critical nutrient involved' (Chapter 4).[7]

But zinc's function as an appetite regulator is complex. Extreme zinc deprivation induces anorexia. This was noted by Dr Archie Kalokerinos in his work with Australian Aboriginal children in remote parts of Australia (Chapters 4 and 5). The introduced diet of tea, white flour and white sugar was low in zinc. When these children developed minor infections, they would quickly lose their appetite. Minor infections sometimes even led to death. Zinc supplementation not only restored appetite, but more often than not it enabled the immune system to fight off the illness.

In a similar manner, Kalokerinos found that it was easier to sober up, and keep dry, Aboriginal adults thus supplemented. He regards the failure to treat this population in such a manner as another 'missed opportunity' of Western medicine.

Tragically, in many areas, this low-nutrient, refined diet is still prevalent today. Along with social deprivation that is the shame of 'the lucky country', diabetes, hypertension, renal failure and addiction affects more than 25 per cent of the Aboriginal population. At Alice Springs, a major indigenous centre, the renal dialysis unit is one of the largest in the country. Renal failure is one of the worst outcomes of metabolic syndrome and subsequent diabetes.

It is almost half a century since Kalokerinos first alerted an uninterested government to the perils of malnutrition in regard to both child and adult health, and the benefits of prescribing supplements as simple as zinc and Vitamin C. In 2006 he was continuing to actively spread this message to a still uninterested medical and political community.

In the midst of plenty, many young people we know are eating poor diets. Junk food renders them both overweight and deplete in nutrients (including zinc). At the same time, there is a cultural expectation of thinness. Often the most nutrient-dense foods are the first to be excluded in any weight-loss diet. Deficiencies of zinc and other micronutrients are quickly compounded. True loss of appetite develops, with all the deranged thinking we now associate with eating disorders. Much of that psychopathology is a result of the deficiencies, but a feedback loop has now been established. No zinc, no appetite, poor diet, no zinc.

'Pica' refers to the habit of eating strange foods, and even dirt. In Western medicine it was often seen as a sign of mental illness. The prophetic truth in this assessment has long been overlooked. Pica is discussed in Chapter 10. Pregnant women often exhibit bizarre food choices which, like pica, may signal an urgent requirement for zinc and other nutrients.

Chromium

Chromium can reduce sugar cravings. When we crave sugar, Mother Nature is telling us we need something like chromium. She is *not* telling us to go out and consume refined white sugar and white flour. Foods that contain chromium include nuts, seeds, whole grains, cereals and legumes, molasses (and dark chocolate). The cravings may signal a need for these nutrient-dense complex carbohydrates. Chromium helps deal with the carbohydrate load that comes with these whole foods through its apparent capacity to increase insulin sensitivity.

In combination with nicotinic acid (Vitamin B3), chromium not only has this vital function, but also produces favourable profiles of blood lipids. Importantly, this has been demonstrated in both Type 1 and Type 2 diabetes, and in hypoglycaemia. Of particular interest has been the potential for benefit in gestational diabetes. Indeed, the cravings of pregnant women may well suggest more than zinc deficiency.[8]

Chromium has even been shown to exert a modest effect in the conversion of fat into muscle, a beneficial feature in the diabetic and obese patient.

Junk food diets produce wide oscillations of blood sugar levels. A drop in blood sugar is read as hunger, although it may simply mean that the blood sugar has fallen from high to normal levels. The hunger signal, however inappropriate, then mobilises adrenalin. In our snack-happy society it takes only a moment to rip the plastic off a candy bar, and we have responded to that alarm signal in a way that perpetuates the vicious fluctuations in the glycaemic cycle.

Therefore, at a time when we are eating less of nutrients such as chromium than ever before, we have a greater need for it, to increase insulin sensitivity so that our metabolism can respond to these unprecedented fluctuations of blood sugar.

(However, nutritional medicine is fraught with controversy. The improved insulin sensitivity, along with the modest conversion of fat into muscle, led to some extravagant claims by promoters of body-building and weight-loss products that chromium was a 'fat-blaster'. Before long, researchers opposed to natural medicine had 'proved' that chromium was carcinogenic. So far, none of these studies have survived closer scrutiny.)

A discussion about appetite control has led us back into the discussion on diabetes. Both chromium and zinc have a role, and this convergence is exactly what nutritional medicine is all about.

Selenium and manganese

Selenium is of crucial importance to the pancreas. It has been shown to prevent pancreatic cancer and to be effective in treating acute pancreatitis. Pancreatitis (which can be fatal) is often caused by alcohol abuse or viral infection, but in many cases the cause cannot be determined.

Manganese deficiency alters carbohydrate metabolism through the destruction of the beta cells of the pancreas. Manganese deficiency has also been associated with pancreatitis. Manganese is found in nuts and unrefined cereals. As with chromium, zinc and selenium, manganese is found in the outer part of the grain, making for deficiency syndromes when grains are refined. Thus, a diet of white bread, white sugar and pasta is, by definition, lacking the very nutrients nature provided to protect us from the pancreatic stress of the starches and sugars of these staples.[9]

The EFAs and vitamins

EFAs reduce cholesterol, bring down blood pressure and favourably affect hormonal disorders (Chapter 5). Vitamin E and Vitamins C, B3, B6 and B12 have all been shown to benefit various aspects of diabetes.[10] Some of these effects are believed to be preventive, as well as having value in alleviating complications.

An iatrogenic disorder?

There is an interesting possibility that obesity may be another problem to which the medical profession itself is contributing. In Chapter 3 we saw that helicobacter, the subject of much medical intervention, has recently been described as 'one of man's oldest and closest friends'. Even more recently, research has suggested that infection with *Helicobacter pylori* in childhood may protect against later obesity by disrupting appetite-related hormones in the stomach. And related studies have shown that people treated to eradicate helicobacter gained weight when cured. The researchers commented on the overall decline of helicobacter in developed countries as a possible reason.[11] The effects of improved appetite when ulcers are cured cannot, of course, be discounted.

THE MEDICAL RESPONSE TO THE OBESITY EPIDEMIC

Mother Nature used mineral-rich and sweet flavours to advertise nutrient-dense foods. When industrialisation made it possible to extract the sugar from the pill, we were confronted by the enticement minus the benefit.

Education about diet and lifestyle is established as a treatment for the metabolic syndrome. Medical institutions are beginning to speak against the advertising of junk food in children's prime television time, for instance. However, political reluctance to upset industry is instanced by the fact that the Australian minister for health was able, at the end of 2005, to say that if people did not like advertisements for junk food they could turn off the television. Emphasis is being placed on exercise. But often diet and lifestyle are given no more than a perfunctory nod. We assume that people already know about them, that they have been tried and failed. We do not take the time to explain that these are the keystones and any other treatment options are merely additive.

Drugs

Like the various mood disorders, the metabolic syndrome has contributed to the phenomenon of drugs in search of a disease. Here are some of the pharmacological 'solutions'.

Preventing the absorption of fat

The drug Xenical is designed to block the enzyme *lipase*. If fats cannot be digested by lipase, then they cannot be absorbed. Patients using Xenical experience gaseous, fatty and foul-smelling stools when they eat fatty foods, which 'reminds' them to eat properly. Unbelievably, this is promoted as a benefit.

But fats, such as the good oils and the omega-3s, are important for health. Many vitamins are fat-soluble. If we argue that compulsive eating may be a sign of nutrient-depletion, artificially purging the body of its ingested fat may only make the underlying problem worse.

A person using Xenical may well lose weight, but may also increase their risk of other problems. We have seen that diabetes is the second commonest cause of blindness in the Western world. Vitamins A and E, which are fat-soluble, are needed for good vision, for preventing the complications of diabetes and so on. The prevention of the *commonest* cause of blindness, macular degeneration, also depends on vitamins such as these. There seems little benefit in substituting one cause of blindness for another. Again, we are playing with the pawns.

Raising the basal metabolic rate

The model for raising the BMR is thyroxin, the thyroid hormone which in excess causes weight loss. A serious attempt to use thyroxin or its look-alikes is regarded as risky, because it has dangerous effects on the cardiovascular system. This has not prevented research into developing a drug along these lines.

Altering fat metabolism

This 'solution' aims to develop a drug to increase the quantity or efficiency of natural molecules, called 'uncoupling proteins'. Enhancing these is supposed to liberate food energy as heat, instead of using it to make fat. Such an approach belongs to science fiction, but scientists are making the attempt.[12] It is easy to hazard the guess that serious side effects would be likely.

And as mentioned at the beginning of Chapter 6, researchers at the Baker Heart Research Institute in Melbourne felt that, as they now understood how *exercise* lowered cholesterol, they could work on a *drug* to do the same thing.

Appetite regulation

With so many hormones, neurotransmitters and nerves involved in appetite control, it is hard to imagine that altering one or two of them will achieve the desired effect. Also, we can assume that those people who eat for comfort would continue to ignore satiety signals. If intake were to be controlled by drugs, consumption of missing nutrients might sink even further.

The drug naloxene has been shown to have some effect in binge eating. (This drug blocks opiate receptors; it is often used by emergency crews for drug overdose.) As with the other drug approaches, one feels that somehow we are missing the crucial issues.

Increasing insulin sensitivity

Drugs such as Metformin (Chapter 7) increase insulin sensitivity. This is not unreasonable, but exercise achieves the same result. Drug prescription should not be the first line of attack.

'Hyperliving': a new disease

The discussion so far has been about prevention of sorts. But the current treatment is to deal with the medical consequences of bad diets.

One of the earliest medications promoted as a treatment for the metabolic syndrome was the class known as ACE inhibitors. ACE stands for *angiotensin-converting enzyme*, and this drug aims to lower blood pressure via part of the adrenal-kidney axis known as the renin-angiotensin system.

One such ACE inhibitor is trandolapril, sold under the trade name Gopten. Its intended market was the overweight, hypertensive patient, who apparently suffers from a condition named, incredibly, 'hyperliving'. As an example of the type of person likely to be suffering from 'hyperliving', the manufacturers used a photograph of a group of executive-type, obese men sharing a joke. The drug is designed 'for those patients who can't or won't change their lifestyle'.

It seemed that the joke was on the executives. The side effects of ACE inhibitors include cardiac arrhythmias, angina, myocardial infarction, cerebral haemorrhage, transient ischaemic episodes, hair loss, bronchitis, and even the often fatal Stevens–Johnson syndrome. There are good indications for ACE inhibitors. We have to ask if hyperliving is one of them.

The statin group of cholesterol-lowering agents can also have severe side effects. Of those who take them, 1 per cent or more experience *each* of the following: arthritic pain, muscle pain, flu-like symptoms, raised enzymes associated with muscle-damage. More rare are severe allergic reactions, hepatitis, and the possibly fatal rhabdomyolysis (Chapter 2). There should be no misunderstanding about these medications — they can and do save lives, but vitamin pills they are not.

Surgery

Surgical measures for obesity include a range of options from 'skin tucks' through to liposuction and stomach stapling. The less said about these the better. I think this approach should be a last resort, given the number of healthier, safer and more effective options.

Nutrition and lifestyle: a better response?

Changing how people live is one of the medical profession's toughest jobs. In Chapter 7 we met Gudrun and Hans, who want a baby. Faced with the option of drawn-out and expensive fertility treatment or no child at all, people are capable of remarkable readjustment.

Exercise
Early in this chapter (Obesity: The Biochemistry) I pointed out that the best place to begin to understand the metabolic syndrome was in the cells of the muscles, liver and fat. This is where excess energy is stored, and the responsiveness of these cells to insulin is at the heart of treatment. Exercise increases insulin sensitivity and gives us an opportunity to break into the vicious cycle in which hyperlipidemia and hyperglycaemia beget further hyperlipidemia and further hyperglycaemia.

A common mistake is to think that large amounts of exercise are required to lose even a few pounds of fat. This is not the point. The aim of the exercise first and foremost is to *correct the metabolic fault*—specifically, to raise insulin sensitivity. This is what obesity clinics are trying to achieve with drugs such as Metformin. Just as fat accumulation was the side effect of bad diet in the first place, the weight loss at this stage should be viewed as a *beneficial side effect* of the exercise.

Exercise on its own is unlikely to solve the problems of the metabolic syndrome. Patients need to understand that it is one of the two main pillars of treatment. The other, of course, is diet. Let us look at some of the proposed diets.

The Stone Age or rotation diet
The so-called Stone Age diet is thought to represent human food intake prior to the agricultural revolution several thousand years ago. It is often regarded as the ideal reference point. The food, of

necessity, is always fresh, always in season. It is picked when there is an abundance, and so you are eating the ripest, and therefore the most nutritious, specimens. They are low in salicylates because they are never harvested when green. And yet there are enough — Nature's aspirin. Particular foods are available for only part of the year. These two features, ripeness and rotational intake, reduce the risk of food allergy.

This diet might have varied from place to place, but if we assume that *Homo sapiens* arose in Africa, the diet would have consisted of fruit, root vegetables, edible plants, nuts and seeds, honey, eggs, and the meat of wild animals. As human migration spread, groups living near the sea added shellfish, fish and sea vegetables.

Over several thousand years and several hundred generations, local adaptations emerged. This was reflected in genetic mutations which either *required* these local conditions to prevail or at least were tolerant of them. For example, the prevalence of the gene for haemochromatosis (iron storage disease) implies that where dietary iron deficiency was prevalent, those with this mutation had a selective advantage.

Therefore, it might be safer to assume that there are several ideal Stone Age diets. With this proviso, it can be useful to consider the Stone Age diet as an ideal norm. This diet is often used by various practitioners to treat a range of medical problems. Absent almost entirely from the Stone Age diet are cultivated cereals, dairy products, alcohol and sugar.

Diets based on the food pyramid

Often, Western dieticians use a food pyramid as their guide when recommending healthy diets. The staples form the basis of the diet (the bottom of the pyramid), and they usually fall into one or more of the following groups:

- the grass family (or cereals) such as wheat, rye, oats, barley, amaranth, quinoa, corn and rice
- starchy roots and tubers such as potatoes, taro, arrowroot, yams and cassava
- legumes such as beans and lentils
- miscellaneous starches such as tapioca and sago (which is derived from the trunk of a palm tree).

In a diet endorsed by the US Department of Agriculture in the 1990s, 6–11 servings a day is the recommended intake from this group. The next group up the pyramid consists of fruit and vegetables. Here the recommendation is for a daily intake of 3–5 servings of vegetables and 2–3 servings of fruit. At the next level, we find 2–3 servings of dairy and 2–3 servings of all other proteins (meat, fish, eggs, etc), lumped together. The small apex for 'sparing use' contains fats, oils and sweets. The placement of the fruit and vegetables is appropriate, but the division of protein into equal proportions of dairy and 'other' is questionable, to say the least. There is a case to be made for accenting fish, nuts and legumes over farmed meats on the grounds of both health and sustainability.

It has been customary for food pyramids to be modelled on American ones, but a 1999 Australian version shows some improvement on the one outlined above. There is now a three-tier arrangement, which sees fruit, vegetables, legumes and nuts moved into the botton layer with the staples. However, in the middle layer, which is protein only, dairy — to my thinking — remains over-represented, and the placement of nuts and legumes in the bottom layer has obscured the fact they, too, are legimitate sources of protein. At the top, all fats, oils and sugars remain a single 'use sparingly' category, with no emphasis on the good oils.

Diets based on these pyramids, with the provisos noted, could be healthy. But there are other problems.

Most Westerners replace the variety of staples with just two: wheat and potato. More often than not, the breads and pastas are made from white flour. Rice, when eaten, is polished. Most potato is consumed as fried potato chips.

In the West, most complex carbohydrates come from the grasses, but these are relative newcomers to the human diet. Of the grasses, wheat, refined as white flour, predominates. Ancient wheats, such as spelt and kamut, were low in gluten. Of the commonly consumed grasses, only corn and rice are gluten-free. In following the current food pyramid, we are adding significant loads of gluten to the human diet. Refinement adds insult to injury.

Chapters 2 and 10 draw attention to the fact that several foods have been associated with the development of Type 1 diabetes. The clearest evidence for this comes from the association between diabetes and coeliac disease. If gluten intake can increase the risk of Type 1 diabetes, there might be implications for Type 2. See comments under: The 'thrifty gene' (in this chapter).

We believe that the genetic distance between any two individuals in a culture is greater than the mean distance between any two cultures. But we don't know how much of this relates to food. Most racial groups have interacted and adopted each other's dietary habits over long periods of time. Particular cultural groups show evidence to suggest medical consequences of dietary differences.

There is a high incidence of coeliac disease in Hungarians and Celts. Aboriginal peoples throughout the world are vulnerable to diabetes and hypertension when they consume a Western diet. This is thought to reflect not just their level of social deprivation but a genetic component as well. We know that many racial groups lose the capacity to digest milk after infancy, while others do not. Genes for salt retention and iron storage suggest an environment in which iron deficiency was a threat, or where salt retention conferred benefit.

In most cultures, diets have been based on what was available locally. The possibility that we should have diets tailored to fit our genetic make-up is discussed in Chapter 10: Blood Group Diets.

Such co-evolution is reflected in the animal world. Alpacas, bred for thousands of years in the Andes by the Incas, have a natural diet low in protein but high in the minerals found in the sedge grasses which grow at high altitudes. Fed a diet high in protein and suitable for horses, such as lucerne hay, they develop liver problems (similar to the metabolic syndrome) and may die. Animals tend to evolve in parallel with their food supply. The difference within a species may be subtle, perhaps the code for just one liver enzyme. But in health terms, this difference may be vitally important.

If we are to have a 'one size fits all' pyramid, one scientist, Walter Willett, chairman of the department of nutrition at the Harvard School of Public Health, has come up with the best one I have seen. (He points out that the food pyramid usually used as the standard is supported and promoted by the US Department of Agriculture.)

Exercise is at the base of his pyramid, reminding us of the role of exercise in achieving insulin sensitivity and healthy cholesterol profiles. On top of that are whole grains (including gluten free cereals such as corn) and various plant oils. Abundant fruit and vegetables make up the next layer (so much for low-salicylate diets, Chapter 10), with legumes and nuts on top of that. Fish, poultry and eggs come next, and above this dairy *or some other* calcium source. At the top, in the tiniest segment, lie red meat, butter, white rice, pasta, sweets and potatoes (so much for the GI diet, below). And he adds 'multiple vitamins for most'![13] My main argument with this pyramid would be the placement of the potatoes, which I would include with all the other vegetables. Nor does it take into account other cultural diets.

Diets based on the glycaemic index (GI)

The GI diet draws heavily on the standard food pyramid, and so my concerns about the food pyramid also apply to this diet. The GI diet is based on the idea that if carbohydrate sits in the gut for long enough before it is absorbed, blood sugar will only rise slowly, and insulin output will be diminished.[14] A food is listed as having a low GI if it has a high ratio of a starch called *amylose* over another starch called *amylopectin*. Amylose is more difficult to digest, and thus is more slowly absorbed.

Also, the process by which some foods are prepared makes them inherently more 'gluey' and thus more difficult to digest. This also contributes to a low GI. Pasta is made from wheat high in gluten (it falls apart in water if it is not), and this gluey ball is harder to digest. (In fact, many patients complain of bloating after a pasta meal. This apparently signifies a beneficial feature.) Thus, pasta has a low glycaemic index and is deemed a good food for people with Type 2 diabetes.

Slowing down absorption reduces insulin output, but we could ask whether we should be eating these foods at all. Put another way, if the Western diet is the problem, why aren't we changing it?

If overeating is in any way a consequence of nutritional depletion, as I have argued, it has to be remembered that white flour and polished rice have lost most of their zinc, selenium, chromium and Vitamin E. What message does the hypothalamus get about nutrient status from this low-GI glue? What capacity is there to make our own dopamine when we are deficient in zinc or selenium? Bloating, as we know, is not a deterrent to ingestion for the morbidly obese.

Gudrun on the GI diet

Gudrun is depressed about her fertility problems (Chapter 7). But the lack of zinc, selenium and EFAs in her diet have not only contributed to her polycystic ovary syndrome, they are also perpetuating reduced levels of serotonin and dopamine. Nature recognises the deficiency and instructs her to seek food. As it's not yet mealtime, she has a cappuccino and a couple of chocolate biscuits. Sugar gives a brief high, the act of eating releases some endorphins, and the opiate-like substances in milk and wheat sustain the repetitive, or addictive, behaviour. The caffeine is addictive in its own right. Only the chocolate has anything going for it (it is rich in chromium and magnesium) and yet this is the bit she will feel most guilty about.

Gudrun's weight remains up, Hans tells her he loves her anyway, and she comforts herself with the fact that most of the women in her family look like her, so it must be genetic. Meanwhile the doctor sends her to a dietician, who gives her a booklet about the GI diet. She stops at the supermarket on the way home, walks past the potatoes and apricots and bananas, and stocks up on pasta, bread, low-fat cheese, and sugar-coated Frosties. They're in the booklet.

A few months later Gudrun goes back to the doctor for a check-up. She has been eating low GI foods and has lost a few pounds. She still is not pregnant, and she is still depressed. At a biochemical level, what is happening? The pancreas, despite the low GI intake, is challenged immunologically by gluten and dairy, and continues to struggle in the face of persisting deficiencies of chromium, selenium, magnesium, zinc and EFAs. The diet has improved her insulin resistance, but there's still no evidence that she is ovulating.

Gudrun doesn't want Metformin or anti-depressants. She is concerned about what these drugs might do to her baby, should she become pregnant. She wants to know if there's something 'natural' that she can try. It seems unfair for us to criticise the advice given by her doctor or the dietician. Both have acted in good faith, relying on the received wisdom. The research behind this wisdom is being conducted at the teaching hospital where they were both trained.

Why did Gudrun avoid the potatoes, apricots and bananas? Because the booklet said that, although these foods (like brown rice) are classified as low-GI, they have a higher GI than the foods she has purchased. But these nutritious foods come with a nice mix of things such as bran, raw starch (slowly absorbed, low GI, ideal substrates for the essential gut flora) Vitamin E, selenium, zinc and chromium. A perfect formula, one might have said, for your average diabetic.

Oddly, Frosties (sugar-coated cornflakes) appear in the booklet's list of 'Top 100 Low-GI Foods'. And M&Ms, candy-covered chocolates, are allowed, so long as they are not consumed more than once a day. In fact, their GI is better than that of the brown rice or the banana. But it gets worse. GI listings are given for: white chocolate, Milky Bar; chocolate butterscotch muffins, made from packet mix; chocolate cake made from packet mix with chocolate frosting; Coca-Cola (which has the same GI as a banana!); Coco-Pops; condensed milk, sweetened—and that's just some of the 'food' that is under consideration.

Now it has to be said that many of these are listed as relatively high GI. My point, if it's not already abundantly clear, is that it is surprising that the authors of this list, who are said to be nutritional scientists, even dignified these products with the title 'food'.

Potatoes, a staple of many cultures since the Stone Age, are off the list unless they are 'small' and either 'new' or 'canned'. Gudrun can have corn (let's hope it's not genetically modified) and the ubiquitous pasta. Or maybe she should just eat Frosties and be done with it.

The booklet favours fructose because it causes only a slow rise in blood sugar. This is not surprising because, as discussed above, fructose is fast-tracked to the liver. Apparently it doesn't matter about the increase in triglyceride production or the risk of fatty liver, just as long as the GI is low. Since this book was first written, the news about fructose has become a whole lot worse. Gudrun may choose the Coca-cola over the banana, not knowing that it is made with high-fructose corn syrup. In 1970, Westerners consumed half a pound of fructose a year. By 2003, that figure had increased to 56 pounds. The use of fructose allowed foods to be labelled 'sugar- free'. What do the authors of the GI diet books have to say about this? Of two books current at 2008, one makes a brief reference to fructose, and the other does not even list it in the index. In view of the growing concerns, this is a serious omission. As well as diabetes, fructose is now linked to heart disease, hypertension, fatty liver and epigenetic changes. Interested readers are referred to the listed references.[15]

To summarise my concerns with the low-GI diet: once again symptoms are being treated as if they are the disease. The Western diet makes us fat; it raises our insulin and blood sugar levels. Fructose raises glycaemic levels only slowly. So we consume fructose, lower the blood sugar, and we've fixed the problem, haven't we? No, we have only interrupted some of the metabolic problems. Jump leads may get the car started, but to fix the problem it needs a new battery.

The CSIRO Total Wellbeing Diet

In 2005 a book by this name was released in Australia.[16] It received a lot of press coverage and quickly went to the top of the bestseller list, where it stayed for a long time. The goal of the diet is weight loss, but as the title implies, the secondary aim is good health. The book was co-written by Dr Peter Clifton, the research director for nutrition, obesity and related conditions at the Commonwealth Scientific Industrial Research Organisation, the nation's chief scientific research body, which endorsed the diet.

Fish appears on the menu about every second day. Meat, as chicken, lamb or beef, appears every day. Bread and cereals (complete with trade names in several cases) appear daily in some quantity. Approximately 400 grams of dairy, often in a concentrated form such as yoghurt, is recommended every day. Tinned fruit is recommended more than once in a one-week plan. On almost no single day does the diet meet the two serves of fresh fruit and five serves of fresh vegetables now recommended internationally. Breakfast is substantial (for further comments on breakfast, see below).

Since first writing this section, I have watched with interest for reactions from nutritional scientists. Among others was a 2008 newspaper article headed, 'CSIRO's best-selling diet ignores cancer concerns'.[17] It revealed that the CSIRO board had received two reports protesting work by three of its own scientists who had established that diets high in red meat and the milk protein casein (promoted by the diet) increased bowel cancer risk. Any assessment of this diet should also take into account the funding acknowledgements (in small print) at the front of the book. Among the six entries are Dairy Australia, Goodman Fielder (makers of bread, breakfast cereals and other farinaceous products), and Meat and Livestock Australia.

Diets based on the 'good breakfast'

Breakfast like a king, lunch like a peasant, and dine like a pauper.

It's common to hear that 'breakfast is the most important meal of the day', that it 'gets your metabolism going'. These mantras have the quality of an urban myth.

One of the commonest problems encountered in the Western lifestyle is eating by the clock. We teach our stomachs to accept food when they are not hungry. Mealtimes are dictated by our busy schedules, so we override the biorhythms that would normally control appetite. And as we are eating to a timetable, we learn to bolt our food. Almost all overweight people are fast eaters.

Researchers, as we have seen, place much emphasis on satiety signals, yet few patients have been instructed in the simple basics of experiencing these: eat only when you are hungry, sit down to eat, chew your food until it is almost liquid, and so on.

When we are seriously hungry, we begin to feel a sense of relief as soon as we start to eat. The sense of urgency begins to abate almost before the food hits our stomach. We might go on to eat quite a large meal, but there is a degree of satisfaction signalled to the brain by the act of chewing itself. Even eating chewing gum can, at least in the short term, alleviate hunger.

Eating to a schedule, particularly eating breakfast, reduces the opportunity for the signals both of hunger and of satiety. The food is not properly digested, giving rise to many gut disorders. Breakfast may have benefited the manufacturers of pharmacological agents used to treat ulcers and indigestion, as well as the dairy industry and the manufacturers of breakfast cereals. I am less certain of the benefit to my patients.

Breakfast has achieved iconic status. If I am to tell patients to ignore what their cardiologist, diabetologist, dietician and family doctor all agree on, I have to give good reasons for doing so.

The biochemistry of breakfast

Insulin resistance is the end result of continuously high levels of circulating insulin. In the West, we rarely fast. Breakfast is meant to be the breaking of a fast. During that fast, our insulin levels should have fallen, stayed low until all the food is absorbed from the stomach, has entered and left the circulation, and has been distributed to the cells of the liver, fat and muscles. During this time, the cells of those organs have minimal exposure to insulin, and thus maintain their insulin sensitivity.

Suppose two individuals eat the same high-calorie diet. One is a grazer and spreads the meal across the waking hours; the other eats it in two sittings, with a long gap between the last meal of the day and the first meal of the following day. The first individual develops insulin resistance and a fatty liver, but the second stands a good chance of avoiding these complications. Why?

Throughout human evolution, hormonal influences developed to tie in with various circadian and diurnal cycles. Hormonal patterns and the impact of various activities can now be studied by laboratory measurement. One of the hormones of interest is DHEA or dehydroepiandrosterone.

DHEA is made from cholesterol, and it is a precursor to all the oestrogens and testosterones we produce (Chart 3.6). Taken as a medication, it is a banned drug for Olympic athletes because it increases their performance and is deemed to give them an unfair advantage. It is also known as a longevity hormone. Pathological states aside, DHEA levels are an indicator of the health of the individual. According to Ray Kearney, an immunologist from the University of Sydney (and a member of the delayed-breakfast brigade), contracting our eating hours by having a late food start to the day improves our DHEA output and appears to reduce cancer risk.

We produce DHEA in opposition to growth hormone and the glucocorticoids. High levels are reached in the early hours of the morning, as these other hormone levels fall. The rise in DHEA production is stimulated by bright sunlight, so it makes sense to be out of doors then. With our first meal, further glucocorticoids are produced and the DHEA surge is suppressed. The longer breakfast is delayed, the longer the DHEA peak lasts and the greater the overall output.[18]

Early-morning urine has a high concentration of DHEA. It is probably for this reason that some monks drink a glass of their own urine first thing in the morning. (Should we suggest this practice to Olympians?)

The health benefits of the overnight fast include both the restoration of insulin sensitivity and the optimisation of DHEA production. Less quirky than consuming odd drinks and easier than undergoing long fasts is simply delaying breakfast until hunger asserts itself. Take a morning jog to complete the picture.

Further support for 'no breakfast' came from a report in *The Lancet* that normal children were unaffected or performed better without breakfast.[19]

This all happened as a matter of course for our primitive

ancestors. They ate at dusk, and finished the meal around the campfire. Without artificial lighting they were finished with food relatively early in the evening. Although they arose with the sun, there is good reason to believe that some time elapsed before they ate. Stored food would be eaten by small animals, or would attract large animals to which the humans were also prey. Almost all food was fresh (with all the attendant health benefits), whole, and acquired by work. They had to find, even hunt, kill and cook breakfast before they could eat. Maybe they snacked on a few nuts and berries as they went. You worked first, ate second. You burnt energy, and then replaced it. We do the reverse. We eat first, pre-emptively fuelling *in case* our supplies run low. The price is called the metabolic syndrome.

Even a few thousand years ago, when many of the storage problems were solved, 'cooking' breakfast meant building a fire in an oven—and maybe finding the wood first. It also meant eating when food was abundant. Always, there would be times of privation, of fasting.

So the 'fast' broken by 'breakfast' was of the order of 15 hours. From a metabolic point of view, this constituted a true fast. As blood sugar levels fell in the early hours of the morning, adrenalin and cortisol surged to give an alarm signal. This is known as the 'morning cortisol surge'. It is often accompanied by a period of intense salivation and hunger. Most people will have experienced this at some stage. As the appetite-suppressant effect of cortisol kicks in, and the glucose-releasing effect of adrenalin mobilises liver glycogen, the ravenous feeling quickly abates.

In nature, this was the signal to get up and commence the business of finding food. Nowadays, such a signal indicates the need to pour boiling water on instant porridge. If people actually listen to their bodies, they will find that this 'hunger' is transient. If they start moving about and delay eating, they often find that the next hunger pangs do not occur until several hours later.

Today we may be eating as late as 10 o'clock at night (snacks before bed), and as early as six or seven in the morning. Many people in the Western world never really experience a fast, or even the sensation of hunger. The signal they interpret as hunger comes from a fall in blood sugar. On a Western diet, it is far more likely to signal a drop from a pathological sugar level to one which is acceptable. Unfortunately, the body will still interpret this as hunger, because in its evolutionary history it has never had to deal with such a situation.

In a primitive society, the baby was usually strapped to the mother's body and slept most of the time. When it became hungry, it woke, cried, was fed, and went back to sleep. It has been said that in a primitive society this cycle might repeat itself more than a hundred times in a day. As the baby grew, the cycles got longer. In today's modern hospital environment, mothers are encouraged to get their babies onto a feeding 'schedule'. The baby — let's call him Harry — may be woken from sleep to feed.

The gastrointestinal tract slows down during sleep. Gastroenterologists suspect underlying pathology if patients have to wake at night for a bowel action. A baby who shows disinterest in feeding during a sleep cycle is labelled a slow feeder, and a bottle of milk (cow's milk in all probability) is thrust into its mouth. Perhaps Harry has 'colic'. Shall we try colic or reflux medication first? So Harry learns to eat by the clock.

Harry grows up and goes to school. There are a few tantrums over breakfast but he will usually eat it if you give him Coco-Pops or Frosties. 'At least the milk will do him some good'. Come the weekend or school holidays however, and it is not until 11 o'clock (with my four children you could almost set your watch by it) that children appear in the kitchen with protestations of being 'starving'. And they seem to be willing to eat food that usually they would reject.

Suppose we feed them, and then wait to see when the next wave of hunger will strike. Usually it will be between four o'clock and sunset. The volumes they can put away at this hour are astonishing, and good food is avidly consumed. We can thank their biological hunger clock for that. But what about term time? Then when they come home from school 'starving' at four o'clock, we fob them off with milk and biscuits (dairy and gluten) so they won't spoil their appetite for dinner. By six or seven o'clock they have gone off the boil, and they only eat their pumpkin and spinach under the threat of missing out on the ice-cream cake (dairy and gluten).

Of course, very young children often need frequent feeding. My point is that if children resist food, at breakfast or any other time, this should be respected. Rather than bribing them to eat with sugary cereals, we should simply wait until they *are* hungry, and offer them only good food.

Many people comment that in modern life it is impractical to 'eat when hungry'. The problem is often one of mindset. I have patients who take rolled oats to the office and cook and eat them at morning tea. Others go to work earlier, do half a morning's work, and then go out for breakfast.

CARDIOVASCULAR DISEASE

Cardiovascular disease covers a wide spectrum of medical disorders. Heart attacks, high blood pressure, aneurysms, clots and strokes are the best-known examples. Nearly all of these problems come down to the same basic pathology. Through one means or another, arteries, veins and capillaries have become diseased. As result, one of two things can happen:

- Normal blood supply to and from an organ can become compromised, leading to injury to the organ.
- A diseased blood vessel may rupture, again causing organ damage and possibly destroying tissues in the adjacent region with leaking blood.

In terms of preventive medicine, the strategy to deal with any aspect of the cardiovascular spectrum is the same: to look after the health of blood vessels.

What can go wrong?

Blood vessels
There are three kinds of blood vessels: arteries, veins and capillaries. Let us look at them in turn.

- *Arteries* can become rigid through a process known as plaque formation. This occurs when there is a build-up of fats, especially low-density lipoproteins, and inflammatory material between the endothelial (inner) lining of an artery, and the adjacent muscle layer (see below). Calcium — often visible on X-ray — settles in these plaques and increases arterial rigidity. The general term for this condition is atherosclerosis, although 'arteriosclerosis' is also used. The arteries become increasingly hardened and narrowed, so that blood has trouble getting through. Sometimes one of the plaques in the wall of the artery bursts, causing clots to form. The debris which is released succeeds in blocking the artery either at the site, or further down.

- *Veins* have much thinner and more elastic walls than arteries. They undergo less wear and tear because venous blood circulates at a lower pressure than arterial blood. But because of this lower pressure, and because of the many alternate routes blood can take when travelling through the venous system, blood flow in the veins can become sluggish. Lack of movement, as in convalescence or long-haul aeroplane journeys, can result in circulation so slow that large clots form in a short space of time, sometimes with lethal consequences. It is probably more appropriate to regard this as a result of the coagulability (thickness) of the blood than as a problem of the vein itself.

- *Capillaries* are the tiny network of vessels where the smallest end-point arteries join up with the smallest of the veins. This is the point, so to speak, where the blood turns around and begins its journey back to the heart and lungs. The capillaries are fragile and easily broken. It is capillary rupture which is responsible for bruising. Certain illnesses, notably diabetes and nicotine sensitivity, may sometimes target these small vessels and produce conditions collectively known as 'microvascular disease'.

Pressure problems

One of the commonest health checks is the taking of blood pressure. It is a quick and simple test and can warn of health risks long before problems occur. High blood pressure, or hypertension, can exist in normal vessels or in vessels damaged as above. This is a highly interactive process. A rigid artery by definition is likely to raise the pressure inside it. As the pressure in an artery rises, wear and tear occurs. Most problems of hypertension relate to arteries, large and small.

Hypertension can be primary or secondary:

- Primary hypertension is sometimes also called essential hypertension. ('Essential' in medicine usually means that we don't actually know the cause.) Essential hypertension seems to be confined to those cultures consuming either a Western diet, or a diet high in salt (sodium). We look at salt below.
- *Secondary hypertension* occurs as a consequence of illness, most notably renal disease. Sitting on top of the kidney is the adrenal gland. This gland is no bigger than the top of your thumb, but it has several functions vital to normal existence. One of these is that it acts as a sensor for blood pressure. When the adrenal gland senses low blood flow to the kidney (say, as a result of atherosclerotic disease in the renal arteries) it interprets it as blood loss. In an ideal world, this would be the most common cause of diminished blood supply to the kidney. On sensing that renal arterial pressure is low, the adrenal gland produces a hormone called *angiotensin*, which redirects blood to vital organs. This ensures that organs that cannot tolerate any diminution of flow, such as the heart and brain, are maintained until the bleeding is staunched. Organs deemed less essential include muscles, skin, and the kidney itself. So when reduction of blood flow is due to causes other than blood loss, the potential exists for a vicious cycle. Renal disease begets reduced blood flow begets renal disease. Many anti-hypertensive agents work by antagonising the effects of angiotensin. Others (the diuretics) aim at clearing the salt and fluid from the circulation, and thus reducing the overall pressure. Still others work by different mechanisms which will not be pursued here.

Salt

Salt is so important that only minor variations are compatible with life. It is as easy to kill a person with *hyponatremia* (low salt in the blood), as with *hypernatremia* (too much). Our bodies have extraordinary mechanisms for salt regulation. When we consume too much we feel thirst and excrete salt through the kidneys. When we are low in the stuff we have salt cravings and renal salt retention.

There are genetic and racial variances in how we handle salt. Often genes are blamed for hypertension, but some interesting studies have indicated that hypertension may result from a genetic predisposition to retain salt. There are various evolutionary advantages to this. Salt retention helps the blood flow respond (haemodynamic response) to physical stress. When blood levels of salt are low, we are less energetic. When the diet was naturally low in salt, salt-retaining genes had a selective advantage.

Salt retention was also an advantage for people in hot climates where a lot of salt is lost to the system through sweat. Australian Aboriginals may well have benefited from such genes in long treks across the desert. On the Western diet, these people suffer from kidney disease and hypertension at a rate unparalleled almost anywhere in the world.

Another advantage in salt retention is that it confers resistance to diarrhoeal disease. Diarrhoea can cause prostration and even death because of loss of sodium. Populations living in the tropics have a long history of exposure to conditions such as cholera and typhoid. These racial groups often share with the Australian Aboriginal a predisposition to salt retention, and the same risk of hypertension.

Australians of Anglo-Celtic descent also seem to have an unexpectedly high incidence of hypertension. This could relate to a cultural indulgence in salty foods. But there is also the interesting proposition that, in the early days of white Australia, the people who arrived had survived the long voyage out from Britain. Death on these sea voyages was most commonly due to diarrhoea, so those who had salt-retaining genes were more likely to survive the journey.

It is generally accepted that salt retention was an advantage because the primitive diet was typically low in salt. In fact, this statement represents only half of the truth. The hunter-gatherer diet was not only low in sodium, it was also high in potassium. Potassium is vital for normal physiology, and is abundant in fruit and vegetables. The ratio of potassium to sodium in a fully natural diet is estimated to be 5 to 1—that is, five potassium atoms to every one sodium atom—*at the very least* (Chapter 3). Unprocessed fish and meat has a potassium-to-sodium ratio of 5 to 1, but most fruits and vegetables are 50 to 1 or even 100 to 1. That is not a misprint. This starts to make sense of the fact that animals find the taste of salt attractive.

Mother Nature wanted to make sure that we got enough of the stuff.

But things have gone badly wrong. In the Western diet, there is a reduction in fresh, potassium-rich foods. Salt is added to most processed foods, even things as basic as bread. So now the ratio of these two elements has reversed and we are eating twice as much sodium as potassium, meaning that, at the *minimum*, our intake is a tenfold alteration from the optimum ratio. Low potassium, as well as high sodium, is believed to contribute to the cardiovascular problems resulting from the Western diet.

Blood pressure tablets which work by enforcing loss of sodium through the kidneys can also cause a loss of potassium. Although most doctors prescribe potassium supplements to go with this medication, this a complicated solution.

Metabolic disorders
Various medical conditions are associated with an increased risk of cardiovascular disease. Some, though not all, of these exert their effects through interruption, partial or complete, of the blood supply. Autoimmune disorders and various hereditary conditions can make the blood thicker (more likely to coagulate). This can result in clots and the complications discussed below.

The effects of diabetes on blood vessels have been mentioned. Raised blood sugar gives rise to a cascade of events involving several hormones and many biochemical pathways, all of which have a negative impact on the cardiovascular system.

Sometimes a noxious agent, such as a virus, a chemical toxin, or even the effects of radiation, damages the heart muscle directly, giving rise to a condition known as *cardiomyopathy*. Deficiencies of essential nutrients can also cause cardiomyopathy. Alcoholism gives rise to chronic deficiencies in B-group vitamins, zinc, magnesium and selenium. Alcoholic cardiomyopathy is the end result of poor diet and alcohol poisoning. Areas where soils are low in selenium have a high incidence of cardiomyopathy, as we saw in the studies on Keshan disease in China (Chapter 4).

Selenium has effects on several metabolic pathways involved with the inflammatory process. Inflammation in heart disease is discussed shortly. Selenium as part of glutathione peroxidase (Chapter 3) is important in heart disease because it helps combat the oxidation of lipids. It is also important to the degradation of hydro-peroxides, which generate dangerous amounts of free radicals and damage the endothelium of blood vessels. When discussing the EFAs in Chapter 5, I commented that the prostaglandins were important in the cardiovascular system. One of these prostaglandins is known as *prostacyclin* which helps dilate coronary arteries (see below, EFAs). The accumulation of hydro-peroxides inhibits the enzymes which produce prostacyclin. High levels of hydro-peroxides also stimulate the production of a substance known as thromboxane, which causes arteries to constrict and platelets to clump together, increasing the risk of clots. Selenium helps prevent these problems.

Magnesium deficiency affects the cardiovascular system at many levels, as mentioned in Chapter 4: Minerals. Once upon a time intravenous magnesium was used in the acute situation to stabilise 'twitchy' heart cells and electrical circuits during a heart attack. Then a wide range of drugs came in and magnesium was all but forgotten. Many of these drugs have toxic side effects, notwithstanding some of their obviously life-saving properties. It is interesting to see that magnesium once again is being used in some intensive care units around the world to treat arrythmias.

Even more interesting is another possibility. Could chronic low-grade magnesium deficiency be unmasking some of the dangerous 'inherited' conduction defects? These defects are responsible for sudden cardiac death in healthy young adults and include syndromes such as 'Wolff–Parkinson–White syndrome', 'long Q-T interval' and mutations in the gene for potassium transport. They may even be responsible for some cases of cot death. These conditions, with a clearly inherited predisposition, are increasingly diagnosed, and represent abnormal genetic variants with life-threatening implications. Are we now diagnosing more of these defects simply because we have the tools and the awareness? Or is the modern diet, deficient in EFAs, magnesium and selenium, along with considerations such as the unbalanced ratio of potassium to sodium, unmasking conditions which in the past were relatively benign?

The harm caused by lowered intake of magnesium is not confined to one aspect of heart disease, such as a conduction defect. Magnesium status affects the production of stress hormones like the catecholamines and cortisol (Chapter 4), and stress has an undisputed relationship with blood pressure and heart disease. Magnesium deficiency is associated with a deleterious effect on the 'bad' fats and their carrier proteins.[20] So it does not make sense to use a drug to lower cholesterol without a full understanding of the status of magnesium and the rest of the biochemistry involved.

Patients with potassium transport defects have been known to benefit from potassium supplements. In a bygone era, when potassium intake was high and sodium intake low, would the gene for this condition have been considered a defect?

Finally, under the heading of metabolic disorders, there is the vexed question of blood fats and related risk factors. High cholesterol, high triglycerides and high plasma homocysteine are all relevant to this discussion. The received wisdom is that the cholesterol and other fats are the noxious agents. But there is a counter-argument that they are only markers for an underlying metabolic problem. Is the underlying problem, in fact, the real 'bad guy'? This will be discussed in more detail presently.

The clinical picture

Cardiovascular disease, if neglected, can wreak havoc either by blocking the blood vessels or by causing them to rupture.

Blockage
A good example of arterial blockage is one type of stroke, known as *ischaemic stroke*. The word 'ischaemia' means 'a lack of blood supply'. In this case, the artery simply closes over, so that blood, and therefore oxygen, cannot get through. The tissue supplied by that artery dies because of lack of oxygen, and because waste products are not removed.

A well-known example of blockage is coronary artery occlusion, also known as 'a coronary'. The artery gradually narrows as plaque builds up. When extra demands are made, as during exertion or emotional events, the heart does not get an adequate blood supply to meets these demands. The patient experiences heart pain, or angina.

Sometimes one of the plaques contributing to the blockage ruptures, turning a relative block into an absolute one as clots form at the site. This leads to what we know as a heart attack. The bit of heart muscle supplied by that artery will be damaged, and may even die. Some parts of the heart are more critical than others. If they contain some of the electrical circuitry of the heart, such injury can quickly lead to fatal arrhythmias. There are various kinds of arrhythmia, but the essence is that the heart beats irregularly, or one part beats out of time with another, and blood flow becomes ineffective. Sudden death is the most feared consequence. This is an example of 'water water everywhere, nor any drop to drink'. The heart, which is pumping blood to every other part of the body, misses out itself.

Sometimes small arteries, such as the tiny vessels inside the kidney, become blocked. This causes kidney damage and eventual failure. This process is the basis of renal failure seen in diabetes. High sugar levels and the poor lipid metabolism which go with the diabetic process often result in atherosclerotic injury to blood vessels, both small and large. Blockage in the arteries of the eye can cause retinal damage and blindness.

Sometimes small vessel blockage is caused by debris (by then known as 'micro-emboli') emanating from a ruptured plaque further back in the artery. This is another cause of stroke and blindness.

In contrast to arterial blockage, venous blockage is usually caused by blood coagulating. The result is known by a variety of names, including venous thrombosis, thrombophlebitis, phlebothrombosis and deep vein thrombosis (DVT). The main clinical problems occur when a piece of the clot breaks off and lodges further downstream, causing a problem such as a clot in the lung (pulmonary embolus). Sometimes the clot can be in a small vessel, such as the retinal vein. Retinal vein thrombosis also can cause blindness.

Rupture
Rupture of arteries can lead to catastrophic blood loss and death. The most obvious example of this is rupture of the aorta, also known as a 'dissecting aneurysm of the aorta'. An aneurysm is essentially a blow-out of the inner lining of an artery, much like the inner tube of a car tyre. Blood tracking between the inner tube and the outer wall is on a path to nowhere. Blockage by the collapsing inner tube complicates things further. There are varying degrees of severity of this condition, but death is a common outcome.

Sometimes the rupture of an artery (usually one much smaller than the aorta) causes local damage. The best example of this is when a small artery in the brain bursts, and the escaping blood puts lethal pressure on the surrounding brain tissue. This is the other major cause of stroke, and is known as a *haemorrhagic stroke*. About 30 per cent of all strokes are haemorrhagic. (There is a rare cause of strokes called 'Circle of Willis haemorrhage', which has a strongly genetic basis. An artery in the brain has a weak structure at a branching point, predisposing the victim to catastrophic bleeds. It is probably the commonest cause of stroke in otherwise healthy young people, especially males.)

High blood pressure and diabetic damage to small vessels can both lead to haemorrhage in the retina. This is a common causes of blindness, especially in older people.

With some exceptions, venous rupture is usually well tolerated by the body. An exception to this occurs with 'portal hypertension'. Portal veins carry blood between the gastrointestinal tract and the liver, and ultimately, the rest of the venous blood. The veins at the base of the oesophagus are part of this system, and when circulation is poor they are referred to as oesophageal varices. Liver problems, caused by alcoholism or viral hepatitis, can increase pressure in the portal circulation. Sometimes large blue superficial veins on the abdomen give a clue to portal hypertension.

An alternative view of prevention and treatment

It is not possible here to give more than an overview of the 'health' approach to cardiovascular disease. However, despite the distinct profiles of various cardiovascular conditions, it is still worth thinking about them in the general terms described above. The rationale is that to prevent or treat one cardiovascular problem is to prevent or treat most of the others.

If we work through the factors leading to cardiovascular illness, it is surprising how much of it is within our control. We will look at these factors under the following headings: genetics; inflammation; EFAs; cholesterol, triglycerides and genes; and B-group vitamins and the homocysteine story.

Genetics
It may seem odd to begin a discussion of controllable factors with genetics. The genetic contribution to cardiovascular disease is real, but I hope the following will show that genes do not write the script.

Inflammation and heart disease
Recent research has moved the spotlight on atherosclerosis away

from cholesterol and onto inflammation. Inflammation is a normal response of the immune system to a wide range of insults (Chapter 4). The inflammatory process underpins every step in the development of atherosclerosis, from the development of plaques which line the arteries through their growth to their ultimate rupture.

A discussion of 'good' and 'bad' cholesterol follows shortly, but the traditional view has been that an excess of 'bad' cholesterol accumulated on the inner lining of arteries, resulting in a fatty build-up on this inner surface. Eventually the artery would become so clogged that blood would not be able to get through. The current view is that the 'bad' cholesterol actually *penetrates* the inner lining, in the process of plaque formation that was outlined at the beginning of this discussion.

It may seem strange for excess fat to do this, until one understands the function of so-called 'bad' cholesterol. This cholesterol, also known as low-density lipoprotein (LDL) cholesterol, transports essential lipids and proteins to any cell within the body which needs them for growth or repair (Chapter 5: Vitamin E). It also combats infection. At low levels, LDL can pass easily in and out of membranes. In excess, it tends to become stuck.

Once stuck, LDL molecules can begin to undergo the process known as *lipid peroxidation*. Discussed in the context of selenium and Vitamin E (Chapters 4 and 5), this term equates to free radical attack, often likened to the rusting of metal on exposure to air and water. The body interprets peroxidation as a danger signal, and other inflammatory cells enter the site to join in the fray. The smooth muscles in the artery wall also engage in the battle, producing further inflammatory chemicals and attracting more immune cells to the site. In short, the LDL, part of a normal repair response, has now become the enemy, and a vicious cycle has begun.

A diet rich in oxidised fats, one lacking in anti-oxidants, or health conditions which increases inflammatory processes *anywhere in the body* — any of these factors can act as precursors to the situation just described. Smoking, chronic infection, raised blood sugar, obesity, and even angiotensin II (the hormone mentioned in association with hypertension) are all well-known agents of the inflammatory process. For these reasons, the measure of an inflammatory marker called C-reactive protein, or CRP, is increasingly seen as a better indicator of cardiovascular risk than

374 THE GOOD BODY GUIDE

such intermediaries as cholesterol readings.

The role of Vitamins C and E and other nutrients as anti-inflammatory and cardiovascular protective agents has already been dealt with.

Essential fatty acids (EFAs)

In cardiovascular disease there are several mechanisms by which EFAs, including the fish oils, can offer a protective benefit:

- They are anti-inflammatory by virtue of the production of the anti-inflammatory PG-1 and PG-3 series (Chart 5.3).
- They provide structural flexibility by their incorporation into lipid membranes, thus resisting the hardening, sclerotic process and facilitating egress of excess LDL from within the intimal lining.
- They act as anti-arrhythmics.[21] This effect is believed to arise from the modulation (decrease) of calcium ion flux into the cardiac muscle cells. EFAs are a simple and productive intervention for both benign and dangerous arrhythmias. One of the commonest causes of death after a heart attack is arrhythmia.
- They have a role in the transcription and expression of many of the genes relating to lipid metabolism.
- They facilitate cholesterol transport.
- The prostaglandin prostacyclin which is released from the lining of arteries acts on the underlying smooth muscle cells of the arteries to induce relaxation.
- Prostacyclin also acts on adjacent platelets, reducing their 'stickiness' and preventing blood clotting. This function in part explains why Inuit people on a diet high in marine lipids have almost no atherosclerosis (but they do have an increased risk of haemorrhagic conditions).

Both of these last effects are clearly protective against the risk of atherosclerosis. Interestingly, this prostaglandin is from the PG-2 series, normally associated with inflammatory disorders, making the point that there is no 'bad' EFA.[22]

Cholesterol

Is cholesterol the 'bad guy' or not?

Cholesterol was introduced in Chapter 3 because it is an important molecule. We make all our sex hormones from it, not to mention other hormones such as cortisol, the stress hormone, and cortisone, our own anti-inflammatory medication. It is structurally important, and can be found throughout the body and the brain. Cholesterol, in fact, is so important to us that if we stop eating it altogether, our liver makes up the deficit by producing more of the stuff.

And there's 'good' cholesterol, and 'bad' cholesterol. Even the most conservative cardiologists agree on that. So what is the issue?

There are many factors in this complex situation, and one is the type of carrier proteins to be found in our bloodstream. These are known as *lipoproteins*, and will be discussed presently. Mutations occur in the genes that code for lipoproteins, or for their relevant receptor sites. These mutations can result in familial lipid disorders, ranging from mild to nasty.

People commonly blame their genes for their risk of cardiovascular disease, but the genes for most of these disorders have been around for a long time. In post-war Britain and Europe the rate of cardiovascular disease plunged dramatically. The rationing of sugar and dietary fats, along with increased exercise as a result of petrol rationing, are good places to start looking for answers.

As many people continue to see cholesterol as the most dangerous substance in the body, it is worth paying attention to it. However, the fats known as the triglycerides share a lot of their transport and chemistry with cholesterol, and should be considered as part of the same narrative. Traditionally they have been regarded as less dangerous than 'bad' cholesterol, but this may be because it is easier to bring down raised levels (see below).

To understand cholesterol, one has to understand the proteins or transport vehicles that carry it, and the other fats, around the body. These proteins, with their attached fats, are the lipoproteins just mentioned.

Lipoproteins were introduced in Chapter 5 in the discussion on Vitamin E, which is important to their metabolism. They originate in the small intestine and the liver, and include VLDLs, and HDLs. Another group are known as *chylomicrons*. Once out in the circulation, lipoproteins can pick up other small protein particles, known as *apolipoproteins*, to become 'mature' forms. From this point, most VLDLs will evolve into intermediate and low-density lipoproteins (LDLs).

Lipoproteins can be divided into two broad groups on the basis of the main apolipoproteins they contain:

- The presence of apo A-1 identifies HDL or 'good' cholesterol.
- The presence of apo B identifies 'bad'.

It is the responsibility of HDL to carry cholesterol *from* body cells back *to* the liver, where excess can be disposed of either directly as cholesterol, or via the formation of bile. HDL is usually referred to as 'good' cholesterol, and is thought to represent the unoxidised form of cholesterol.

VLDL and LDL are responsible for carrying cholesterol and the other lipids *from* the gut and liver *to* the cells in the body as needed for various functions. An excess of such molecules indicates an increased cholesterol burden. In this form cholesterol is likely to be in the oxidised form, increasing the risk of free radical damage to tissues which come into contact with these molecules. Thus, the theory goes, high levels of HDL indicate that disposal function of the system is working.

High levels of the other two mean that a lot of cholesterol is being absorbed from the gut, or that an overloaded liver is spilling excess cholesterol into the circulation. As generalisations go, these would seem to be reasonable assumptions. But as always with something as complex as biochemistry, separating cause and effect can be difficult.

Many studies have shown that high levels of 'bad' cholesterol do not always correlate with ill-health. Conversely, heart attacks and strokes can occur in people with normal blood lipid levels. In fact, most heart attacks occur in people with normal lipid levels.

Furthermore, some cultures with a diet high in saturated fats do not have high rates of atherosclerotic disease. The French diet is one such, with a high content of butter, cream and cheese. What is often overlooked in such an analysis is that high dietary intake of fresh fruit and vegetables potentially provides all of the anti-oxidants needed to protect the cholesterol from becoming oxidised. When there are high levels of LDL, if most of it is carrying fats that are not oxidised, the risk is lessened.

Even oxidised cholesterol may serve a purpose. Such molecules are the source of free radicals. In excess, free radicals have undesirable effects but, as we have seen, free radicals are also one of the means by which pathogens, and even cancer cells, can be 'nuked' (Chapter 3). Time will tell whether the use of lipid-lowering agents give us problems other than those already discussed (see above, Obesity, and Chapter 2).

Stress increases our risk of cardiovascular events, and it also raises cholesterol. This is because our stress hormones, cortisol and cortisone, are made from cholesterol (Chart 3.6) Raised cholesterol may be telling us about a nutrient deficiency as outlined in Chapter 3, and also about our stress levels. In both cases, by focusing on the cholesterol levels we are at risk of shooting the messenger. This is another problem stemming from the fixed-name disease approach to medicine. High cholesterol signals a problem: the high cholesterol itself is not necessarily the problem.

Cholesterol, triglycerides and genes

Several well-known genetic conditions affect cholesterol and triglyceride levels. Blood cholesterol can be high as a result of defects in a single gene or in multiple genes.

There is a condition known as familial hypercholesterolaemia (FH). It occurs in the heterozygous form (that is, with a bad gene from only one parent) in about 1 in 300–500 individuals. This gene causes a reduction in the number of receptors for LDL. The result is high levels of 'bad' cholesterol. Levels of 'good' cholesterol and triglycerides are usually normal. A double dose of this gene (homozygous, one from each parent) can cause atherosclerosis, and even death, in childhood.

Another single-gene abnormality results in a mutated form of apo B. This is inherited as an autosomal dominant gene. Like FH, it results in isolated raised LDL levels.

Genetically determined high cholesterol levels usually come about as the result of the actions of *several* 'rogue' genes. The manifestations of cardiovascular effects in these cases are much more dependent on environmental factors than the single-gene problems.[23]

Often patients have increased levels not only of cholesterol, but of triglycerides as well. Triglycerides are energy-dense molecules, consisting of three fatty acid chains linked by a sugar molecule. They are carried in the bloodstream as VLDLs. Elevation of triglycerides is associated with obesity, metabolic syndrome, excess consumption of sugar, fat and alcohol and inactivity. It can usually be managed by lifestyle adjustment, but the consumption of omega-3 fatty acids can lower levels by up to 65 per cent. Vitamins E, C and carotene, and the minerals selenium, zinc and manganese can protect the fats in the triglycerides from oxidation.[24] Genes for isolated raised triglycerides (without elevation of cholesterol) are not clearly in evidence.

A dominant gene results in yet another lipid disorder. In this case, both cholesterol *and* triglycerides are raised. The condition is called familial combined hyperlipidaemia (FCHL). This condition is thought to occur in as many as 1 in 50 or 1 in 100 Americans, and is the most common inherited disorder found in the survivors of heart attacks. A second condition in which both lipids are raised is a rare disorder affecting 1 in 10,000 people. This is due to a mutation affecting the gene for apo E.

There are other genetic variants, such as one which codes for lipoprotein apo A, and which increases the risk of raised LDL.

Overall, the devastating effects of genetic disorders of lipids seem to be rare. Far more common are the genes which predispose to illness, but interact with the environment. In other words, a good diet coupled with a healthy lifestyle has a real modifying effect on the 'bad' genes.

A dramatic study from The Netherlands demonstrates this concept. A large pedigree in a family known to be carrying the mutation for FH was traced back to a single pair of 19th-century ancestors. The researchers estimated how likely the descendants were to carry the mutation and charted it against the age of death. They concluded that mortality was not increased among carriers in the 19th and early 20th centuries. After 1915 it rose, peaked between 1935 and 1964, and fell again thereafter. The benign outcome before 1915 was thought to be due to the pre-industrial diet and lifestyle. The improvement after the 1960s was put down to the increased awareness of lifestyle factors in the development of heart disease in at-risk families.[25]

B-group vitamins and the homocysteine story

Homocysteine is derived from an amino acid, methionine. Because of the importance of homocysteine and methionine, these amino acids were introduced in Chapter 3. Before discussing what happens when homocysteine metabolism goes wrong, we will go back a few decades.

In the 1960s, a graduate of Harvard Medical School, Kilmer McCully, was studying a rare genetic disorder called homocystinuria. (Two homocysteine groups join together and appear as homocystine in the urine — hence the name.) Children who inherited two copies of a particular faulty gene often died of heart attacks and strokes. McCully examined autopsy specimens of the plaques that lined the arteries of these unfortunate children. There he found characteristic plaque lesions under the microscope, but no fatty deposits. He wondered if the raised levels of homocysteine might be the culprit. And if so, what might this mean to the understanding of atherosclerotic disease in the general population?

At that time the genetic defects responsible for the disease were not well understood. We know now that they are mutations in the genes which code for the enzymes that handle the amino acids methionine and homocysteine. McCully's work was focusing on the action of these enzymes.

Meat and dairy products are rich in methionine. Homocysteine is produced in the body as a breakdown product of methionine (Chart 3.4). Either faulty enzymes, or a deficient production of normal enzymes, could result in accumulation of certain metabolites. In homocystinuria, homocysteine was accumulating, with devastating results.

McCully came to realise that, even under normal circumstances, these enzymes depended on the presence of Vitamins B6, B12 and folic acid. Perhaps a diet rich in animal protein and low in fruits, vegetables and whole grains, the source of such vitamins, was mimicking the severe genetic condition. Perhaps the high fat and cholesterol inherent in such a diet were the last straw for these plaques. McCully's work gained further significance as he became aware that homocysteine was one of the amino acids to be found in the lipoprotein LDL. Could it be the *homocysteine*, and not the cholesterol, that was the 'bad guy' in LDL?[26]

But the drug companies had just discovered cholesterol, and his work was thought to be heretical. The funding for his research ceased, and McCully lost his job. Although homocysteine levels now constitute a respectable part of a cardiac work-up, the name of McCully goes unsung. And you are more likely to know the levels of your 'good' and 'bad' cholesterol than you are to know your (plasma) homocysteine.

Several milder conditions can result from a couple of other mutations in the genes which code for the enzymes necessary to methionine/homocysteine metabolism. The commonest of these is the *methylenetetrahydrofolate reductase* enzyme which we met in Chapters 3 and 5. This enzyme determines how well we handle folic acid. The means by which raised homocysteine might contribute not only to heart disease but also to birth defects (including spina bifida), Alzheimer's disease, dementia, cancer and diabetes was discussed in Chapter 3: Biochemistry.

Once again, it is better to regard these as polymorphisms, or gene variants, rather than faulty genes. As up to 50 per cent of the general population is thought to carry a homocysteine variant (Chapter 3), up to 50 per cent of people have a risk factor for cardiac and other problems that can be reduced by adequate intake of B-group vitamins.

Since McCully's early attempts to engage the medical profession in the homocysteine debate, many other implications of raised homocysteine have come to light. The transcription of many genes is known to be turned off during development by the process of methylation (Chapter 3) of their promoter regions. That means that if raised homocysteine during pregnancy is a marker for low levels of Vitamin B12 or folic acid, 'bad' genes that otherwise might have been switched off will remain switched on, permanently affecting the foetus.

Tumours are known to exhibit altered gene methylation in certain cases.[27] Whether homocysteine itself acts as a carcinogen, or is simply a marker for folic acid deficiency, is unknown. The association between some of the heritable cancers and raised homocysteine, and the risk reduction (bowel and breast) with folic acid supplementation, will reward further research.

Before leaving the subject of B-group vitamins, we should note that the other members of this group make contributions to cardiovascular health. This was discussed in some detail in Chapter 5, but here is a quick recapitulation.

- *Vitamin B1 or thiamine:* Gross deficiency of this vitamin causes beriberi, with symptoms that include salt and water retention leading to tachycardia (rapid heart rate), enlarged heart, eventual heart failure, and even death. Moderate deficiency may cause a sub-clinical picture which is not easily identified as B1 deficiency.

- *Vitamin B3 or niacin:* Prior to the development of the statin medications, B3 was the only known treatment for severe elevations of LDL cholesterol. It has been proven effective and (with a few provisos) safe. The main reason patients (and doctors) give for not using it is that many people complain of a red flush in the early stage of treatment, which is visible and can look quite dramatic. There are several simple strategies for avoiding this annoying side effect. It is not an allergy, and it is not dangerous.
- *Vitamin B5 (pantothenic acid):* Several studies have reported the effect of B5 in lowering both LDL and triglycerides, while at the same time increasing the levels of HDL.[28]

Treatments

A staggering array of drugs is available for the treatment of cardiovascular disorders.

- Drugs for heart failure include those known as cardiac glycosides, the oldest being digoxin, derived from the foxglove plant.
- Drugs for high blood pressure block angiotensin, or cause diuresis, as already discussed.
- Calcium channel blockers are also used to treat high blood pressure. Magnesium acts as a calcium channel blocker, and the very response of a patient to calcium channel blockers should alert the physician to the possibility of a magnesium deficiency.
- Nitrates dilate coronary vessels. The inbuilt mechanisms for achieving the same end were discussed in Chapters 4 and 5.

Drugs to lower cholesterol work by interfering with one of the most crucial pathways in human metabolism. Drugs that interfere with the absorption of cholesterol also interfere with the absorption of some of the fat-soluble vitamins most essential to the prevention of heart disease. Yet after 30 years of all these medications, treatment for uncomplicated hypertension is no better with the newer drugs than with the old-fashioned diuretics.

Indeed, in a five-year study on 40,000 people in the United States it appeared that people on diuretics were much *safer* than those on the newer treatments. Patients treated with calcium channel blockers had 38 per cent more likelihood of heart failure, and those on ACE inhibitors had 15 per cent greater stroke risk and 19 per cent increase in heart failure.[29]

Drs Matthias Rath and Linus Pauling argue that the many genes which seem to predispose us to cardiovascular disease and death must have served an evolutionary purpose or they would not be so persistent and pervasive in the human genome. They suggest that the process of thickening the arteries might be a defence against scurvy, which otherwise *weakens* connective tissue and would normally increase the risk of arterial rupture. Rath goes further, and suggests that it may be lipoprotein (a) which gave humans planetary dominance, since it is important for tissue differentiation, fertility, and the development of the human brain.[30] The implication for lowered consumption of fresh fruit and vegetables causing heart disease through low Vitamin C levels is unavoidable.

Chapter Nine
MENTAL HEALTH AND NEUROLOGICAL DISORDERS

If the doctors of today do not become the nutritionists of
tomorrow, then the nutritionists of today will become the doctors
of tomorrow. —Anon

AS MENTAL ILLNESS ASSERTS ITSELF as one of the main concerns of
Western medicine, it takes on the problems of the fixed-name
approach to disease. The international standard text, *The Diagnostic
and Statistical Manual of Mental Disorders*, is now in its fourth edition,
known as *DSM-IV-TR*. Over time, *DSM* certainly has served a
purpose, but its approach highlights the pitfalls of semantic
determinism.

For example, if 'depression' appears to respond to an anti-
depressant, and that anti-depressant happens to raise levels of
serotonin, then depression becomes a serotonin-deficiency disorder.
Doctors note the effects of Prozac and other SSRI medications, but
this reductionist approach bypasses the complex workings of the
brain. The following trenchant commentary by Californian
philosopher Dominic Murphy applies to physical medicine as much
as to psychiatric medicine:

> The DSM is designed to be atheoretical. It doesn't talk about
> causal theories of particular disorders. It doesn't say that there
> isn't a theory of what a mental disorder is, but it is designed to
> avoid causal theories. People sometimes use the phrase 'Chinese-
> menu approach' to characterise the DSM: to meet a certain
> diagnosis, you have to have two out of four from list A, three out
> of six from list B plus either C or D, and so on. *I think that*
> *philosophy of science suggests that you really can't have a satisfactory*

classification without it being based on some causal understanding of
what you're classifying... These false distinctions result from the divorce
between psychiatry and neuroscience [my italics].[1]

There are many categories of mental illness. They are defined by terms such as depression, bipolar disorder, obsessive-compulsive disorder, attention deficit disorder (with or without hyperactivity), personality disorder, eating disorders, substance dependency, schizophrenia. Historically, bipolar disorder and schizophrenia have been regarded as psychoses and the rest either as neuroses or personality disorders. *DSM IV* gives the current definitions of these conditions.

Personality disorders and psychoses often threaten the society in which the individual lives, as well as the well-being of the sufferer. Neuroses primarily afflict the individual, although it is rare for those close to the sufferer to remain unaffected.

Other diseases of the central nervous system, such as Parkinson's, Alzheimer's and multiple sclerosis, are classified as degenerative diseases, and are discussed in the second part of this chapter. However, because they share much of the physiology and biochemistry of mental health problems, many of the comments made here apply to these conditions as well.

It is nowadays generally accepted that both life events and genetic factors lead to the development of mental illness. In this context, the term 'life events' is usually interpreted as the emotional and psychological impacts on the individual. Only recently has serious attention been paid to dietary and environmental influences on the brain.

It is sometimes thought that the brain is 'hard-wired' to develop a pattern of behaviour, and that the reversal of that process can be difficult. Until we know more about neurochemistry, the whole area of human emotion, thinking and behaviour remains, at best, an educated guess.

Neurotransmitters

There are thought to be about 500 messenger chemicals in the brain, usually referred to as neurochemicals or neurotransmitters. These act on receptor sites, which may be specific to a particular neurotransmitter. However, we now know that one receptor site may be acted on by more than one neurotransmitter, with similar or even contrasting effects. And indeed, one neurotransmitter can act at more than one type of site, where it may have differing effects, determined by the structure of the particular site. The best-known of these neurotransmitters are serotonin, dopamine, gamma amino butyric acid (GABA) and cortisol.

Many of the drugs currently used to treat mental health disorders target one or more of these neurotransmitters or their receptor sites. In the case of Parkinson's and Alzheimer's, enzyme systems within the brain are also targeted.

Drugs affecting neurotransmitters can act in various ways. They can act to block receptor sites, to delay or promote the destruction of the neurotransmitter, to stimulate its release, or even to mimic its action. Most naturally-occurring psychoactives also use one of these mechanisms.

Cholesterol, essential fatty acids and interesting molecules known as sphingomyelins, all form part of the structural components of the brain. These nutrients are derived from diet, and it is only recently that their impact on mental health has received attention. One reason for looking at them was because cholesterol-lowering drugs seemed to be associated with an increased risk of depression and suicide. The possible role of the essential fatty acids will be discussed presently. The lack of benefit to vested interests once again may account for the slow rate of research into the nutritional aspects of mental health.

To some, the ability to manipulate neurotransmission is the wonder of modern psychiatry. Others are more cynical. For example, an article in *Time* magazine in 1997 said: 'So far, the tools used to manipulate serotonin in the human brain are more like pharmacological machetes than they are like scalpels — crudely effective, but capable of doing plenty of collateral damage.'[2] And later in the same article, 'A person's mood is like a symphony, and serotonin is like the conductor's baton.' If serotonin is the baton, who is the conductor? Prozac? The doctor who writes the script? The patient who takes the drug?

MENTAL HEALTH

Overview

History

Psychiatry is often thought of as one of the newest of medical sciences, which began with Freud's attempt in the early 20th century to understand the mechanisms of psychological processes. The *art* of psychiatry, by contrast, is one of the oldest medical disciplines. Prescriptions to treat hysteria date back to ancient Egypt. And the four 'humours' of Galen (CE 131–201) gave rise to the terms 'melancholic', 'choleric', 'sanguine' and 'phlegmatic', all still in use today. These humours were thought to be the basis of all disease, and are profoundly psychologically referenced.

Hippocrates (460–377 BCE) is usually regarded as the father of modern medicine, and it is probable that, despite Freud, he should also be regarded as the father of psychiatry. Hippocrates dragged medicine away from the idea, prevalent in both ancient Egypt and ancient Greece, that all disease was caused by demons and evil spirits. He deemed both physical and mental ill-health to be the result of natural causes which could be studied and thereby understood.

Hippocrates' enlightened views did not always prevail. Throughout the Middle Ages the mentally ill were often maltreated in order to 'drive out demons', and luckless schizophrenics and psychotics were subjected to merciless 'witch hunts'. Tragically, present-day practices sometimes seem to show little improvement.

In modern times, few would doubt Freud's contribution. Once described by Auden as not just 'a person but a whole climate of opinion', his ideas have permeated medical, sociological and artistic thinking. The revisionist criticisms of his work are valid only because they assess Freud by his own criteria. Freud wanted to make psychiatry a scientific endeavour. While there is 'science' in what he did, it is not the sort of science which lends itself to random controlled trials. Freud's observations of his patients allowed him to draw conclusions about what worked. Talking in an unstructured way about their deepest fears and anxieties seemed then, as now, to work. That it did not, or does not, work for all does not invalidate his findings. Few treatments in medicine have anything near a 100 per cent success rate, whatever the context.

There was no lack of historical precedent for talk therapy. Almost every society had wise men and women, and confessional priests and priestesses or oracles. Freud's attempt to unravel the *processes* of what worked was his greatest contribution. On the downside, this also laid the foundation for a doctrine from which rigid and unproven dogma was able to arise. Psychiatry might better have been served had Freud proclaimed talk therapy for the art that it is, rather than restraining it with inappropriate 'scientific' law.

Although there are regular challenges to the alleged success of talk therapy, the evidence to support such challenges is as difficult to produce as the contrary. At this point in time, it seems reasonable to regard it as one valuable tool in the available range of treatment options.

As we begin to understand the biochemistry of neurotransmitters, it seems possible that we might be able to quantify human feeling. With improvements in measurement techniques, we may be able to demonstrate that a patient talking to a trusted therapist experiences a reduction in stress hormones such as cortisol and adrenalin, and a rise in the feel-good hormones such as serotonin and dopamine. Although revisiting harrowing events may cause a temporary rise in stress hormones, we may find an overall reduction of them over time, and an increase in the hormones associated with positive mood.

If this were the case, what would we do with this knowledge? Undoubtedly it would be used to measure the effectiveness of one therapy over another. What if it is used to measure the effectiveness of one *therapist* over another? Is talking to a trained therapist any more effective than talking to a caring family doctor, or a close friend? What about an untrained member of the public who is a good listener? Or the clever charlatan who can guarantee a favourable neurotransmitter level? Is it always appropriate to make someone feel good? Is the *art* of therapy knowing when to face bad feelings?

Encounter groups, which were popular in the 1970s, fell out of favour when some participants decompensated rather badly after the encounter was over. Some of the leaders of these groups had few qualifications other than charisma.

Whatever the biochemistry of mental ill-health turns out to be, there can be no doubt that the pharmaceutical industry will continue to show a significant interest in adding to the already staggering pharmacopeia of drug treatments.

The size of the problem

The World Health Organisation has predicted that by 2020 depression will be the second most common cause of disease worldwide.

In the US and UK the number of adults who suffer from depression is estimated to be about 10 per cent of the population with women almost twice as likely to suffer as men. In 1998–99 the prevalence rate of depression Australia-wide was estimated at 3.4 per cent of all men and 6.8 per cent of all women.[3]

In Australia, Post-natal depression was thought to afflict approximately 10–15 per cent of all women. At that time depression was the third leading cause of disease burden in Australia, and the leading cause of non-fatal disease. The direct cost of treating depression was estimated at $500 million annually. (Such estimates do not take account of indirect costs such as time lost from work.)

Intentional self-harm accounted for 5.3 per cent of all hospital admissions and 1.8 per cent of all deaths. Depression was estimated to be the fifth most commonly treated disease in general practice. Other mental health problems that overlap with depression, such as psychosis, alcoholism, ADD, ADHD and autistic spectrum disorders, all add to the mental health burden.

Mental ill-health, if its spectrum is increased to encompass problems other than depression, is rapidly approaching the status of the greatest disease burden of the Western world.

The medical approach

The pharmaceutical industry has jumped eagerly into this yawning market opportunity. It has provided programs to 'educate' doctors with pseudoscientific journals such as the *Depression Awareness Journal*, or with free counselling like that which at one stage was offered with scripts for Aropax.

In criticising this approach, a degree of caution is in order. There are no rewards for suffering. Mind-numbing and soul-destroying, depression is as destructive as any physical illness. If anti-depressant medication works for even some of its sufferers, it is a valid treatment option. But it is also true that a bit of misery is part of the human condition, and may even build character. Depression, for some at least, seems to be part of the growth process. Youthful idealists may well feel despair on realising that they live in a world where

Darwinian survival of the fittest can be enshrined (albeit in disguise) in government policy.

One study purported to show an association between the suicide rate and the political persuasion of the government of the day. Under conservative governments it rose, but fell with an increase in socialist leanings.[4] This, of course, caused an outcry, and the refutations were predictable. At least, however, it helped focus the debate on the *society* in which the depression statistics occur.

Lost opportunities?
Medication becomes a problem when it is seen as the first or *only* treatment option. Patients complain that they were unable to talk about their problems because the doctor had already reached for the script pad. If you are being bullied at work or at school, or sexually abused, or have been abandoned by someone who you thought was your lifelong friend, the first-line treatment is *not* an anti-depressant. This should be stating the obvious, but indications are that it is not.

If someone has a life in which everything seems ideal but they lack the will to continue, 'true' depression will probably be diagnosed. Anti-depressant medication may buy time in such cases—suicide can claim lives while professionals decide which diagnosis to attach. But those professionals should ask why someone whose personal life is in good shape would find life itself pointless. Is the person in denial over some major life event? Is it genetic? If it is genetic, how does this gene survive and flourish? Is it biochemical? If there is a lack of serotonin, how did this come about? If people are failing to produce adequate serotonin, what other health implications might this have? After all, there are serotonin receptors all over the body. Maybe the altered biochemistry explains the high co-morbidity seen in depression. But will Prozac address all these other problems?

Mary in Chapters 1 and 4 was suffering depression *and* painful periods. There was a possibility that both were the result of magnesium deficiency. What might a magnesium deficiency do to her mother, Fran? Fran, we have seen has alcohol intolerance and mild hypertension (Chapter 6). With the approach of menopause, mood swings have been a problem. Magnesium deficiency has a role in all of these disorders. Does this explain the statistic that mood disorders and depression go with menstrual disorders and such like? If we treat Fran's mood swings with Prozac alone, what will that do for her blood pressure or her menopausal problems?

What about the essential fatty acids and B-group vitamins? EFAs have important therapeutic effects in depression, cardiovascular disease *and* menstrual disorders. B-group vitamins play a part in depressive illness, cardiovascular disease, alcohol metabolism, gynaecological disorders. If there is deficiency of B-group vitamins and/or magnesium and/or EFAs, we should not be surprised that depression and cardiovascular disease appear together—we should *expect* it.

In this way, the treatment of one condition becomes the treatment of the other, because we are addressing an underlying biochemical disorder. There is little likelihood of unwanted side effects and a good chance of a positive outcome. The EFAs we give Fran for hypertension stand a good chance of moderating her mood swings and preventing them leading to depression. By stark contrast, the selective serotonin antagonists, especially if combined with some other medications, may actually *increase* her blood pressure. This is how polypharmacy, or the use of multiple and often conflicting medication, starts. One drug is introduced to compensate for the effects of another.

A patient I saw recently—let us call her Betty—was suffering from insomnia and probably from an anxiety disorder, which may have been severe at some stage. She was also taking medication for arthritis, hypertension, high cholesterol and an irritable bowel. Her list of prescription medications included Somac, Celebrex, Avapro, Pravachol, Stelazine, Tofranil, Valium, Sinequan, Hypnodorm. If you saw Betty sitting in my waiting room, would you recognise her as an invalid, a walking textbook of human illness? She looks like any other middle-aged woman.

A depressing number of people consume this type of pharmaceutical cocktail. We may know the individual actions of all of these medications, but we cannot know how they interact. The hypertension, arthritis, raised cholesterol, insomnia and anxiety disorder in this patient are all amenable to simpler treatments, particularly by magnesium, B-group vitamins and the EFAs. Supplementation would certainly have been a more rational starting point. Maybe some medication would still be required, but surely not this appalling list of pharmaceuticals. And despite this impressive intake, she was still sleeping badly!

In fact, Betty later reported that she felt magnesium had transformed her life. She remains on some medication, but the list is shorter, and the patient much happier. Like Fran, Betty was never suffering from a drug deficiency.

Toxins

Pollution, as most people are all too well aware, is ubiquitous. Early symptoms of lead and mercury poisoning include depression, learning difficulties and behavioural changes. The effects of pesticides and herbicides are not fully known, but many of these chemicals are soluble in fat, and therefore can pass from the blood into the brain. Agricultural chemicals are one of the strongest environmental correlates with the development of Parkinson's disease.

The use of recreational drugs has been associated with the promotion of mental disorders in the young. Unfortunately, it is the most vulnerable who are drawn to this form of self-medication.

And then there is the question of iatrogenic disease — the harm done to patients by the medical profession itself. Mental health is an area where the risk of iatrogenic illness is considerable.

This book cannot cover in detail the appropriate response to mental health problems such as depression, autism and insomnia. Instead we will look at some interesting ideas, which, with some exceptions, have *not* been proved by random controlled trials. Although we focus on one particular diagnostic category, the implications are there for all aspects of mental health.

Anti-social and criminal behaviour

A double-blind study was undertaken in Britain on a prison population. The aim was to determine whether providing supplements of vitamins, minerals and essential fatty acids made any difference to the behaviour of the inmates. A system of documenting offences within the prison already existed, and so it was a good setting for such investigation.

The study, undertaken by the Department of Physiology at Oxford University, showed dramatic results.[5] The 231 young offenders were divided into a treatment group and a control group. For nine months their behaviour was documented to provide a baseline. For the following nine months, the treatment group received a commercial preparation called Forceval, a multivitamin-mineral tablet (including the full range of vitamins, with minerals such as selenium, zinc and magnesium); and Efamol capsules containing a mix of essential fatty acids (see Appendix 1).

The treated group were involved in 35.1 per cent fewer

disciplinary incidents than previously, while the control group showed only a 6.7 per cent reduction. If only violent incidents were included, the treatment group showed a 37 per cent reduction as against 10 per cent in the control group. The leader of the study, Bernard Gesch, suggested that poor diets may also influence criminal behaviour in the community, remarking that 'the brain required nutrients in common with the rest of the body, and it was not unreasonable to believe that anti-social behaviour could be caused by a lack of them.'

It is always difficult to say how far one should extrapolate from any study. The discussions in Chapter 2 on the hazards involved in interpreting clinical trials are relevant, whether the treatment is a natural product or a pharmaceutical. However, in defence of studies such as the one just discussed, it has to be said that the university department had little to gain from investigating natural substances other than the academic kudos of good research.

When diet has been shown to be responsible for so many physical ailments, it is not difficult to make the case that behavioural and mood disorders may have similar origins.

It could be argued that the prison diet is a particular case. In fact, it was reported that good food was available in the prison, but prisoners were no more likely to choose it than anyone else in the general population.

It could also be argued that a prison population is a small and rather specialised group, and that the findings would not apply to the broader community. However, there is little doubt that the mentally ill are over-represented, and that depression and suicide are significant health problems in gaols. Behaviour is widely considered to be a measure of a person's well-being. The results are all the more remarkable for being demonstrated in this situation.

The daily cost of these supplements was just one pound. If supplementation were to be extended to every prisoner in British jails, the cost benefit could be significant. New Scientist reported that a criminologist from California State University had completed three trials apparently with similar results.[6]

Depression

An inflammatory disorder?

A study reported in New Scientist explores the possibility that depression is an inflammatory disorder, mediated by cytokines.[7] Cytokines were discussed in Chapter 3 as chemicals which, in excess, are normally associated with diseases such as rheumatoid arthritis. In recent years mood changes have been linked to changes in cytokine production.

Depression has been noted as a side effect of drugs that stimulate the immune system in order to treat such chronic diseases as cancer and viral hepatitis. These drugs are designed to increase the production, or mimic the actions, of inflammatory cytokines. They include medications such as alpha interferon and interleukin-2.

By contrast, some of the more specific *anti*-inflammatory medications, those targeting the prostaglandins-2 pathway (see Chart 5.3) have been reported to induce a feeling of well-being. St John's wort historically has been used against both inflammation and depression. Support for the theory that inflammation and depression might be connected also comes from the typical co-morbidity of certain conditions. For example, depressed people have up to a threefold risk of death from heart disease, an inflammatory disease. Depression is a well-known complication of cardiac surgery. Cardiac surgery is very invasive, and significant inflammation is an inevitable part of the process. Post-viral depression is so common as to be considered a normal part of viral illness. Part of the immune defence against viral (or indeed, bacterial) infection is to release inflammatory cytokines.

Perhaps the co-existence of inflammation with depression is non-causal, but there is the opposite case to be made. What evolutionary advantage might accrue if infective disease or (surgical) wounds result in depression? One characteristic of depression is the desire to withdraw from the world. In the case of infection, such withdrawal would automatically protect vulnerable members of the group (children, pregnant women) from exposure to the germs.

One of the researchers quoted in the *New Scientist* paper, a neurobiologist called Dantzer, makes the point that 'sickness behaviour' (which he was able to elicit in experimental rats by injecting them with parts of bacterial cell walls) serves another purpose. Sickness behaviour includes a rise in body temperature (also observed in depressed patients), altered sleep patterns, a drop in sociability and loss of appetite. 'Sickness behaviour is like fear. It makes the animal reorganise its priorities.' Cytokines, in short, make the animal withdraw and conserve its energies to fight the infection

394 THE GOOD BODY GUIDE

or heal the wound.

Dantzer maintains that it is not the bacterial cell walls, themselves harmless, which cause this change. Rather, it is the *immune response* to the injected material which is responsible. Cytokines, such as interleukin-1, when injected cause a similar response. Interferon, for example, is one of the earliest of the cytokines to be produced against viral infection, and is one of the most important anti-viral defences. Interferon is maximally produced when an animal is at rest. The 'depressed' mode therefore is not only a side-effect of the cytokine: it actually enhances its production.

Similarly, whether infection is present or not, a major wound or surgical procedure such as cardiac surgery releases many inflammatory cytokines as part of the healing process. The patient is immobilised by depressive responses so that reserves may be focused on the business of wound healing.

In summary, an underlying inflammatory condition could contribute to the development of more than one co-existent disease, such as heart disease and depression. In the case of an individual who is not recovering from a viral or surgical condition, the inflammatory reaction becomes pathological. This is where the Western diet may exert its depressant effects. Inflammation is exaggerated by the consumption of saturated fats and refined carbohydrates. It is reduced by nutrients such as selenium, magnesium and omega-3s.

Mood change in response to certain medications has also been mentioned. Certain anti-depressant medications do not seem to work by altering neurotransmitter levels. Some even seem to lower serotonin, and still produce a 'get up and go' response. The possibility that the effect is due to their anti-inflammatory actions is under investigation.

The pity will be if this new knowledge leads to another explosion in psycho-pharmaceuticals and fails to address the simple questions of dietary inadequacy. In 2002, the *Journal of the American Medical Association* reported a study on a selective serotonin re-uptake inhibitor (SSRI) which not only acted as an anti-depressant in heart attack victims but also reduced the incidence of further adverse events.[8] The hypothesis was that the SSRI blocked serotonin receptors throughout the body, thereby increasing circulating levels of serotonin. This reduced platelet aggregation, which in turn reduced clot formation.

There are two interesting aspects here. The study was funded by Pfizer, the manufacturers of sertraline (Zoloft), the SSRI in question. Although the study included just 369 people and was carried out over a relatively short period, it was published in a prestigious medical journal and also received a full page in the international magazine *Time*. Would this study have been deemed newsworthy without the publicity machinery of the pharmaceutical giant behind it? The second interesting point is that, if the result of this study *is* significant, there should be a debate about the adequacy of dietary anti-inflammatories. Are we really to believe that we are succumbing to heart attacks and depression because no one had the foresight to prescribe Zoloft for us? And will the overall risks of taking SSRIs outweigh the benefits? The widespread use of SSRIs barely spans a decade; their long-term effects are unknown, but their use has already been linked with an increased risk of conditions such as Parkinson's disease. In adolescents and children, whose brains are still undergoing development and maturation, they pose a different range of risks.

Does EFA deficiency contribute?

Joseph Hibbeln is a psychiatrist and biochemist from the National Institute of Health near Washington, DC. Struck by the fact that the brain is almost entirely made of fat, and that dietary changes could alter the composition of those fats, he began to investigate the possible role of the essential fatty acids in mental health.[9]

The different types of EFAs were discussed in Chapter 5. There is general agreement that the Western diet has an excess of the omega-6 arachidonic acid over either the omega-3s or the anti-inflammatory omega-6s. In contrast, Hibbeln focused on the balance between the two *anti*-inflammatory EFAs (Chart 5.3).

The switch from a diet high in omega-3s to one which favoured arachidonic acid began with the agricultural revolution. The advent of industrial technology in the food industry pushed that balance even further. Soy, corn palm and cottonseed oils were favoured because of their long shelf life. These oils are rich in both kinds of omega-6, and the balance between omega-3s and omega-6s is lowered even further when, for commercial reasons, the oils are hydrogenated.

Hibbeln estimated that the average annual consumption of soy oil in the United States stood at 11 kg, accounting for 83 per cent of all fats eaten. This represented a startling thousand-fold increase in the last century. Fewer of the foods containing omega-3s are now consumed. Diets which a century ago had contained an equal amount of omega-3s and omega-6s now have a *16 to 1* ratio in favour of omega-6. 'Nobody could adjust that fast', he says, in what seems to be a masterly understatement.

There is a whole pizza generation who have never ever eaten a can of sardines, whose closest contact with fish has been the occasional fish finger. This is the generation in whom the depression and suicide rate is rising at an alarming pace.

Hibbeln asserts that fats are important for brain signalling. Neuronal cell membranes are 20 per cent EFAs. The composition of the fats determines the ease with which signals are transmitted. There is no point in having high levels of serotonin if the nerve cells fail to adequately transmit the message signalled.

Furthermore, in a way not yet fully understood, the actual *levels* of serotonin, both in humans and experimental animals, seem to be paralleled by the levels of omega-3 fatty acids in cerebrospinal fluid.

Moreover, omega-3 supplements 'promote brain cell and synapse growth and seem to protect those cells from dying'. Neuronal damage has been linked to depression, especially, but by no means exclusively, in the elderly.

Cultures with low fish intake have high rates of depression, post-natal depression, bipolar disorder and homicide. The flaws in extrapolation to any one factor or in 'guilt by association' are obvious, but there are clearly grounds for further research. It is reassuring to see that there are no fewer than ten ongoing clinical trials to assess the role of omega-3s in mental disorders which include schizophrenia, depression and attention deficit disorders.

The role of minerals
Could mineral deficiency contribute to depression, dementia and other mental disorders?

In selenium-deplete states, it seems, the brain receives priority supply, a sure indicator that selenium has a key role in brain chemistry. The turnover rate of some neurotransmitters is altered when selenium is low, and in three separate studies 'low selenium state was associated with a significantly greater incidence of depression and other negative mood states such as anxiety, confusion, and hostility'.[10] In one of the studies, those who showed considerable mood benefit were consuming approximately 226.5 mcg daily of selenium. In another study (double-blind), those consuming as little as 100 mcg a day also benefited.

The average daily intake of selenium in Britain is between 29 and 39 mcg. Because of lower soil levels, this figure may be even lower in Australia. Selenium deficiency may contribute to Australia's unenviable status of having one of the highest suicide rates in the world.

The effects of low selenium may apply to other aspects of mental health. Low plasma selenium is associated with senility and accelerated cognitive decline, and the selenium levels in the brains of Alzheimer's patients was found to be just 60 per cent of that in a control group.[11]

We have already discussed the roles of minerals such as magnesium, zinc and copper in mental health (Chart 3.4; Chapter 4).

It should be noted that none of these studies meet the criteria for the gold standard RCT, yet the ideas are simple and rational, intuitively appealing. It is a great pity that we are not working actively to test these hypotheses. At best, they are seen as adjunctive or complementary therapies. It seems difficult for the profession to make the conceptual shift from treatment as a means to *bypass* biochemical dysfunction to treatment as *correcting* such dysfunction. The problem with the accepted approach is that it treats symptom, not cause.

Childhood disorders: fact or fiction?

Now we look at a group of childhood disorders which can be classified under all manner of headings. I choose several broad categories, but again argue that they are both arbitrary and overlapping:

- autistic spectrum disorders (ASD)
- specific learning difficulty/disorder (SLD)
- attention deficit disorder and attention deficit accompanied by hyperactivity (ADD, ADHD)
- behavioural disorders: a variety of titles from ODD (oppositional defiant disorder) to 'psychotic'
- depression
- obsessive and compulsive disorders (OCD)
- addictive disorders.

Parents usually find it useful to regard these conditions in separate diagnostic categories, and further sub-classification is not unusual. It is valid to take a descriptive approach to any illness, but both physical and psychological disorders can have multiple causes and considerable overlap. A factor that causes one kind of illness in an individual may cause a different condition in another. Given our rudimentary knowledge of how the brain works, it may be as helpful to understand what injures the brain, or what factors keep it healthy, as to investigate the various descriptive 'categories' and the pharmacological manipulation thereof.

In paediatric mental health, conditions once regarded as 'non-existent' or 'exquisitely rare' are now frequently diagnosed. Perhaps these conditions have always been with us and only now are receiving recognition and treatment. Still, the rise in diagnosis seems to reflect a true rise in incidence, which is alarming. Let us look at some figures.

- It is estimated that up to 10 per cent of children in the UK and Australia have been diagnosed with one of the forms of ADD or SLD, and a significant percentage of these are being treated with one of the two major stimulants.
- In the UK and Australia 1 to 2 per cent of all children are thought to be autistic or to suffer from an autistic spectrum disorder.
- In the United States it has been estimated that 25 per cent of all children, and 8 per cent of all adolescents, are depressed.
- In January 2003 the US Food and Drug Administration for the first time approved prescription of Prozac for either depression or OCD in children.[12]

What is causing this extraordinary deterioration in children's mental health? To answer this question, we need evidence. Sometimes evidence threatens to be politically uncomfortable, as the measles vaccination saga so aptly demonstrated (Chapter 2). Sometimes evidence is simply lacking. When researchers in 2002–3 wanted to compare mercury levels in the hair of children diagnosed as autistic with similar studies, the only other published study they could find dated from 1985.[13]

There is unlikely to be one single cause for any of these problems. This is what makes cause and effect so difficult to establish. It may be that a 'toxic' assault on the developing brain is toxic only if other conditions such as a vitamin or mineral deficiency are also present.

Here I will examine only the mysterious condition of autism. I choose it because the rise in the diagnostic rate reflects a rise in the incidence of the condition. Because autism is so devastating, it cannot be blamed on over-anxious parents or the pressure of psychosocial change. If we can understand something as complex as autism, perhaps we will gain some understanding of the relatively more straightforward diagnoses such as depression and ADD.

Autistic spectrum disorders (ASD)

There are many theories about the causes of autism. In fact it may be a paradigm for multiple causation.

The genetic theory

There is little doubt that autism has a genetic component. Currently, researchers believe that autism is a collection of disorders involving between 12 and 15 genes. The focus is on chromosomes 7 and 17. The estimates of population incidence vary but are consistently rising. In the United States in 2000, it was thought that 16 in every 10,000 children had one of the autistic spectrum disorders. In New South Wales in 2003, the estimate was 10–60 in every 10,000.[14]

Seeming to confirm the genetic theory, other genetic disorders sometimes confer an increased risk for the development of autism. These include tuberous sclerosis and phenylketonuria (PKU).

At the time of the American estimate, the risk of developing autism was assessed at 3 to 8 per cent for siblings of affected children, with a concordance rate of 60 per cent for identical twins. This makes a case for heritability, but indicates that other factors, such as environmental influences, affect the expression of the relevant genes.

The birth-defect theory

About 5 per cent of thalidomide victims are autistic.[15] Using the statistics current at the time of this assessment, that was 30 times higher than the population norm for autism.

The minor physical changes which are seen in many autistic

children, such as ear and mouth shape, occur very early in the development of the embryo, about 20 to 24 days after conception. Neurological abnormalities characteristic of both autism and the autistic thalidomide victims would have occurred at approximately this stage. The major part of neurological development at this time involves the cranial nerves and the brainstem. Abnormalities of eye movement, eye focus, and facial expression seem to be defining characteristics of autism, which supports the idea that the actions of the cranial nerves indicate damage at this early, and very specific, stage.

The possible effect on the developing brainstem is even more interesting. Neurobiologists usually associate brainstem activity with the most basic functions. Hypersensitivity to touch and sound, excessive wakefulness, and major sleep disturbance are well-known aspects of autistic spectrum disorders and can easily be related to brainstem malfunction. The case for birth defects as a cause is augmented by the observation that exposure during pregnancy to alcohol, German measles and valproic acid (an anti-epileptic) all increase the risk of autism.

Toxins
For some time now mercury, even at quite low levels, has been thought to damage the developing brain and nervous systems of foetuses. Estimates of 'acceptable' mercury levels in adults and children are always a cause for contention among environmental scientists. From time to time there is a call for these levels to be revised downwards, but this challenges the interests both of big industries and of the politicians they support.

Recent studies have looked at mercury levels in the baby hair of children later diagnosed as autistic with startling results.[16] It might have been expected that, if these children differed from the norm, their levels would be higher. Instead, children with autism had a mean level of 0.47 ppm; the normal group's mean level was 3.63 ppm. And the greater the degree of impairment, the *lower* the levels.

The researchers concluded that mercury in samples from the newly born was primarily derived from the mothers. Suspected sources were dental fillings, high fish consumption during pregnancy, and thiomersol, a mercury-based preservative in the injection given to Rh negative mothers.

In the normal group, the baby's mercury levels reflected those of their mothers. In the autistic group, however, the baby's levels remained low, independent of the mother's reading.

Possible explanations for this phenomenon remind us of the difficulty of statistical interpretation. We could even argue that such data suggest that small doses of mercury are good for us, for it was the children with the lowest levels who were most at risk. The lines of thought offered by the researchers included:

- Low hair levels are indicative of an inability to excrete toxic metals. These children were storing mercury in vital organs such as brain and nervous tissue, rather than passing it out of the body in hair, urine or skin.
- Autistic children have a problem with the absorption of metals. As a result, they are deficient in metals necessary for normal brain development, such as iron, copper and zinc. The low levels of mercury are simply a marker for metal malabsorption, and could be regarded as a beneficial side effect of the problem.

Another kind of toxin

Gluteomorphine and caseomorphine are opiate-like peptides found in milk and gluten-containing cereals (Chapters 2 and 10). Their 'numbing' effects on the brain are thought by some to contribute to ASD.[17] A trial elimination diet is a simple intervention and, many of us believe, quite promising. A higher rate of autism (and schizophrenia) in coeliacs is now accepted as fact.

Nutrient deficiency

Another study that compared hair mercury levels of an autistic group with those of a control group found no difference. However, 'lower levels of calcium, copper and chromium ... were so distinctive that they could be used as a "diagnostic tool for autism".'[18]

When an essential mineral is lacking, the body may substitute a toxic mineral which occupies the same receptor sites. Were these children autistic because they were poisoned with a heavy metal other than mercury? Or was the problem a lack of copper, chromium and other essential minerals? Perhaps neither explanation is correct. However, in a society where the rise in autism is paralleled by rising pollution and falling nutrition, further study of these questions seems urgently indicated.

At the end of Chapter 4, I mentioned emerging theories of iodine and bromine. Iodine deficiency affects half of Western school children, and may affect any aspect of their mental health. The Western diet is lacking in iodine-rich foods, such as sea vegetables and seafood. Salt in processed food is not iodised, and there is the complicating factor of bromine. Like iodine, bromine is a halogen. In trace amounts, it may be valuable; in quantities found in processed foods, substitution can occur. It may become toxic in its own right, and it may replace iodine.

The debate is beyond the scope of this book, but the interested reader would be advised to follow the unfolding research.

There is an interesting genetic footnote on the subject of nutrient deficiency. An article in *New Scientist* cites the rising incidence of both asthma and autism as a possible example of epigenetic inheritance.[19] Epigenetic inheritance refers to those factors which are outside the DNA molecule, but which alter the way in which it is read or have some other powerful influence on inherited characteristics. Diet, by providing methyl, acetyl and other chemical groups, may influence epigenetic processes. If this is so, the article proposes, any modification of intake of the sources of those groups, notably vitamins, could switch genes on and off. In other words, the autism genes may not be new, but the ability to suppress them may be affected by a diet deplete in the foods which supply nutrients such as methyl groups. Specifically for methylation, this includes Vitamins B6, B12 and folic acid (Chapter 3).

Immune disorder

It is both intuitive and predictable that immune dysfunction might be associated with the development of autism spectrum disorders. This line of thinking was at the heart of the debate as to whether MMR vaccination in some children triggered both inflammatory bowel disease and autism (Chapter 2).

Immune disorders manifest themselves in every aspect of human biology. Earlier in this chapter the discussion of depression as an inflammatory (and therefore immune) disorder explored this theme. The success of the essential fatty acids in treating conditions from asthma to arthritis suggests that the prevalence of such conditions may be in part due to the known reduction of EFAs, especially omega-3s, in our diet.

Doctors who see a lot of autistic children observe that they often suffer from asthma, eczema and irritable bowel. This may not constitute scientific proof of immune dysfunction as a cause of autism, but it is hard to ignore. Many doctors see positive effects from supplements of anti-inflammatory omega-3 fatty acids in autistic children.

As one researcher in the area of autism as an immune disorder comments, 'Arguments over autism and MMR have overshadowed this important line of research.'[20]

Savant theory

Although autism appears to occur across the whole IQ spectrum, impairment of function is such that the autistic child is more likely to be assessed in the lower IQ range. Asperger's syndrome is generally regarded as a mild form of autism, and the term is usually confined to those of normal IQ. A lack of learning difficulty, in particular, characterises Asperger's children, whose main difficulty lies in relating to the feelings of others.

'Savant syndrome' describes a related and extraordinary phenomenon. People who have brain damage, mental retardation, major developmental disorder or autism may retain 'islands' of special knowledge or skills. If the talent is not particularly valued by the community, such as memory for sports trivia or car number plates, it may go unremarked. Sometimes the talent seems noticeable only in comparison to the other areas of deficit in that person. Sometimes however, the skill is so extraordinary that it would be outstanding in even the most able member of society. Calendar calculating, prodigious musical performance, linguistic and artistic achievements are some of the skills displayed by savants.

Of all known savants, at least half are thought to be autistic, and the remainder have some kind of brain damage or developmental delay. In some cases, 'normal' individuals have developed outstanding talents *after* brain injury. Recently, a similar phenomenon has been observed in elderly people who suffer blindness or dementia.

It has been estimated that 1 in 10 of all people with autism, and 1 in 2000 of those who are brain-damaged, have savant skills. Savant syndrome in the younger age group is usually seen in the IQ range 40–70, although higher levels exist. In this group, males outnumber females up to six to one. This is reflected in the higher ratio of male to female autistic children. The 'toxicity' of testosterone has sometimes been implicated in this regard.

It has been proposed that both Einstein and Isaac Newton may have been suffering from either autism or Asperger's. They were not savants because their talents were not isolated, and they were capable of normal function in society. However, they had certain personality traits which have led some to speculate that they were so socially inept that they may have been high-functioning Asperger's individuals.

The rare condition of savant syndrome may have only curiosity value. But the overlap between extraordinary ability, autism and brain damage is such that Darold Treffert, a neurobiologist and one of the world's leading authorities on savant syndrome, has said, 'No model of brain function will be complete until it can explain this rare condition.'[21]

Outrage: the changing picture of mental health in children

Children today are being medicated at a rate that would have seemed incredible just a few decades ago. It has been estimated that upwards of 50,000 children in Australia in 2002 were being prescribed medication for ADHD. The commonest drugs used were methylphenidate (Ritalin) and dexamphetamine. An unknown number have been treated with anti-depressants for a wide variety of conditions.

If it is true that so many children 'need' medication, what has gone wrong in our society that this type of medical condition is so common? There cannot have been a change in the gene pool in so short a time, despite immigration. Are we to accept this rate of pathology? Are we honestly addressing the possible causes? Perhaps we need politicians with the courage to make breast-feeding obligatory, to ban pesticides, to prohibit junk food and mandate dietary supplements.

If we seek a psychosocial explanation for the learning difficulties in our children, we must be brave enough to challenge the status quo of a success-driven society. We must ask whether it is desirable to incarcerate children as young as four in an enclosed environment for up to seven hours a day. Perhaps this creates an environment which will produce obesity, learning difficulties, behavioural problems and even visual disorders. Multiple studies suggest that exercise is one of the most potent of all anti-depressants. By prescribing medication for conditions known to respond to exercise, the medical profession is failing these children.

What do we really know of the long-term effects of medication? The results of severe autism are so devastating that any medication which demonstrates value must be considered; but for every child who is truly autistic, many more are receiving some form of drug treatment.

There are still unanswered questions about the safety of these medications in the adult population for whom they were designed, and yet wide use in young and developing brains has, until recently, gone largely unchallenged. Studies have already suggested that, although medication quietens the children diagnosed with 'attention deficit', they do not learn any more than if they were not treated. Even worse, we may be setting up these children for addictive or other problems in later life.

The psychoactive medications most commonly prescribed for children fall into four categories:

- tricyclic anti-depressants
- selective serotonin re-uptake inhibitors (SSRIs) and serotonin and noradrenalin re-uptake inhibitors (SNRIs)
- stimulants such as Ritalin and the amphetamines
- anti-epileptics.

The tricyclic anti-depressants have been used in low doses for several decades as a treatment for bed-wetting in children. These seem to have been effective, and low-dose usage appears to have relatively few complications. Because they were introduced at a time when psychotropic medication was used rarely and with considerable caution in children, prescribing seems to have been mostly uncontroversial.

The advent of the SSRIs and SNRIs was hailed with a fanfare of publicity. These drugs were no more effective than the earlier anti-depressants (although this fact was not part of the publicity machine's proclamations), but they had the enormous advantage of being relatively non-toxic.

The prototype, of course, was Prozac, and the word came rapidly into common usage. Before long, not only was this wonder of the pharmaceutical industry prescribed (unofficially) for children, but veterinary surgeons were giving it to pets. Was this another example of the growing phenomenon of a drug in search of a disease? The list of indications for Prozac seemed to be growing longer by the day.

As I was writing the first draft of this chapter, a circular arrived on my desk. Dated 28 August 2003, it was written on the letterhead of Wyeth, a major drug manufacturer, and it warned about Efexor, one of its products in the SNRI family of anti-depressants. It read:

> Wyeth wishes to inform you about important safety
> information on the use of Efexor (venlafaxine HCL tablets)
> and Efexor-XR (venlafaxine HCL modified-release capsules)
> in children and adolescents. Efexor and Efexor-XR have not
> been, and are not now, approved or recommended for use in
> children and adolescents below the age of 18 years.

Notice the subtlety of the wording: 'have not been, and are not now, approved'. It went on to say that young people on Efexor-XR showed increased hostility, and had thoughts of suicide and self-harm; this was in addition to the side effects also found in adults, which included 'decreased appetite, weight loss, increased blood pressure and increased serum cholesterol'.

It is odd that *MIMS* (the advertisers' handbook directed to doctors) gives only a 'precaution' about use in children and does not mention adolescents, effectively leaving the choice to doctors. And what demarcates a child from an adolescent, or an adolescent from an adult? The instructions on many over-the-counter medications such as cough mixtures divide children at age 12, and some in effect advise doubling the dose on the child's 12th birthday. Is the girl who has breast development and is menstruating at 10 a child, an adolescent, an adult? Is a drug which is not safe for 16-year-old Mike, who has the build of an athlete, all right for his underweight, depressed, 18-year-old cousin? Am I happy about giving this medication to his sister Mary, well into her twenties, given the *known and accepted* side effects listed above?

The use of Prozac and similar drugs in young children is worrying enough, but it is outstripped by the use of amphetamine analogues for the attention-deficit spectrum of disorders. Ciba–Geigy first approached the US Food and Drug Administration in 1961 for approval of the use of the amphetamine-like drug Ritalin for the condition then known as Minimal Brain Dysfunction. It was originally rejected, but was then approved in 1963. In 1980 the *DSM III* of the American Psychiatric Association reclassified this condition as 'attention deficit disorder, with/out hyperactivity'.

The rationale for using an amphetamine analogue (although this was probably not understood in 1960) is easy to comprehend. Like amphetamines, Ritalin works as a stimulant; and while this may seem paradoxical in hyperactivity, it is thought to bring patients into focus and reduce restless behaviour.

But let us take a closer look at this drug. Ritalin's listed side effects include 'dependency'—in other words, it is addictive. It cannot be prescribed by the local family doctor without a special approval authority. Alarm bells should ring. Sales in the school playground are notorious—this drug gives 'highs'. If regulations protect most patients from current addiction, we still must ask what we are teaching the developing brain. Remember that we do not fully understand how addictive drugs can be used socially by some people, while others are destroyed by them.

How the brain learns addiction

Like all drugs of addiction, amphetamines interact with, or in some way simulate, the effects of the body's own neurotransmitters. Although many of the addictive drugs increase arousal, it is the effect on the sense of *pleasure* that underpins the addictive properties. Any of the neurotransmitters may be involved in the complex pathways which lead to feeling pleasure; but certain ones, notably acetylcholine and dopamine, seem to be central to the processes.

At all times the body is striving for an optimal balance between the need to feel good, and the level of stress and anxiety necessary to keep the organism alert and out of danger. The balance between the two is a fine one. Naturally, people and other animals prefer pleasure over stress. Unfortunately, some stress is required in a world where only the fittest survive.

Psychoactive drugs can act on the brain in several ways:

- *Mimicry:* Morphine mimics the actions of the endorphins produced by the brain. Morphine is principally associated with the reduction of pain, but the body's response to it is more complicated. As with nitrous oxide (laughing gas), the patient often reports that they still feel the pain, but they have such a sense of relaxation and well-being that they feel totally detached from it.

- *Neurotransmitter accumulation:* Another pathway to addiction is to inhibit the destruction of the feel-good neurotransmitters. These then accumulate, producing a heightened sense of well-being. This is how cocaine works and, some might say, the SSRIs and SNRIs also.
- *Up-regulation:* Stimulating the body's own production of a particular neurotransmitter can also lead to addiction. Amphetamines are in this category, increasing the output of nor-adrenalin, and its precursor dopamine, a major feel-good neurotransmitter. These neurotransmitters are associated with focus and a heightened sense of purpose. Nicotine acts at one of the receptor sites for acetylcholine. Although acetylcholine can work at several receptor sites, nicotine works at just one of these. What happens after that has yet to be elucidated, but it is generally thought that the release of dopamine is increased, or that there is heightened sensitivity to this chemical.

Whether psychoactive drugs are addictive or not, they interfere with the chemistry of a complicated system and raise the spectre of iatrogenic illness in the immature brain. This is why a sense of outrage at these developments is understandable.

Adult sleep disorders

Sleep disorders are one of the commonest problems seen by general practitioners. Patients typically see themselves as having a medical condition, a fixed-name disease: they say things like 'I've got insomnia', or maybe 'I can't sleep, doc. Could I have depression/ sleep apnoea?'

Of course, all possibilities need to be considered. If the doctor replies, 'Yes, I think you are depressed, here's a script for some anti-depressants', the patient might reasonably ask if something else could be tried. But if the doctor were to say, 'I think you have a disruption of your circadian rhythms, and I want you to change your job and get a whole new lifestyle', would the patient opt for the anti-depressants after all?

Circadian rhythms are discussed in Chapter 10, but let us look for the moment at the contrasting lifestyle of a representative of our earliest ancestors. Let us call him Otto. How will he prepare for sleep?

To begin with, he will probably have eaten two meals that day, as dictated by his biological hunger clock (Chapters 8 and 10). The evening meal is prepared around dusk, and is eaten as the light fades. As the meal is digested, there may be storytelling and music around a campfire. The scene is peaceful. And the biochemistry?

Otto is sitting down to eat, a fact which gives his digestive processes a head start on his counterpart in the 21st century. He will not leap up and rush out to a meeting, except in the unlikely event of enemy attack. Thus the opiate-like peptides and neuroactive amines in his food will undergo full digestion to amino acids. These amino acids will help, not hinder, his ability to sleep.

As daylight fades his pineal gland starts to produce melatonin. He has adequate precursors for this in his diet. Vitamins and minerals will be available to catalyse the amino acid tryptophan through serotonin to melatonin (Chart 3.3). By the time the light has gone altogether, he is already becoming sleepy, but not through drugs, alcohol or sugar. These things produce 'dopiness' rather than healthy somnolence. Otto is sleepy because has been physically active during the day, and now has an abundance of circulating melatonin.

As he watches the embers of the fire, the flickering induces alpha wave patterns in his brain. Alpha waves are the slow waves associated with relaxation in the conscious state. (Watching television can also produce alpha waves. Do people become addicted to television because the ancient part of their brain is hungering for the flickering pattern of the fire? This whimsical thought has been the subject of serious consideration.)

Otto's modern counterpart could not conduct his evening more differently if he tried. Let us take the case of John, whom we met in Chapter 6. At dusk he may just be coming home from work. He gives Junior a quick cuddle, eats a rushed meal and heads off to a meeting. On a quiet night he spends a bit more time with Junior, eats with Jean, and goes to his study to do several hours more work. There's an important deadline to meet. His focus on the office problems puts his brain into a state of high alert. He may drink tea, coffee or some other stimulant to keep himself going. He is on a proton pump inhibitor to deal with his irritable bowel and associated digestive disorder. Fatigue is one of the side effects of this drug, but its not the sort of fatigue conducive to sound REM sleep. John sleeps but awakes unrefreshed.

Perhaps the person who comes closest to his caveman ancestor is Fred, slumped in front of the television. At least he has a few alpha waves on his side. On the other hand, if he has a coffee or a beer in his hand, his sleep will not be normal. Fred, like most people, has noticed that his sleep problems are worse if he drinks coffee at night. He prefers a beer. However, while this helps him to nod off, he often finds himself awake several hours later.

Maybe this is due to the two-phase action of alcohol. Sedation is the initial response of the brain but a few hours later, depending on how much alcohol has been consumed, there may be a phase of excitation. Unfortunately, this stage is often reached just when deep REM sleep should be cutting in.

What about melatonin? John has recently read an article in the paper about it. Should you be able to buy it over the counter, as you can in the United States and Britain? Melatonin is a natural, and therefore, presumably, safe product. It may help John sleep, but will it fix his gut problems, his chronic stress? Will it help his relationship with Jean or with Junior? Perhaps his insomnia is a timely warning to look at his lifestyle, his diet, his priorities, before he joins the ranks of those with premature heart disease and his marriage becomes just another statistic.

Sleep disorders in infants and young children

Cot death

Cot death is, of course, a tragedy rather than a disorder, but it is convenient to group it here with other disturbances of sleep. Putting a baby to sleep on its back has reduced the risk enormously. However, babies still die from this condition. What other factors influence risk?

We might expect that cot death would appear in cultural myths and ancient texts, but mentions are so infrequent that we can infer that this is predominantly a disease of civilisation. Cot death seems commoner in the babies of smokers than in babies from non-smoking households. It is commoner in bottle-fed than breast-fed babies. It is also more common in developed and affluent societies than in crowded, poor communities. Over the years, several interesting theories have emerged.

One is that the combination of urine and PVC mattresses produces toxic fumes. Such mattresses did not exist until the last half of the 20th century. Maybe sleeping face up provides air circulation to dissipate the fumes.

Another theory is 'forgetting to breathe'. The idea is that a human baby at birth is an embryonic life form. This is the price of our big brains; a larger head could not navigate the birth canal. Perhaps this 'embryo' has not fully developed its 'automatic breathe' function. In sleep, breathing may slow so much that, unless it is kick-started, it may cease altogether. In a 'natural' environment, it is argued, the sounds or movements of parents in the same bed or siblings in the same room will serve to start it. Some studies have shown that infants who sleep in their parents' bed have an increased risk of cot death. Other studies show that this applies only when the parents are smokers; once smoking was factored out, co-sleeping appeared to be protective.[22]

Bottle feeding is thought to contribute to cot death in one of at least three ways:

- Plastic bottles when heated emit toxic PVC fumes, a risk which is increased when these containers are microwaved.
- Cow's milk lacks some essential nutrients and immune globulins, normally found in breast milk.
- The clinical picture of cot death resembles death by anaphylaxis (allergic shock), raising the possibility that the babies die as a result of anaphylactic shock in response to bovine protein in cow's milk.

Even the hygiene theory (Chapter 6) has been raised. Independent of the role of vaccination, an immune system not matured by the exposure to common germs may be at increased risk from some of these factors.

It is easy to see how one medical problem can have a complexity of possible contributing factors. Unravelling these can be impossible. This is the weakness of single-cause theories for fixed-name disorders. The example also shows the many ways in which deviation from simple lifestyles might contribute to the medical problems most commonly feared in 'civilised' cultures.

Unremitting and relentless infant crying

Family doctors often see babies that cry excessively. This is associated with post-natal depression (cause or effect?), and there is a real risk that a despairing parent may injure the baby.

Locked in her hermetically sealed modern home, alone with her newborn, the mother relates with anguish the stories of a baby who simply won't stop crying. These mothers often say that the only thing that pacifies the baby is to put it in a pram and wheel it into the street.

What is more natural—the 'white noise' generated by street sounds, the continuous movement of the pram on the pavement, or the deathly stillness of the lonely cot without sound or movement? Babies are primed by nine months of movement and the rhythmic sound of a heartbeat, not to mention thousands of years of human evolution, to sleep through noise, activity and human presence. Perhaps they are screaming in panic at the bizarre situation they find themselves in.

If post-natal depression is linked to the crying, what clue might this give? One possibility is neglect by a depressed mother, and her depression may be the result of deficiencies in zinc, magnesium and essential fatty acids. But if the mother is deficient, there's a good chance that the baby is as well. This will lead to poor sleep, a twitchy nervous system, an irritable infant. Forget the psychology for a moment—this may be a biochemical disorder.

Even in babies whose mothers do not show clinical depression, a marginal deficiency may be enough to trigger a state of chronic irritability. If this seems fanciful to the reader, I offer the personal experience of seeing babies settle miraculously when a breast-feeding mother is supplemented with B-group vitamins, zinc and magnesium.

Summary

Both bedwetting and night terrors show a genetic predisposition, but both are also subject to the considerations just explored. It would be interesting to know whether they are prevalent in tribal settings. Avoiding food allergens and supplementing with essential nutrients has produced promising results in my experience.

Maturation of the central nervous system requires the B-group vitamins, zinc, selenium, essential fatty acids. Magnesium is important in neurotransmission. We know that omega-3 fatty acids concentrate in breast milk, so they must be important. We know the changing status of magnesium, selenium and zinc in the diet. Poor sleep affects not only the child, but the whole family.

Ask whether the department of paediatrics at the university nearest to you is studying these questions. If not, why not?

NEUROLOGICAL DISORDERS

Any disorder which afflicts the brain or the central or peripheral nervous system can be classified as neurological. As with any other organ or organ system, dysfunction can arise in multiple ways. Some conditions are genetic, although these are relatively rare. Some are caused by illnesses such as meningitis and encephalitis. Toxic chemicals and ionising radiation can cause DNA damage, resulting in malignancies. And poor blood supply due to diabetes and vascular disease can cause nerve damage (neuropathies) and brain injury (stroke).

It is hard to do more than generalise. And yet, in terms of prevention and treatment, generalising may be the most valuable thing we can do. I will look briefly at just four neurological disorders: Alzheimer's disease, multiple sclerosis, Parkinson's disease, migraine.

Alzheimer's disease

Dementia refers to loss of brain function, and can be due to many causes. Brains damaged by alcohol, accidents, birth injury or vascular disease can all produce cognitive and emotional responses which could be recognised as 'demented'.

Alzheimer's is in some ways the left-over category. In this condition there is no obvious injury or neglect, just a brain losing its higher functions. Further subdivision recognises that some forms of Alzheimer's can strike at an early age, or they may have a hereditary component, as with the dementia associated with a particular allele of one of the lipid-carrying proteins known as apo E (Chapter 8).

This variant can be associated with both sporadic and with late-onset familial cases, but is not considered to be sufficiently predictive to be used as a screening tool.

A link between Alzheimer's, untreated coeliac disease and Down syndrome raises the fascinating question of gluten sensitivity and the brain (compare gluten and autism above). Another aspect of this linkage will be mentioned shortly.

Let's return to our 'typical' family.

Fran's mum, Mary's grandmother, is called Sarah. She is in her early 70s, and since her husband Edward died a few years ago she has been depressed, sleeps badly, and is not eating very well. Her memory recently has been so poor that the family has begun to worry about her. Her skin is dry, and she does not look well. Is she suffering from depression? Or does she have early dementia?

When she begins to have 'accidents' on her way to the toilet, a geriatrics team decides she needs residential care. This is difficult for her and the family, but is felt to be for the best. Sarah's signs of dementia were at first thought to be due to depression. There is, indeed, much overlap between the two conditions — sleep disturbance, lack of interest in food and, of course, short-term memory problems.

But the either-or nature of this question, depression or Alzheimer's, shows how easy it is to fall into the traps of diagnostic categories. Sarah may well have suffered from depression after Edward's death, considering that she and Edward had almost never spent a day apart in the past 50 years.

Sarah found that, once she was cooking only for herself, she now lacked the motivation to make the meat and three vegetables which had been the mainstay of their meals; soon, an egg on toast was enough. Gradually, except for the once or twice a week that she ate at Fran's, the egg was left out, and it became just tea and toast. Fish on Friday had been a ritual, but now it was too much trouble. Fran tried to keep an eye on things, but she didn't see what got thrown out. Sarah had always been rather independent. Fran felt she was intruding.

After the 'accidents' become obvious, Fran accompanied Sarah to a routine doctor's visit. The question of bowel problems was broached with a very defensive Sarah. Was there a bowel infection or, worse still, a bowel cancer? Thyrotoxicosis (an over-active thyroid gland) can cause diarrhoea, but the tests were negative. Pellagra was not on the list of possibilities.

Pellagra, or classical Vitamin B3 deficiency, was discussed in Chapter 5 as part of the three Ds: dementia, diarrhoea and dermatitis. Does this sound like Sarah? Could a Third World disease really exist in the midst of plenty? Sarah has been well looked after, taking diuretics for hypertension, anti-depressants since Edward died, and a mild sedative for sleep. She has had something to lower her cholesterol (a disorder that responds to Vitamin B3), something to 'firm up' her bowel, and a variety of skin lotions. Now the geriatricians are talking about a (very expensive) drug called Aricept.

Aricept is described as a 'gift' by its promoters, although it is one of the most expensive drugs on the market. Along with cholesterol-lowering drugs and a few other medications, Aricept helps blow out health budgets throughout the Western world. And yet the summary by clinicians of the efficacy of this drug, subsidised by the government, is 'disappointing'. At best, it delays the progression of dementia by about six months.

If the doctor prescribes selenium, Vitamin B3 or B12, who will pay? The pensioner medical benefits do not as a rule cover vitamins and minerals.

If we take the view that fixed-name disease treats symptoms not causes, Sarah demonstrates many missed opportunities here. First there was her depression. Loss of appetite is common in depression and also during mourning. Perhaps a vicious cycle set in. Zinc deficiency is a recognised problem in the elderly.[23] Low zinc levels in turn produce anorexia. As tea and toast becomes the mainstay, a cycle of vitamin and mineral deficiencies is set in train. This in turn leads to sleep disturbance and deepening depression. After all, the production of serotonin, melatonin and dopamine all depend on a range of enzymes, which require Vitamin B6, B12 and folic acid (Chart 3.3).

Then there were Sarah's other medical problems. After Edward had his first heart attack, Sarah had testing that showed mild hypertension, raised cholesterol, and raised homocysteine. The diuretic for her hypertension removes not only sodium from the body, but other valuable trace elements. The cholesterol-lowering drug produces gastro-intestinal disturbance as well as many other side effects. Did this affect her appetite or contribute to her 'accidents'? And would it be churlish to mention that cholesterol has both structural and biochemical roles within the brain?

The fact of raised homocysteine was noted at the time, but no specific treatment was thought necessary. Now we know that raised homocysteine is associated with an increased risk of Alzheimer's, heart disease and cancer, and that folic acid and the B-group vitamins are the best way of bringing it down. Would a multi-B vitamin have slowed the onset of Sarah's dementia? Current evidence suggests that it would.

Here are the nutrients that are thought to benefit dementia and Alzheimer's: Vitamin C, Vitamin E, B-group vitamins, folic acid, zinc, magnesium, selenium, copper and omega-3 fatty acids.[24]

Here is a list of nutrients which are connected to the treatment of Sarah's other problems (again, not comprehensive). What does the overlap tell us?

- *hypertension:* omega-3 fatty acids, magnesium, Vitamin C, Vitamin E, zinc, selenium
- *raised cholesterol:* omega-3 fatty acids, Vitamin C, B-group vitamins, especially B3 and B5
- *depression:* B-group vitamins, zinc, selenium, omega-3 fatty acids, magnesium.[25]

So we can begin to make a case that, even before Edward died, Sarah's diet was subject to all the problems discussed throughout this book. After his death the limitations increased, and the brain began to pay the cost. Do we have any clinical evidence for this? There is one interesting bit of corroborative evidence.

The risk of dementia is known to be high in people with coeliac disease and in those with Down syndrome. Down syndrome, in turn, is strongly associated with coeliac. In coeliac disease, one of the earliest abnormalities is the malabsorption of vitamins, minerals, and fats. There is the tantalising thought that the link between coeliac and Alzheimer's, possibly even between Down syndrome and Alzheimer's, is not genetics but a nutrient deficiency (see also Chapter 10).

Multiple sclerosis (MS)

MS seems to correlate with the adoption of the Western diet, among other factors. It afflicts the young, and thus hurts people at the most productive time of their lives. (It usually makes its first appearance between the ages of 20 and 40, and rarely after the age of 50.) And finally, it appears to be on the increase throughout the world, even in cultures where it was relatively rare before.

Pathology

When one part of the body wants to 'talk' to another part of the body, it can do so in many ways, but most of them fall into one of two categories:

- chemical messengers, such as hormones and neurotransmitters, in the bloodstream
- electrical messages sent via nerves.

For rapid transmission, the nervous system is the most effective. We withdraw our hand from a hot stove before our brain has consciously registered that it is hot. We respond to pain even when we are asleep or in a coma. (The speed of response to pain is one way, in fact, of measuring the depth of coma.)

Nerves can transmit messages with such impressive speed because of the myelin sheath which is wrapped around nerve cells within the brain, the spinal cord, and the peripheral nervous system. The myelin sheath is like the insulation around electrical wiring. Electrical insulation is vital for protecting us from electrocution, but its primary purpose is to prevent leakage of electrical energy. Without insulation the signal would be delayed, severely weakened, or lost altogether.

MS results in patchy removal of the myelin sheaths of various nerve cells. Sometimes certain sheaths recover, only to have others succumb. Once the demyelination becomes permanent, the function of that nerve cell is effectively lost.

Theories about causes

MS has long been regarded as an autoimmune disease. As with most autoimmune diseases, there appears to be a genetic predisposition. Recently, there has been a challenge to the autoimmune theory,[26] and it will be interesting to see this line of inquiry unfold. But it is the identification of common factors in MS patients which has made it a fascinating subject for neurologists and epidemiologists alike.

From the earliest recognition of MS as an entity, it became apparent that there was a clear global variation according to latitude. In the northern and southern hemispheres there were typically 50–100 cases per 100,000 population, compared with 5–10 cases in the tropics. With this kind of distribution, and in the absence of an obvious causative agent, theories abounded. Suggestions included viruses, ethnic variance, geography, diet, and a lack of minerals and vitamins. Let us look at each of these.

The regional predictability typical of MS is commonly associated with a virus or a parasite such as malaria. Certain viruses have been shown to cause other demyelinating diseases, but with MS no such culprit was found. Many viruses have been suggested, most prominently measles and herpes, but these infections are not confined by latitude. Still, many feel that a virus may play at least some role in the illness.

With regard to ethnic variance, as so often happens, it was the exceptions which proved to be most interesting. Scots are by far the most vulnerable group, with an incidence of 153 per 100,000 in the Orkney and Shetland Islands. In Japan, where the latitude leads one to expect an intermediate incidence, the figure was just 2 per 100,000.

Racial and sex variations were also noted, in that Caucasians were more at risk than Asians, and Black races least of all. Caucasian women were found to be twice to three times as susceptible as Caucasian men. The disease is almost unknown in Australian Aboriginals, particularly those living most nearly the traditional lifestyle. But these racial variations still did not explain the latitude effects, or the exceptions.

Was it the Celtic gene? Many Scots and other Celts migrated to similarly cold climates. Did they simply take the gene with them? Were the victims of MS in *warmer* climates typically of Celtic origin? Some epidemiologists traced the movements of thousands of Scots who had migrated around the world, including Scots living in warm climates such as Australia. It seemed that moving from a low-risk area to a high-risk area made a difference *only* if the move was made before the age of 15. Whatever the detrimental effects of living in a risk zone, it appeared that they exerted their influence early in life.

So if we are looking for a single agent, we still do not have the answer. These are some of the other correlates:

- European diets may be classified as either 'beer and butter' or 'wine and oil', typical of Germany and Scandinavia and of Greece, Italy, Portugal respectively. The wine and oil food cultures confer a significantly lower risk of developing MS.
- Cultures which consume a diet based on dairy and gluten are associated with greater risk than those with a high rice and vegetable intake. In keeping with the autoimmune theory, these foods may be acting as antigens. However, it is also true that the dairy-gluten diet has more saturated fats. The role of dietary fats in MS will be discussed shortly.
- Minerals and vitamins, as we would expect, have a role to play. Another correlate which emerged was an association between thyroid problems and MS, and Parkinson's disease and MS. In this case, the link seemed to be iodine deficiency. Other studies showed that living in low-selenium areas increased the risk. Compared with a typical Western selenium intake of 30–50 mcg per day, the protection provided by a traditional Japanese diet (over 200 mcg) is not hard to grasp.
- Levels of Vitamin B12 have been implicated. Certain dietary, metabolic and digestive factors can lower B12 levels. Occasionally these can be genetically determined, in which case cause and effect may be difficult to separate. Whatever the genetic picture, intramuscular injection of B12 in the form of methyl cobalamin can have dramatic benefit in acute flares.[27] My own experience of this has been very positive.
- Attention has recently focused on Vitamin D. Sun exposure may explain the latitude correlations, and this effect may also operate at high altitudes. In Switzerland it has been shown that the risk of MS decreases with increase of altitude, where ultraviolet radiation, necessary for the conversion of Vitamin D, increases.[28]
- The protective role of fish, in terms of its EFA content, is discussed shortly. Cold-water fish, such as sardines and herrings, are rich in Vitamin D.
- MS appears to be associated with heavy metal poisoning. Heavy metals such as lead and mercury have direct

neurotoxic effects, and they also compete with desirable minerals like selenium by occupying the same receptor sites (Chapter 3: Chemistry).

- Chemical poisoning has also been implicated. Formaldehyde exposure has been linked to various neurological conditions, including MS. And studies comparing the blood of MS patients with that of controls have shown significant differences in the levels of toxic chlorinated pesticides, volatile aromatic hydrocarbons, volatile chlorinated hydrocarbons, and volatile aliphatic hydrocarbons. In one such study the MS patients had no less than 14 different intracellular minerals, including potassium, chromium, calcium and magnesium, which were abnormal, along with an overall deficiency of B-group vitamins. The epidemiologist concluded: 'All of these abnormalities suggest membrane damage, which is usually triggered by pollutants.'[29]

Membranes and essential fatty acids

How do these various findings fit in with the geographical distribution of MS? If membrane damage is a common factor, then the ability to *repair* damaged membranes becomes relevant. (Membrane physiology was discussed in Chapter 5: EFAs.) What dietary influences are peculiar to high-risk and low-risk areas?

Overall, dietary fat seems to emerge as one of the most important factors in the vulnerability to MS. This is not surprising, as between 70 and 80 per cent of the myelin sheath is composed of fat. Dietary lipids are directly incorporated into lipid membranes. In Norway, Scotland and other high-risk countries, the level of risk in genetically-close groups is closely linked to the amount of fish consumed.

EFAs help to keep the structure of the membrane healthy, but they also have functions which go beyond scaffolding. The omega-3s are necessary to the biochemical elongation of other fats integral to the structure of normal myelin. Deficiency of omega-3 interferes with that, independent of the structural role of the omega-3 itself.

Omega-3s also control the production of inflammatory prostaglandins. Saturated fats and those EFAs which end up as arachidonic acid, all promote inflammatory pathways (Chart 5.3). MS is certainly an inflammatory disease. Hence the benefits of steroids in acute flares.

The functions of omega-3s have been discussed in Chapter 5 and do not need repetition, but two important points are:

- EFAs are significant in modifying any potential for autoimmune disease.
- EFAs help to determine how the genetic code is read.

These points may have a bearing on the age of migration and its effect on susceptibility to MS.

So what implications are there in EFA consumption and the prevalence of MS at extreme latitudes? Many of these nations eat a lot of cold-water fish. Certain racial groups are more vulnerable, and the fairer the skin, the weaker the resistance. Perhaps the groups whose diets naturally contain cold-water fish, those in the higher latitudes whose skin is naturally fair, somehow genetically have less tolerance of omega-3 deprivation?

Many of the plants which are naturally rich in omega-3s come from cold climates. This makes sense. Omega-3s, with their anti-freeze function, are protective against cold. With fish, flaxseeds, walnuts, algae and leafy greens, those who evolved with this kind of diet would rarely have lacked these EFAs. Of course, people from warm climates also need omega-3 fatty acids in their diet. But as with many things, there may be variable degrees of tolerance to deficiency states.

Genetically, we know that some people have sluggish delta-6 enzymes (Chart 5.3). Which enzyme system you have inherited will determine the facility with which you convert EFAs into protective PG-1 and PG-3. Unless you eat appropriate foods in sufficient amounts, there is an increased risk of inflammatory disorders. We might conclude that MS is one of those.

Digestion has a role in most illnesses, and MS is no exception. If membrane damage is a factor, then the membranes lining the gut are as likely to be affected as any other membranes in the body. Damaged gut membranes make for a leaky gut, impairing the absorption of protective vitamins, minerals, and EFAs. And if MS is an autoimmune disease, absorption through a leaky membrane of large protein particles will favour the development of an autoimmune process. All of which highlights yet again how inappropriate it is to look for single agents in fixed-name conditions.

Parkinson's disease

Parkinson's disease is a relatively common condition afflicting more than 1 per cent of people older than 55. After the age of 85, this figure rises to more than 5 per cent, indicating the degenerative nature of the problem.

Parkinsonism is a collection of problems rather than one entity. There are certain characteristic symptoms, and post-mortem shows characteristic damage to certain nerve cells in the brain. The classic symptoms include:

- *Gait:* Loss or reduction of arm swing when walking, shortened but often accelerated stride, and impaired balance.
- *Tremor at rest:* This is often an early diagnostic sign, most noticeable in the hands, and usually asymmetric at first. Conscious movement of the affected limb will often stop the tremor for the duration of the action.
- *Rigidity:* When a limb is passively moved by another person, there is a 'cog-wheel' resistance as the rigid limb gives way in short bursts.
- *Akinesia:* This refers to the difficulty such patients have in initiating a movement. It is like watching a person who is anxious about escalators trying to judge when to put their foot forward onto the moving steps.

The underlying damage to brain cells varies according to the different types of Parkinsonism, but it is often divided into two groups, idiopathic and atypical.

Idiopathic Parkinson's
This form is characterised by the features listed above, and symptomatically at least, responds well to treatment with the drug levodopa, which is converted to dopamine in the brain. Post-mortem examination shows the normally dark *substantia nigra* in the mid-brain is pale, signifying loss of dopamine-producing neurones. The remaining damaged neurones contain abnormal structures known as Lewy bodies and neurofibrillary tangles.

Strictly speaking, diagnosis can only occur after death, because this degree of accuracy is not possible on a living brain. Up to 10 per cent of people with this form of Parkinson's are thought to develop symptoms before the age of 40, but this is only recognised retrospectively. Studies of twins indicate that there is a strong genetic component to early-onset Parkinson's.

Besides levodopa, a wide range of other medications is employed in the treatment of Parkinson's. None are able to halt or even slow the disease, but all give symptomatic relief. Many have side effects which are prohibitive in individual patients.

This illness has been labelled idiopathic, the term used to represent a fixed-name disease which has no known cause. Yet for many years now, researchers have shown connections between the risk of Parkinson's and environmental factors.

- One study demonstrated that people who used pesticides in the home had a 70 per cent higher risk of getting the disease.[30]
- In another study on rats, the common pesticide Rotenone gradually destroyed the dopamine-producing neurones, resulting in a clinical picture of Parkinsonism. This natural plant product acted by inhibiting one of the mitochondrial enzymes. The enzyme is also inhibited by a chemical called MPTP, a known contaminant of heroin. Some heroin addicts developed Parkinson's after exposure to this chemical.[31]
- A study published in *The Lancet* threw light on the role of poisons and the genetic aspect as well.[32] Of the many genes involved in the production of enzymes to detoxify poisons, one important enzyme called GSTP is known to be polymorphic. The allele (gene variant) known as GSTP1 seemed to be protective against developing Parkinson's. A person who had only one, or no, copies of the GSTP1 allele had an increased risk of Parkinson's, but only if they had handled pesticides.
- Other research has shown that the combinations of lead and copper, lead and iron, and iron and copper, increased the risk of developing Parkinson's disease up to fivefold.[33]
- In a 1996 study in Germany of 380 patients, there was a significant over-representation of people who had had occupational exposure to organochlorines and alkylated

phosphates. Wood preservatives and general anaesthesia also appeared to be risk factors.[34]

In his book on chemical sensitivity, William J. Rea lists the following chemicals as being associated with the development of Parkinson's:

- 1-methyl-4-phenyl-1,2,3,6,tetrahydro-pridine (MPTP)
- organophosphate pesticides
- petroleum derivatives plus pesticides
- carbon tetrachloride and carbon disulfide (CS_2)
- *Cycas circinalis*, a neurotoxic plant from Guam
- hexachlorobenzene (a fungicide).[35]

Many of these studies go back to the 1970s and 1980s, yet 30 years later we are still describing Parkinson's disease as idiopathic. Neurotoxins may not be the only things to trigger Parkinson's and they may not even be the cause, but as many of them are ubiquitous in the environment it is hard to understand the lack of interest in them in the assessment of this disease.

Research has long indicated that oxidative damage to the cells of the substantia nigra is one of the most significant initiators of Parkinson's disease. In the early 1970s, Gerald Cohen and Richard E. Heikkila from the Mount Sinai School of Medicine in the United States found that a synthetic toxin could produce Parkinsonism in animals by the formation of at least two different kinds of free radical. One of the 'fingerprints' of free radical damage is the formation of lipid peroxides (Chapter 5: Vitamin E), which they were able to demonstrate.[36] The high fat content of the brain makes it particularly vulnerable to lipid peroxidation.

Oxidative damage can occur in various ways. An overload of metals such as iron and copper can act as a source of free radicals. Chemicals can do this, too. Alternatively, these substances may damage the redox enzymes. Even a simple deficiency of the anti-oxidants required to support those enzymes could result in lipid peroxidation. These are not either-or options. Probably a complex of insults triggers the events which lead to the diagnosis of Parkinson's disease.

Although Parkinson's is a fixed-name disease, or even a fixed-name syndrome, perhaps it is actually another free radical disorder. It is different in presentation, but not in kind, to other free radical diseases such as arthritis, heart disease and cancer.

Atypical Parkinson's

Atypical Parkinson's refers to a collection of other syndromes which have clinical and pathological similarities to each other, but vary to a greater or lesser extent. Notably, Lewy bodies are not usually a feature of these other forms.

It has been estimated that up to 25 per cent of Parkinson's disease is misdiagnosed because many other conditions can mimic it. These include Wilson's disease (an inherited tendency to copper overload) and cerebrovascular disease. There is also a form of dementia which can be accompanied by Lewy bodies and can mimic Parkinson's.

Perhaps best-known in the category of the atypical forms is drug-induced Parkinsonism. Many prescription medications actually work against the effects of dopamine (usually unintentionally), and in certain people Parkinson-like effects can be seen early in treatment. The vulnerability to this side effect is unpredictable, and it may have a genetic basis. Early withdrawal of the medication is mandatory in order to avoid long-term damage.

Some recreational drugs have been associated with the development of Parkinson's disease. In recent times a scandal erupted when there was evidence of tampered results in studies purporting to show that the drug Ecstasy could induce the illness.

Treatment

Three senior neurologists have said 'no treatment has been shown to arrest or slow the neurodegenerative process' of Parkinson's.[37] But a wide range of nutritional treatments for Parkinson's have shown varying degrees of benefit. On theoretical grounds alone, this should not be surprising. Oxidative damage can be halted, and sometimes reversed, by appropriate anti-oxidants.

Vitamin C is a chameleon, as we have seen (Chapter 4). It can act as an anti-oxidant, and by donating electrons it can act as a catalyst to enzyme reactions. Interestingly, it is also a competitive antagonist at dopamine receptor sites. This means it can mimic or block the action of dopamine, in a manner analogous to the phyto-oestrogens when they occupy oestrogen receptor sites. Vitamin C has been shown to antagonise the effects of amphetamines, and to enhance the effect of the anti-psychotic drug haloperidol. (Psychotic illness such as schizophrenia is associated with excess dopamine production.) There is a role for Vitamin C in schizophrenia, autism and Parkinson's. Used early in Parkinson's, it is claimed that it can delay the need for levodopa.

There are positive reports on the use of other nutrients as well. However, the trials are marred by following the methodology of the standard drug trial. Trials on single nutrients, such as folic acid and Vitamin E, have unsurprisingly been disappointing. When they are used in consort, we could reasonably expect a favourable outcome.

Various nutrients, such as the omega-6 fatty acids, Vitamins C, E, B3, B6 and beta carotene, and minerals such as magnesium and iodine, have had apparently beneficial results. A recent trial of co-enzyme Q10 has confirmed a role for this nutrient in Parkinson's.[38]

Migraine

It is Friday morning, and there are two migraine patients in the waiting room. One is Louise, aged 17, and the other is Astrid, who turned 50 on her last birthday.

Louise is in her last year of school, and is a good student. She works hard, and if her grades are good enough, she hopes to study medicine. Louise has been suffering from what is known as *classic migraine* since puberty. Classic migraine is characterised by aura, visual disturbance, severe pain, photophobia and vomiting, although not all attacks show all of these features. Louise's headaches are often associated with her periods and always seem to come at the worst times. Today she has a major assignment due and has been working hard on it because the marks will go towards her final assessments. She is in the throes of an attack and looks wretched. She is holding a plastic bucket because she feels she might vomit. Her mother is outside parking the car, having taken the morning off work to bring her to the surgery.

Astrid, by contrast, is flipping idly through a woman's magazine. Today is a routine appointment not specifically related to her migraines. She heard Louise checking in and offered her place in the queue. Astrid doesn't usually get as sick as Louise does with her headaches, but it has happened a couple of times. She knows why people say that if it were a dog, you would shoot it. Astrid can have a headache twice within a week. They are more frequent during times of stress and before her period. With simple painkillers she can get through the day. At night she will take an anti-histamine and go to bed early. She fits the typical profile of someone suffering from *common migraine*, where the symptoms are similar to classic migraine, but much milder. She is pleased to note that as she approaches menopause, the headaches seem to be lessening.

Who gets migraine?

The medical literature is full of stories of people like Astrid and Louise. As women outnumber men three to one in this condition, the typical patient is likely to be female. The headache was first described in ancient Egypt, and there have been many well-known victims, including Charlotte Bronte, van Gogh, and possibly Charles Darwin.

Because it is common, migraine receives a lot of press. Louise feels that if she ever studies medicine, she may specialise in migraines! She has read how, once a migraine is triggered, a whole set of biochemical and neurological events known as the 'migraine cascade' are set in train. This may then lead to the full catastrophe of pain, vomiting and visual disturbance. With all that knowledge about the trigeminal nerve, neuropeptides, serotonin, and so on, surely there's an answer?

The treatment

Louise will be treated for her acute attack with injections for pain and nausea. She has already had several consultations and tried a range of preventive medicines. These have made her sleepy or forgetful, and in most cases have been ineffective. The newer triptans are not recommended for people under 18. Her doctor, like many of his colleagues, finds that his patients complain that triptans only delay the headaches, and many say they cannot afford the medication. Yet they were introduced with such a fanfare: 'The end of the headache that has lasted thousands of years!' After a few deaths, cautions were issued against their use in patients with cardiovascular disease. They were found to be risky when used in conjunction with one of the commonest migraine treatments, ergotamine. All in all, Louise and her doctor would prefer another option.

So why do I and my colleagues feel a sense of despair when we see Louise and others sitting there with their plastic buckets? Menopause may bring relief, but that is a long way off for Louise.

Research into migraine has brought forth many drug therapies, but no cure. What's more, migraine seems to be on the rise. The former estimate of 1 in 10 has been revised to 1 in 6.[39] And more children and teenagers are developing migraine in its various manifestations.

The research

Is migraine another fixed-name disease? Perhaps we have failed to make a difference because we have focused on the symptoms rather than the cause.

Researchers have been looking at neurotransmitters for decades now. Everything from the trigeminal nerve to the brainstem has been studied. PET scans have made all sorts of observation possible. Migraine has been painstakingly classified into a catalogue of variants; impressive as an exercise in taxonomy. Yet in 2002, Ninan Mathew of the Houston Headache Clinic told *Time* magazine what any migraineur knows: 'At one time people thought that migraine was a disorder all its own and that tension-type headache was totally separate. Now we know that headaches are not all that clear cut.'[40]

More than 50 per cent of migraine sufferers have a family history of the condition. Could there be a 'migraine gene'? Common migraine has a complex inheritance pattern which suggests the involvement of several genes. There is a nasty form of migraine known as familial hemiplegic migraine (FHM), in which there is an increased risk of strokes during an attack. The first FHM gene was located on chromosome 19 and seemed to implicate calcium channels.[41] But some people with FHM did not have this particular gene. And then, in February 2003, a mutation in the gene for sodium and potassium channels was found.[42] A second gene had been implicated.

Nutritional deficiency

Magnesium has been shown to be reduced in blood, saliva and cerebrospinal fluid of migraineurs. This may be a cause, rather than an effect, of the migraines.

Magnesium is a smooth muscle relaxant, and part of the migraine cascade involves spasm of the cerebral vasculature. Migraineurs are acutely aware of the throbbing of scalp arteries, and vascular spasm is a significant aspect of the strokes which occur during migraine. Arteries are contracted into a spasm by the smooth muscles which control their diameter.

Magnesium also modifies the functions of hormones and neurotransmitters. Demands on magnesium supply reach a peak in the premenstrual phase of the female cycle. Women with symptoms of premenstrual tension, including headache, have been shown to have lower than expected blood levels of magnesium. And low levels of magnesium increase the sensitivity of blood vessels to the neurotransmitter serotonin.

As we have seen, one of the 'migraine genes' had to do with calcium channel dysfunction. Magnesium is the other half of the story. Magnesium and calcium are like twins, always requiring an equilibrium throughout the body.

A study observed the effects of supplementing migraine patients with high doses of oral magnesium.[43] Before the end of the second month of supplementation, therapeutic benefit was statistically significant; it included a reduction in both the frequency and the severity of attacks. A separate group of women with 'menstrual migraine' were also shown to respond. Yet to my knowledge, no migraine clinic in Australia has trialled magnesium, or routinely incorporates it into its treatment regimes. Some hospital departments claim to use intravenous magnesium in the Emergency Room for acute migraine. The pain and risk of stroke are both derived from arterial spasm, so the benefit of releasing spasm does not need to be spelled out.

One of my patients went to the Emergency Department of a large teaching hospital suffering severe migraine. She was injected with pethidine and sent home. When the effects of the pethidine had worn off, the migraine returned. She was frightened because there was a family history of migraine and of stroke at a young age, and she was feeling numbness and weakness on one side. I phoned the hospital and spoke to a neurological registrar. Yes, he thought intravenous magnesium would be a good idea. I sent her in. When I phoned him back, he said that he had not given her the magnesium because she was 'too sick for that'. He'd given her pethidine again.

As well as magnesium, B-group vitamins have a role to play. More than one study has shown that supplementation with Vitamin B2 has reduced the frequency of migraine by up to 50 per cent.[44] The list of foods rich in B2 is extensive. Notably absent however, are milk, white flour, sugar, refined carbohydrates, saturated fats — the backbone of the Western diet. Vitamin B6 is another key nutrient. Many of the drugs used to treat migraine actually perpetuate the problem by depleting central nervous system endorphins (nature's own pain relievers), and by suppressing the receptor sites for them.[45] B6 is probably the single most important tool for reversing this situation.

Part of the migraine cascade involves the swelling and inflammation of blood vessels when inflammatory mediators are released into the circulation. As our bodies experience a fall in the ratio of omega-3s to omega-6s, another defence against migraine is lost. The efficacy of fish oil as a treatment for migraine has been shown in several small studies.[46]

Migraine clinics could conduct large studies of combinations of these nutrients, but they resist treatments not involving the pharmaceutical industry.

Diet

That the modern diet seeks out and reveals our genetic weaknesses is, of course, a central theme of this book. The 'genes for migraine' provide examples. Magnesium deficiency can result not only from an absolute deficiency, but also from imbalance relative to calcium. High dairy consumption, calcium supplements taken without equal amounts of magnesium, and other aspects of the Western diet, certainly promote this disequilibrium.

We have also seen that sodium and potassium pumps are implicated in the cast of migraine genes. The ratio of sodium to potassium in the Western diet was discussed in Chapters 3 and 8. If the migraine cascade results in part from genetic vulnerability in the ion channels, such alteration in the ratios of calcium to magnesium and sodium to potassium may affect people with genes that cannot meet the challenge.

Genetic sensitivity might be unmasked in other ways also. Some people are especially sensitive to the 'warning' chemicals embedded in our food. Foods high in natural chemicals which affect blood vessels and act like neurotransmitters are often associated with migraine. These chemicals include tyramine, histamine, salicylate and amines. Is increased sensitivity to such chemicals an asset or a liability? Are genes for this sensitivity a 'disease' or an adaptive advantage?

- *Tyramine* is found in chocolate, Vegemite (and all its relatives), pickled herrings, red wine (especially Chianti) and cheese. One patient of mine, a refugee from an illustrious migraine clinic, lost all her headaches and was able to cease taking the powerful drug methysergide when persuaded to give up her Vegemite habit. The eminent professor had told her that migraine had nothing to do with food.

- *Salicylates* are found in fruits and vegetables. They are at their maximum in fruit and vegetables which have been picked before they are ripe.
- *Histamine* is found in cheese, salami, sausage, and wine. Histamine headaches are well established in the medical literature.

People who have a genetically determined deficiency of the enzyme *phenolsulphotransferase* cannot metabolise dietary amines as well as others. Some food additives and some dietary phenols (such as in red wine), are known to actually inhibit this enzyme. It's too bad if you weren't born with a lot of it to start with.

Monosodium glutamate (E621–623) and the E numbers 102, 110, 210–219 (benzoic acid derivatives) and 220–227 (sulphite and metabisulphite derivatives) have been shown to precipitate migraine. Proteins in milk, wheat and other grains are strongly associated with migraine headache. But is that because we eat too much of them, or do not digest them properly? Suggest removing them from diet and many people are convinced that there is nothing left to eat.

Environmental factors

Besides stress, most migraine patients report a range of environmental triggers for their headaches. Predominant among these are pollution, petrochemicals, perfumes (a spin-off of the petrochemical industry), glare, flicker, strobe lighting, and even stripes. The last three of these may be compared to the way in which epilepsy and its auras can be triggered by strobe lighting, and motion sickness is related to visual perception. It seems reasonable that similar cues might trigger the migraine cascade. Flickering on the periphery of the visual field can provoke unease, which in evolution may have been protective against being stalked by predators.

Pollution and petrochemicals are poisons and their role in migraine is simple. Volatile agents go straight up the nostrils, through the cribriform plate, and into the brain. It is an instant warning system for toxic gases. The air is not good, move on, the volcano might erupt. At the same time, these poisons can saturate or even inhibit many of our detox enzymes. These enzymes then are left with no capacity to detox the natural food chemicals involved in migraine.

In summary, the fixed-name disease of migraine is probably nothing more than the cumulative effects of a stressful life lived in a polluted environment. The word pollution encompasses food, air and water. The immune system, to deal with these multiple stressors, struggles on a diet deplete in magnesium, B-group vitamins, essential fatty acids, and all the rest.

Migraine is a common, but eminently treatable, condition. The diagnosis, however, should be made by a trained medical practitioner, because migraine can mask brain tumours, epilepsy, strokes and several other neurological disorders.

Chapter Ten
SOME CONCLUSIONS

I am a little world made cunningly
Of elements, and an angelic sprite.

JOHN DONNE, 1572–1631

How wisely Nature did decree,
With the same Eyes to weep and see,
That, having view'd the object vain,
They might be ready to complain.

ANDREW MARVELL, 1621–1678

THE METAPHYSICAL POETS of the 17th century, of whom Andrew Marvell and John Donne are representative, had an intensely spiritual view of the natural world. Of particular interest was the way in which Nature mirrored itself at every level. Indeed, the image of the mirror was central to their poetry. So, too, was the idea of the universe as an infinity which could be contained (mirrored) within a drop of dew or a teardrop.

It is unlikely then that these metaphysicists would have had difficulty with the concept of themselves as a coral reef (Chapter 6: The Gut). In fact, this is an intensely metaphysical concept. Startling though the image may be, it is a way of saying that we provide a habitat for the many micro-organisms which live on and within us, and in turn we depend on them for health. Just as we see ourselves as a species within a larger ecosystem, so another species may live within us, our bodies constituting their habitat. Infinity expands inwards as well as outwards.

Even more confronting than sharing our bodies with gut and

434 THE GOOD BODY GUIDE

other bacteria is the fact that the very cells of our body, our DNA, host the remnants of the viruses that once invaded our ancestors and are now part of our own genetic makeup. Infinity stretches outwards and inwards in space, forwards and backwards in time.

This is both metaphor and reality, whether metaphysics or particle physics. We do not simply live in our environment, past, present and future — we are part of it, and it is part of us.

Since the term metaphysics is often used to denigrate something which is not adequately 'scientific', perhaps it is an unfortunate framework for this discussion. After all, nutritional and environmental medicine is often criticised for its lack of 'science'. But it is the thesis of this book that we spend a lot of time finding good 'scientific' answers to the wrong questions. Perhaps there is something to be learned from these 17th-century metaphysicists who saw all life as connected, not only to other life forms, but to the soils, the oceans, the planets and even to a drop of dew. Now, through human ingenuity, even that drop of dew, a symbol of pristine purity, may have a molecule of PCB in it.

The extension of human exploration into outer space and into the deepest of ocean canyons encourages fallacious conclusions: if we can conquer these physical barriers, surely a cancer cure must be just around the corner. But to pursue a cure for cancer while we release more and more carcinogens into the environment is worse than bad science: it is no science at all.

COMMUNAL HEALTH PROBLEMS

Health for each one of us depends on the genes we received in the gene-lottery, and what we do with those genes throughout life. However, as cancer rates rise and epidemics like SARS and HIV-AIDS emerge, we realise that it is not enough to take care of our own genome. We need to put it into the broader context of how we live. We sometimes feel powerless when we think about this, but I would argue against this.

Public health

We take it for granted that governments in modern nations have departments of public health. Often these have responsibility for such matters as housing, sanitation, water supply, immunisation programs, food and drug regulation and other related issues because there is no point dealing with health problems if their origins are neglected.

Public health as a concept probably goes back to the Industrial Revolution, although sophisticated ancient cultures, such as the Greek, Roman and Mayan civilisations show clear evidence of public health measures. The idea of public health is often associated with germ-based epidemics, such as bubonic plague in the Middle Ages and the attempts to control it by collecting and burning the dead. Although *Yersinia pestis*, and indeed germs themselves, were yet to be recognised, there was a sense that the disposal of diseased material, or the avoidance of certain areas, might affect the spread of the disease.

Other theories abounded, of course. These were sometimes bound up with concepts of sin, mysterious vapours, and the more prosaic observation of the associations between disease and vermin such as rats.

Epidemics

Traditionally, epidemics were diseases caused by germs. The term is now generalising to include a whole range of modern health problems, but let us start with the germ model.

'Old' germs

Although germs were not identified until the work of Lister, Pasteur, Koch and others in the mid-1800s, our ancestors noticed that certain patterns of behaviour would render an epidemic of say, measles, predictable. It was obviously highly contagious. Children were the typical victims, and once infected, demonstrated immunity to further infection. Some children died, but most were better within a week or so. In some years the disease demonstrated greater virulence, with greater morbidity and mortality.

Other diseases did not come in waves, but seemed to be continuous. Venereal disease is a good example. Rife at various times in human history, it was not seen as an epidemic. In this sense, it could be regarded as endemic, a medical problem demonstrating both predictability and persistence.

When explorers took their illnesses, both venereal and other, to unexposed populations, epidemics of a different intensity occurred. The decimation of populations like the Australian Aboriginals and the Easter Islanders was as much to do with measles and venereal disease as it was to do with the effects of conquest and confrontation.

The idea that epidemics shaped history has been explored in the well-known *Guns, Germs and Steel* by Jared Diamond. An earlier text on the same theme, *Rats, Lice and History*, was written by Hans Zinsser in 1934. From the discipline of public health grew the related field of epidemiology around the middle of the 20th century.

'New' germs

The emergence of the HIV virus as a virulent and widespread cause of death and disability in the early 1980s caused shock waves in a world where the eradication of smallpox, and the success of the polio vaccine and other vaccines, had caused many to believe that science was rapidly winning in the war against germs. The response to AIDS was as superstitious as the response to the Black Death in medieval Europe. Indeed, Gothic images of the Grim Reaper appeared on Australian television to the chagrin and embarrassment of Australians world-wide.

For a long time, debate about AIDS reflected people's fear of the unknown. It was a disease of homosexuals; it was God's judgement on 'unnatural' sexual behaviour; it was caused by the amyl-nitrate used as an aphrodisiac in the gay community; it was a germ made by Russians (or others) for the purpose of germ warfare; it was an unfortunate by-product of the polio vaccine

AIDS demonstrates that germs can jump species. This fact is implicated in most of the emerging 'new' infectious diseases, abnormal proximity between two species being a key consideration.

Many of these 'new' diseases are not new at all. They are old germs behaving in new ways, adapting to new environments, finding new hosts. Some have undergone mutation, but many have not mutated much at all. Infections such as Ebola virus and rabies, once contained in the forests, affected animal populations able to deal with them. As forests are cleared, animals are driven into contact with humans and bring with them diseases to which humans have little natural resistance.

Humans can acquire the diseases of other species where animals are farmed intensively. Disease spreads rapidly where the animals' immune system is weakened by poor housing and lack of fresh air and sunlight. In the presence of a weakened immune system, more virulent viruses can evolve. The most intensive farming takes place in the poorest parts of the world, where there is close contact between the animals and their carers, who often themselves have weak immune systems. In short, the ideal conditions for jumping from one species to another are created.

Intensive farming will almost certainly be the cause of the next influenza pandemic, which will probably kill millions and will not spare the First World. It could be avoided if humans chose to eat the food normally fed to animals instead of pursuing wasteful and unsustainable meat-based diets. The traditional Asian diet used meat only sparingly. The West is exporting its carnivorous ways along with its consumer lifestyle. As the result of unfair trade agreements and continued exploitation, poor nations are forced to cut corners to survive in the global economy.

Western farming practices are just as reprehensible. Wealthy countries have more choices, but we still dose factory-farmed animals with antibiotics to minimise the effects of poor animal husbandry. We do not always use agricultural chemicals wisely. We feed animal products to vegetarian animals that have no gut capacity to process meat. The BSE crisis—mad-cow disease—bears testimony to the dangers.

New germs: the future

The potential disasters which loom with genetically modified organisms, and worst of all, xenografts (Chapter 2: Vaccination) have been judged unlikely by 'experts'. Fortunately, some scientists are more cautious than others. Jeffery Platt, director of the Mayo Clinic's transplantation program, has said that recent findings in their clinic showed that 'human and animal DNA can fuse together naturally'. As such, 'the finding explained how a retrovirus could jump from one species to another and might help uncover the origin of AIDS and SARS.'[1]

In *The Coming Plague*, Laurie Garrett quoted some speakers at a conference in Washington in 1989:

Nature isn't benign ... The survival of the human species is not a preordained evolutionary program. Abundant sources of genetic variation exist for viruses to learn new tricks, not necessarily confined to what happens routinely, or even frequently. ... It is, I think, worthwhile being conscious of the limits of our powers ... It is worth keeping in mind that the more we win, the more we drive infections to the margins of human experience, the more we clear a path for possible catastrophic infection. We are caught in the food chain, whether we like it or not, eating and being eaten.[2]

Epidemics: the non-germ model

As public health authorities took on the responsibility of dealing with epidemics, the number and scope of epidemics grew. There is now a danger of the word losing its meaning. We have the obesity epidemic, the heart disease epidemic, epidemics of depression, breast cancer, babies born by caesarean section, precocious puberty. Since the terrorist attacks of September 11, 2001, there is now an epidemic of fear.

These are all real health issues, but in naming them we risk falling into the traps of the fixed-name disease — that is, we identify a symptom and set about treating that, instead of looking at the collection of causes that may underlie this epidemic of epidemics.

If I were to add one epidemic to this list, I might call it the epidemic of greed. Many of the problems hinted at above come from national and commercial greed. The maldistribution of wealth results in a world where those not starving to death are at risk of dying of obesity. People eking out an existence in Asia or Africa cannot spare a thought for emerging avian viruses when they are worrying about providing the next meal for their children.

Climate change

Faces along the bar
Cling to their average day:
The lights must never go out,
The music must always play,

(from 'September 1, 1939', W.H. Auden)

In 2008, climate change sceptics are going the way of the dinosaurs. Climate has become one of the greatest threats to our health (not to mention civilisation itself).

In Australia, the draft report of Ross Garnaut (2008) follows the example of Sir Nicholas Stern's in the UK. Garnaut's plan is to address macroeconomic costs of action, medical and societal consequences of inaction, costs of mitigating the effects and, finally, costing the un-costable: damage to places of natural beauty, like the Great Barrier Reef.

A group called Doctors for the Environment Australia, endorsed by the Royal Australian College of General Practitioners, notes that climate change will increase the incidence of death and debility from heat stress, cardiovascular disease, respiratory illness and trauma from extreme weather, as well as from infectious diseases, such as Ross River fever, Dengue fever, malaria and gastroenteritis. Problems with supply of fresh food and water speak for themselves. Climate change anxiety is also appearing in the consulting room.

The great irony in this debate lies in politicians protesting the increased cost of petrol. Here is an unparalleled opportunity to institute positive change — better public transport, reduction in greenhouse gases, cleaner air — that many diseases, not least asthma, depression, diabetes and cancer would benefit from.

FOOD, GLORIOUS FOOD

Let food be thy medicine, and medicine be thy food.
— *Hippocrates*

Food is more than fuel. We talk about needing 'comfort food' when we are miserable. Food nourishes us in a way that goes beyond biochemistry. In a scientific age this may seem to be 'soft' science, yet science itself has produced the evidence. For instance, if we eat in stressful surroundings we may not produce enough acid to digest protein; the peptides pass through the system undigested and contribute to mental problems, allergic disorders, irritable bowel.

Humans are designed to enjoy food. We have been programmed

by nearly 200,000 years of evolution in which one major preoccupation was the seeking and enjoyment of food. Food was fuel, medicine and nourishment, both physical and emotional. Yet we have created a world in which we gobble down fast food, convenience food, so that we have more time for 'important' pursuits.

Avoiding bad food

Toxins

Once avoiding poisonous food was straightforward. People did not eat rotting food or food which did not smell appetising. Nature has many built-in warning systems. Animals in the wild have an instinct for what is good for them to eat.

Many old cultures had means of both identifying and dealing with marginal foods. They had highly sophisticated means of removing toxic substances. Australian Aboriginals removed alkaloids and other toxins in foods by thorough soaking in water. The Moreton Bay Chestnut is an example of a toxic legume rendered edible in this manner. Other plants were used sparingly as a food, but were employed for their medicinal properties in indigenous medicine.

Nowadays, food poisoning is far more likely to come from other sources.

Micro-organisms

Governments enforce strict hygiene rules in factories, shops and restaurants. However, this hygiene can be the lesser of two evils. To kill germs, moulds and fungi, preservatives are added to food. Old cultures often preserved food with salt or sugar, which are non-toxic, although they both pose health threats for the modern Western diet. Today's preservatives pose different risks. Metabisulphite and benzoates adversely affect a small but significant percentage of the population.

Often toxins are signalled by other visible signs, themselves unappetising but not dangerous. This is a natural process, and we have an instinctive response to it. We may avoid food because of visible mould. One of the accepted methods (in some countries) of providing food hygiene is gamma radiation, which can prevent the growth of spoiling moulds, while more sinister germs and moulds survive. The threat does not arise from the radiation, but from what the radiation may mask.

Other additives

As well as preservatives, commercially prepared food such as bread may contain traces of herbicides, pesticides (including rat poison), bleach (to turn the flour white), anti-caking agents, and even axle grease from the dough mixer. Axle grease, rat poison and herbicides are additives which can escape labelling because they are incidental, as opposed to deliberate, additives. The only restraint is that they must fall within 'allowed limits'.

In addition to all these potential toxins are the food colourings to be found in most foods, especially sweets and soft drinks. These do not always appear on the labels because some products escape regulatory control. Imported whisky, for instance, often contains unlabelled food colouring. Well-known vitamin products like Berocca may contain E110. Other products have enough tartrazine (E102) to cause migraine, asthma and even anaphylaxis, but escape labelling through a 'grandfather clause' in the laws.

Missing in action

'Bad' food can also be defined by what is not in it. This was discussed in Chapters 4 and 5.

GM food

Foods may be genetically modified to meet agricultural or commercial needs rather than to improve their nutritional content. Constituents such as essential fatty acids may be collateral damage. Cold-climate legumes and nuts, when bred to grow in warm climates, may show reduced levels of omega-3 fatty acids. We do not yet know about all the factors in our food which are important, so such variables are rarely measured.

Another concern with GM food is the introduction of novel proteins. Allergic reactions may occur because we are unaware that these proteins are present. When a tomato contains fish protein, those who are allergic to fish may get a nasty surprise.

If world production heads towards wide-scale GM foods, we shall lose much genetic diversity. The 19th-century potato famine in Ireland should remind us of the vulnerability of monocultures.

Other considerations

Just as the developed world takes on the message that omega-3 fatty acids are vital for health, we learn about the dangers of mercury in seafood. Waters throughout the world are being overfished, yet if we choose farmed fish we worry about antibiotics and other aspects of their diet.

To avoid bad food, we seek out organic food. But if it has been grown far from home, we have to take account of the increased burden of global pollution imposed by the transportation of this food.

Eating good food

The subject of a 'good' diet was introduced in Chapter 8: Obesity. As we learn more about genetics, we realise that, of the many 'good' diets, some may apply more to one individual, or one racial group, than another.

Having said that, many benefits are conferred by the traditional Japanese diet. They include not only lower risks of most cancers and cardiovascular disease, but a significantly lower risk of neurological disorders. Multiple sclerosis has been discussed, but recent analyses seem to indicate that only the Japanese among the industrialised nations have avoided the alarming growth in Parkinson's, Alzheimer's and such degenerative brain disorders. Even supposedly genetic disorders, such as polycystic kidney disease, have been found to progress more slowly in Japan. These protective effects are lost when a Japanese individual migrates to another culture and adopts its customs.

Features of the Japanese diet include low calories, wide variety, great diversity of vegetables (seaweed, ferns, fronds, lotus and bamboo), and a high intake of fish, fruit and soy products. On the other hand, sugar, gluten, beef and milk are all but absent.

Until we know more about genetic factors which might dictate how we should eat, broad principles are safest. Fresh, unprocessed and organic seem to be good starting points. The food that our ancestors ate in the rainforest included fruits, berries, tubers, vegetables, herbs, spices, honey, nuts, seeds and eggs. Of meat, fish seems to be the most protective. This ancient diet is easy to emulate, even from today's supermarket.

Food as medicine: nature's pharmacy

At this point, I would like to develop a theme introduced earlier in this book, one that is likely to appear increasingly in the scientific literature. At its heart is the idea of diversity. The study of a wide variety of food chemicals has begun to uncover the reasons behind the value of the diverse diet. Without diversity, we can survive — many people manage on an extraordinarily narrow diet. When they succumb to ills such as arthritis, diabetes or cancer, we blame their family history or point to the bad factors in their environment. Attention is now turning towards factors which may not be essential to life, but which evolved with us to offer protection against genetic and environmental threats.

A decade ago only botanists had heard of phyto-oestrogen, yet now the word is commonplace. It and others — polyphenolic compound, lutein, glycosaminoglycans — belong to the vocabulary of people who have never studied botany, pharmacy or organic chemistry. To me it is thrilling that there are compounds in nature which can not only be employed as medicines when we are sick, but which as part of a diverse diet may prevent illness or the expression of our 'bad' genes.

In a culture where 'meat and three veg' and 'drink lots of milk for your bones' have been the most important food wisdom, this idea is radical. Yet I remember my grandmother saying that fish was brain food and that we should eat vinegar with fried potato chips because it 'cuts the fat'; 21st-century science is proving what she already knew. The folk wisdom of other cultures tells of foods to be eaten to achieve pregnancy or treat a fever, much as one might be told to consume a herb for the same reason.

Some people find it fanciful to think that 'the right medicines just happen to be out there'. But if we take a current example, the phyto-oestrogens, we can see how this might work. Mother Nature has 'just happened' to make chemicals look like hormones, but if we move away from the anthropomorphism, there are some basic considerations:

- *The natural limitations of organic chemistry:* There are many variations on a chemical structure or molecule, but there is a finite number of the basic units which can form stable molecular structures. As a result, there is an inevitable overlap of molecular configuration in the natural world.

- *An ancient immune system:* Some of the 'coincidences' in living forms are the result of common ancestry. One aspect of the human immune system can be traced back to an ancient immune system used by the ancestral life forms which gave rise to both plants and animals. Under attack, tissues release hypersensitivity enzymes which set up a cascade of events. The release of nitric oxide leads to programmed cell death, and balancing mechanisms are essential to ensure that it does not damage the organism. In both plants and animals, the chemical which can control nitric oxide is salicylic acid. Salicylic acid is widely distributed in nature; long before we 'discovered' aspirin, it was consumed as both food and medicine by most of the animal kingdom. Other common aspects of biochemistry, including the existence of seleno-enzymes and omega-3 fatty acids in the most basic life forms, were discussed in Chapters 4 and 5. Still others are under study.
- *Co-dependency:* Through simple Darwinian principles, co-evolution may lead to mutual benefit, or even co-dependency. Plant sterols are a good example. A degree of mutual benefit is conferred when a sheep eats clover: the sheep gains nourishment and at the same time helps disperse the seeds. A plant may 'say' to the sheep, 'Eat some of me and that's okay, but eat too much and I will stop you.' In some cases it achieves this by killing the animal, but a less drastic response is better all round. In the case of the clover, its oestrogenic nature means that in excess it has a contraceptive effect.

Co-evolution: the plant's view

If it is in the interest of a plant to be eaten, it can protect itself from over-consumption in various ways. To utilise its phyto-sterols is one, as we have seen. To fill itself up with bitter chemicals is another. Some of these, such as salicylates, are at a maximum as the fruit is developing, which keeps predators away until the fruit and seeds are fully matured and abundant. The unpleasant taste of unripe fruit is a deterrent. Once it has ripened, the salicylate levels fall and the sweet and aromatic compounds increase. Eaten at this stage, they both nourish the consumer and ensure seed dispersal.

Other plants have low levels of toxins, enough for the consumer to voluntarily limit intake. Some foods contain sugars known as oligo-saccharides, which cause farting. Legumes when consumed by humans are notorious for this. Legumes also contain a toxic chemical called phytohemagglutinin, which belongs to a class of chemicals known as lectins. Lectins are interesting substances which have been associated with the development of certain autoimmune diseases. Their potential both to prevent and treat medical conditions is an area for future exciting research.

The ability to tolerate various lectins is associated with blood groups, indicating possible racial and regional variations. This fact also lends some credence to the various blood-group diets (see below). Toxic lectins are usually present in tiny quantities, although they are thought to be at a maximum in red kidney beans. Every now and then a rogue crop of legumes turns up with levels sufficiently toxic to cause vomiting, diarrhoea and blood changes.[3]

The chemicals in some foods, such as mushrooms and nutmeg, can produce hallucinations. In small doses this might be fun, but animals and humans learn to be wary of large doses.

Co-evolution: the animal's view

If the plants have learnt to protect themselves, so have the consumers. Restriction of intake and avoidance are two mechanisms. Preparation techniques such as soaking, cooking or mixing with clay have been employed to detoxify foods. These methods are not confined to humans; they have been observed in various animal species.

At a biochemical level, many species have developed specific liver enzymes to detoxify common poisons. Alcohol dehydrogenase is an enzyme which we have already discussed in Chapters 3, 4 and 6. Other enzymes detoxify the chemicals known as pressor amines. Some pressor amines, such as serotonin, tyramine, noradrenalin and dopamine, are made within our own bodies, and some are ingested in food. Amines occur in high levels in foods such as pineapple, banana and avocado.

Medications often mimic the actions of these amines. Perhaps in taking the medications we are simply using a drug where once we would have used a food. Unchecked, amines can cause high blood pressure, headache and other unpleasant symptoms. The enzymes we have developed to keep things in balance are called monoamine oxidases.

Mutual benefit

Over long periods of time, and with the benefit of a broad diet, plants and animals have become mutually beneficial members of a complex ecosystem. Seed dispersal, the activities of elephants 'logging' forests and beavers damming rivers, are well known. Recently it has been shown that reef fish selectively 'cultivate' the kelps that they prefer, rooting out undesirable plants and leaving others to grow to maturity.

The benefits of this interaction are often obvious, but sometimes they are subtle. For example, when moose graze on plants, substances in their saliva actually heal the bitten surface in such a way that fungal and bacterial infections cannot gain entry to the plant. With the marvellous economy so often observed in the natural world, the anti-bacterials that exist in saliva to protect the mouth are pressed into service to protect the animal's food source.

Accessing the pharmacy

The foods which seem to be outstanding in terms of their nutrient properties include fish, algae and seaweed. Their content of essential fatty acids and minerals such as iodine, calcium, magnesium, selenium and zinc is in almost perfect proportion to the requirements of both the plant and animal kingdoms. This may reflect the aquatic origins of life on this planet. As an island nation with limited arable land, the Japanese have long had a diet based on the sea, which may explain some of their extraordinary health benefits.

There are other ways in which we can access Nature's Pharmacy. What is needed, perhaps, is a change of mindset. If we look at the properties now being ascribed to some of the foods listed below (and these are but a sample of those under study), the division blurs between medicine as food and food as medicine.

In the animal world this food–medicine spectrum is demonstrated over and over. Animals grazing on new pastures seek out the novel plants. They always seek variety. On mixed pasture, few prefer toxic weeds in any significant quantity. Sick animals have been shown to seek medicinal herbs appropriate to their particular illness, plants which at other times they ignore.[4]

It is likely that humans have these same instincts, but they have atrophied through conditioned neglect. Notwithstanding, many people still report cravings in pregnancy or when recovering from an illness. I treat those cravings with an interest and respect that was lacking in my earlier days as a medical practitioner.

Here is a list of foods that demonstrate 'food as medicine'. It is not comprehensive, but there are plenty of books on this subject (Further Reading).

Nature's Pharmacy: specific food chemicals

- *Alkaloids:* These are chemical compounds with potent pharmacological activity. In quantity they may be toxic, but in small doses the boundaries between natural toxins and valuable medicines are blurred. Nicotine, atropine and caffeine are some of the better-known alkaloids. Some, such as theophylline and theobromine, have been shown to have therapeutic value in conditions such as asthma.[5] These stimulants can be found in beverages such as coffee, tea and cocoa. In moderate consumption they are a pleasant stimulant. Asthmatics often comment on a reduction in symptoms with usage, but for insomniacs and those with an anxiety disorder they can be, literally, a nightmare.

- *Allicins:* These sulphur-based compounds, also known as thioallyl compounds, are found in garlic, onions and other members of the allium family. They are believed to reduce blood clotting by inhibiting thromboxane synthesis, and to lower blood lipid levels by their action on the enzyme HMG-COA reductase. They are thought to have anti-cancer properties. They are the main biological active in garlic.

- *Anthocyanins:* These are the red pigments that give colour to foods such as apples, beetroot, eggplant, radish, plums, blueberries, cranberries and other berries. They are anti-oxidants, with impressive health cred. They are in the flavonoid family of chemicals.

- *Aspirin:* A common anti-inflammatory first derived from willow bark, in the body it is rapidly converted to salicylic acid, a substance also found in fruit and vegetables. Salicylic acid is produced by plants as a defence against disease and stress. As such, levels in foods grown organically can be as much as six times higher than in those foods protected from weather extremes and by pesticides.[6] Studies on Buddhist monks confirm other findings that vegetarians have unusually high levels of salicylic acid in their blood.[7] Salicylic acid inhibits COX-1 enzymes, producing an anti-thrombotic effect. It also inhibits the transcription of genes responsible for the production of COX-2, thus making it an anti-inflammatory.

- *Capsaicin:* This is the chemical which gives the 'bite' to chillies. It is anti-bacterial. Poultry exposed to *Salmonella enteritidis* reduce their risk of infection by 50 per cent if they have eaten capsaicin or chillies.

- *Flavonoids and bioflavonoids:* These anti-oxidants are found in fruit and vegetables and in plant-derived beverages such as tea and wine. They have anti-cancer properties and are also active in preventing cardiovascular disease. They are particularly effective at reducing the symptoms of hay fever. (Pollen is hardly a new threat to the human population.) The best-known flavonoids are quercetin, catechin and luteolin. They are richly concentrated in the pith of citrus fruits and capsicums, which affluent societies usually throw away.

- *Glucosinates:* These compounds give pungency to some cruciferous vegetables, such as mustards and radish and, to a lesser extent, the other brassicas (cabbage, broccoli, cauliflower, brussels sprouts). They protect against cancer but can contribute to goitre, highlighting the fact that foods are rarely all good or all bad. The ideal diet is balanced and varied.

- *Glutathione peroxidases:* Anti-oxidant enzymes

important in tissue repair and cancer prevention, made in the human body and found in some foods as well. Asparagus is a particularly good source.

- *Lycopene:* A carotenoid found in tomatoes and thought to have anti-tumour properties in cancers such as prostate.

- *Phenyl ethylamine:* This neurotransmitter has been dubbed 'the love molecule'. High circulating levels are associated with states of both love and lust, and it is present in significant amounts in chocolate.

- *Phyto-oestrogens:* Better referred to as phyto-sterols or phyto-chemicals, these molecules have a structure that broadly mimics some hormonal rings. They have many actions, but because they look like many of the body's own hormones they can act as useful buffer molecules. Thus they provide protection against the symptoms of both hormonal excess and hormonal deficiency. Phyto-sterols come in three main classes: isoflavonoids (principally genistein and daidzein), lignans and coumestans. The major sources of the phyto-sterols are fruits, vegetables, nuts, seeds and legumes. (These are the foods which also assist in balancing hormones by stimulating the production of SHBG; see Chapter 7: Fertility.)

- *Polyphenolic compounds:* This is the generic name for a range of molecules sharing some common structural features. Polyphenolic compounds appearing on this list include tannins, flavonoids, alkaloids, and phyto-oestrogens.

- *Polysaccharides:* These molecules are found in a range of plant foods. Of clinical significance are the glucans and proteoglycans found in algae, seaweed and a variety of mushrooms. They have been found to boost production of immune cells and enhance the invasion of tumour cells by the dendritic and cytotoxic T-cells. Thus they are active against cancers of the stomach, colo-rectum, oesophagus, nasopharynx and some breast and lung cancers.[8] Other polysaccharides include the type found in starch. Particularly important in this regard is 'resistant starch', found in legumes, root vegetables and bananas.

- **Resveratrol:** This is a compound known as a 'stilbene', which is a nonflavanoid phenolic compound nonetheless related to the flavonoids. You can forget the chemistry but do not forget that in at least 18 test tube studies it showed cytotoxic effects against a variety of cancer cell lines.[9] Another researcher was able to show in both animal and test-tube experiments that it inhibited the initiation, promotion and progression of tumours.[10] A non-alcohol component of wine, especially red wine, it has strong anti-inflammatory activity. It is also found in grapes.

- **Salacinol:** This is the active ingredient in *Salacia reticulata*, a plant used in India for more than 3000 years to treat diabetes. Salacinol blocks a gut enzyme known as alpha-glucosidase. This enzyme normally helps digest the disaccharides, sucrose and maltose, hastening absorption. Slowing such absorption reduces rapid rises in blood glucose.

- **Tannins:** Most of these are flavonoids and are usually a catechin derivative. They are found in a wide range of plants, from tree bark to cocoa beans. Tannins block the oxidation of low-density lipoproteins (and are therefore anti-oxidants), thus reducing the formation of 'bad' cholesterol. The huge quantity of catechins in red wine (800 mg per litre, compared to 50 mg per litre in white), is one of the proffered reasons for the 'French paradox', the good health of the French despite their high consumption of animal fats (see also Chapters 1 and 8). Tannins also have actions against parasite infection.

- **Zeanthin and lutein:** These carotenoids specifically protect against macular degeneration (Chapter 7) via anti-oxidant and blue-light-filter functions. Lutein has also been associated with reduced cancer risk. It is found principally in the cabbage family, but also in corn, eggs and certain fruits.

Nature's Pharmacy: sample foods

- *Algae:* They are high in omega-3 fatty acids and share the benefits of seaweed. The consumption of spirulina has been associated with health by many tribal cultures. Algae also produce substances known as furanones, which have the primitive but effective ability to stop aggregation of pathogenic bacteria. Furanones have the potential to treat bacterial infection both by application to the skin and by ingestion.

- *Apples:* It may be true that 'an apple a day keeps the doctor away'. Studies have shown that apple consumption has a positive association with several indices of good health, including reduced cancer rates and good lung function.[11] Apples contain fibre, Vitamin C, flavonoids such as quercetin and various trace elements, and are rich in salicylic acid.

- *Asparagus:* This vegetable is rich in beta-carotene, Vitamin C, selenium and glutathione, all important anti-cancer nutrients. It is mildly diuretic and laxative and contains the soluble fibre used by gut florae for their own energy source, with the beneficial short-chain fatty acids as a by-product.

- *Bananas:* When green, bananas provide ample supplies of resistant starch. They are free of fat, rich in Vitamin B6 and contain tryptophan, a precursor to serotonin and melatonin. They are a candidate for the fruit of temptation in the Garden of Eden, although in fact they are not a fruit but the product of a giant herb.

- *Blueberries:* Blueberries topped the list of the flavonoids responsible for anti-oxidant and protective effects on the brain in a Tuft's University trial.[12] The specific reference for this trial was the prevention of conditions such as

Alzheimer's.

• **Birch:** Reminding us of the vast untapped pharmacy in the natural world, some cultures have made great use of the birch tree. Birch wine is made from the sugary sap of the tree, Native Americans make a paste from the buds for sores and ringworm, and a brew from the silver birch treats cystitis.

• **Carrageenan:** A derivative of seaweed, it is thought to inhibit HIV and the genital herpes virus from binding to cells and infecting them.

• **Chocolate:** Originating in the South American jungle, chocolate was brought to Europe after the voyages of Columbus and Cortes. Mayans and Aztecs regarded it as a food from the gods and often consumed it in a drink with starch and chilli peppers; chocolate with chilli is still a popular mix in South America. Chocolate contains Vitamin A and small quantities of B1, B2, B3 and potassium. It also contains copper, a natural antibiotic, which is essential in forming bone, cartilage and connective tissue. Chocolate has anti-bacterial action against the germs which cause tooth decay. It contains anti-oxidant flavonoids, and it is a good source of magnesium with all the attendant benefits. It releases serotonin, thus elevating mood, along with various endorphins which have a comforting effect. It releases theobromine, giving increased alertness. In an experiment at Middlesex University in London in the late 1990s, the odour of chocolate was found to significantly increase both alpha waves (relaxation) and beta waves (alertness), while suppressing theta waves (stress).[13] At Westminster University, also in Britain, researchers found that the smell of chocolate increased levels of an immune globulin, secretory IgA, leading to the attractive conclusion that the smell of chocolate could boost the immune system.[14]

• **Eggs and corn:** Both these are high in the carotenoids

specific to the prevention of macular degeneration
(Chapter 7).

- **Figs:** A revered food which has been part of the
  Mediterranean diet since ancient times, figs are full of
  vitamins and minerals and are a particularly good source
  of calcium. The preference of birds for figs is thought
  to relate to their calcium content. Figs are the most
  frequently mentioned fruit in the Bible, but they were
  not healthy for Cleopatra, to whom the fatal asp was
  brought in a basket of figs.

- **Fish:** Many of the health benefits associated with a
  fish-based diet are attributed to its omega-3 fatty acid
  content. Fish is also a good source of selenium and zinc.
  When whole small fish are eaten, the raw material of
  bone and cartilage is consumed, enhancing repair and
  maintenance of these tissues. The liver of such fish is also
  a good source of Vitamins A and D. Fish is one of the
  most protective foods we have.

- **Garlic:** A historic plant medicine with a reputation for
  reducing inflammation, protecting against cancer and
  lowering cholesterol.

- **Ginger:** Long thought to have medicinal properties,
  ginger in recent times has been shown to be an effective
  anti-emetic and anti-inflammatory. The compounds in
  ginger have been named gingerols, and in a 2001 study
  at the University of Sydney, were shown to be effective
  COX-2 inhibitors.[15] They prevent platelet accumulation
  in a manner similar to that achieved by aspirin, but
  with a milder effect and therefore less risk of unwanted
  bleeding. As the inflammatory pathways are also the
  starting point for many cancers, the reputation of ginger
  as an anti-cancer agent may be further promoted in
  future trials.

- **Honey:** Demonstrated to be effective in surgical wounds,
  burns, abscesses, boils, eczema and skin grafts, honey

acts against *E. coli, Salmonella, Helicobacter* and even the
much feared MRSA (multiple resistant *Staph. aureus*),
often referred to as a superbug.[16] A couple of varieties
of wild honey are now receiving international attention.
Notable in this regard are Manuka honey from
New Zealand and tea tree or 'jelly bush' honey from
Australia (derived from pollens of leptospermum trees).
An enzyme in the bees' saliva called glucose oxidase
converts glucose into gluconic acid, with the release of
hydrogen peroxide. As hydrogen peroxide breaks down
it releases free radicals in the form of hydroxyl radicals,
which damage the bacteria. On contact with the
moisture in the mouth, gut or a wound, glucose oxidase
in the honey is activated to produce a regular supply
of hydroxyl radicals, a process which is dormant while
the honey is sitting in the jar. It has been suggested
that honey is probably active against *Streptococcus mutans*
(dental decay), but this remains to be fully established.
When eaten, honey is believed to treat gastroenteritis
and help restore normal bowel flora balance.

- *Legumes:* These protein-rich vegetables include
beans, peas and lentils. They are a source of soluble
fibre converted by gut flora to short-chain fatty acids,
including butyric acid. The anti-cancer effect of these
substances has been discussed. Legumes also contain
substances known as protease inhibitors which are
believed to inhibit the growth of cancer cells.

- *Macadamia nuts:* This bush food has proven efficacy in
lowering 'bad' cholesterol. In one study all three of the
inflammatory markers—leukotriene LTB4, prostacyclin
PGI-2 and thromboxane TXB2—were lowered by
a statistically significant level, simply by the daily
consumption of a handful of these nuts.[17]

- *Nuts:* One of nature's most nutrient-dense foods, nuts
contain protein, good oils, vitamins and minerals.

- *Okra:* A source of soluble fibre, this versatile vegetable is also rich in many nutrients and acts as a laxative through its mucilage content. Its seeds are rich in good oils, and it is thought to slow the absorption of sugar, thus reducing insulin resistance.

- **Olive oil:** One of the key ingredients of the Mediterranean diet, it is a good source of anti-oxidants and one of the major contributors of monounsaturated fats in the human diet. These fats have been associated with reduced cognitive decline. Researchers have proposed that monounsaturated fats may be important in the maintenance of brain cell membranes. Italian research appears to have demonstrated the effectiveness of olive oil in lowering blood pressure. Olive oil may also reduce breast cancer risk.[18] It has been proposed that the anti-oxidant phenols in olive oil might be responsible for this effect.

- **Oysters:** A mineral-rich dietary supplement, they contain copper, selenium and zinc in good quantities.

- **Plums:** Dried plum extract has been shown to kill food-borne pathogens such as *E. coli, Listeria, Salmonella* and *Staph. aureus*. This effect has been produced even when using only the smallest amounts. The widespread use of plum sauce in Asian food may be taking advantage of this preservative function, not to mention the anthocyanin content and the delicious taste.

- **(Brown) rice:** Rice is an accessible staple which has the benefit of being gluten-free. In its brown form it is a good source of selenium, zinc, chromium and Vitamin E, all of which are lost during polishing. It is also a source of soluble fibre or resistant starch.

- **Seaweed:** This is a rich source of omega-3 fatty acids and of minerals, especially calcium, magnesium, selenium and zinc. On a weight-for-weight basis, it outstrips other sources of these minerals such as milk, meat, and even nuts. Seaweeds are also rich in the polysaccharides that are thought to be potent anti-cancer agents, and which promote insulin sensitivity in diabetics.

- **Shiitake and maitake mushrooms:** These mushrooms contain glucans and proteoglycans which inhibit plaque formation, increase insulin sensitivity, and are believed to have direct anti-cancer and anti-viral properties.

- **Sweet potatoes:** Members of the morning glory family, they are not potatoes at all. But they are rich in phyto-sterols, and the yellow varieties are important in providing Vitamin A and preventing blindness in some developing nations.

- **(Green) tea:** While there is an ongoing debate about the risks and benefits of coffee, there seems to be wide acceptance that tea, rich in polyphenolic compounds and anti-oxidants, is well placed in the ranks of health foods with medicinal properties.

- **Turmeric:** A member of the ginger family, it has an established anti-cancer function.

- **(Red) wine:** Red wine is rich in polyphenolic compounds and therefore anti-oxidant and anti-inflammatory. It causes vasodilation and mental relaxation. It contains resveratrol. Consumption of two standard drinks a day is associated with greater longevity than either total abstinence or greater intake.

Clearly, this list is not complete as it does not include foods such as the brassicas and capsicum, or the more exotic ones such as lotus roots and bamboo shoots. It is meant only as a starting point in understanding the wealth of nutritional options that we might seek out.

Food as culture

The culture of food brings us back to where this chapter started. Food is more than fuel. Orthodox Jews keep kosher and Muslims follow halal practice, obeying the laws set down in scripture. Most food customs are based on hygiene, humane slaughter, or some philosophy other than rote religious observance.

In tribal Aboriginal society, people had a totem animal assigned to them. One did not kill or eat one's totem animal. This engendered both respect for living creatures and contributed to the survival of species now endangered. Many animals, after all, were someone else's totem, if not your own.

Most societies have recognised foods for specific festivals, such as Easter bread, Christmas pudding, the Thanksgiving turkey. In Japanese culture, a dish called *oyako*, containing both chicken and egg, parent and offspring, is served when absent children return home. In temperatures of 40 degrees Celsius, generations of Australians have sat down to Christmas meals based on English winter food. For some, even those who have never visited England, this ritual is so important that it does not feel like Christmas without the historic culinary trappings.

It is hard to over-estimate the psychological value of culture in food. Foreign aid workers comment that malnourished children may refuse to accept food that is not familiar, even when they are very hungry. A friend returning from a refugee camp in Africa described children refusing to eat meals not drenched in the fiery chilli sauce used in that area. Food is such a part of our psyche that 'nursery food' or 'comfort food' can really give relief when we are anxious or depressed. Homesick people often seek out a familiar meal as a way of dealing with their unease. One can only pity those generations whose memories of special occasions are associated with fast foods and junk foods.

Some of the rituals associated with eating serve more than their overt purpose. Prayers of gratitude and formal expressions such as *bon appetit* encourage people to sit down before they start to eat, thus initiating and facilitating the complex process of digestion. So much of our food today is eaten on the run or timed to television programs. It is not surprising that digestive pills and ulcer medications are among the largest-selling pharmaceutical agents in the Western world.

Some food practices seem odd to those not used to them. Fermentation to produce alcohol is a familiar practice in the West, but Anglo-Celtic cultures have only recently adopted (or rediscovered) fermented milk products such as buttermilk and yoghurt. The health benefit of these as a source of good bacteria for the gut is now widely appreciated, and a generation of young people express surprise that their parents did not grow up with these foods.

Asian cultures ferment legumes to produce miso and tempeh, which are rich in the phyto-sterols associated with preventing cancer and hormonal disorders; they are even believed to be a source of Vitamin B12, long held by Western nutritionists to be obtainable only from animal products. Much ancient wisdom is available for our understanding.

FUNNY DIETS

Many people attempt to help their various medical symptoms by invoking particular diets which they feel will make a difference. Sometimes these are based on simple observations that when they eat, or avoid, certain foods they feel better. It is difficult to argue with this approach. Some people adopt a diet that they have found in a book or magazine. These range from the good to the bizarre.

Under Agriculture in Chapter 1 and Obesity in Chapter 6 I discussed the Stone Age diet, hunter-gatherer diets, diets based on the so-called food pyramid, and the glycaemic index diet, and I have mentioned a diet that avoids cholesterol. Now I look at some other popular diets.

The dairy-free diet

Milk is a complex substance, which is not surprising, as it is a complete food for the baby animal in its first weeks or months of life. The macro ingredients are protein, fat and sugar. The micro ingredients include vitamins and minerals, essential fatty acids, hormones, and other small molecules such as immune globulins. Casein and albumin are two of the predominant proteins in milk. Lactose is the name of the main sugar in milk. The mineral which most people think about in relation to milk is, of course, calcium.

If milk is a problem, just exactly what is the nature of this problem? The milk, the cholesterol, or something to do with the cow itself?

Honorary 'cows'
In discussing milk, we usually refer to cow's milk because the cow is the greatest provider of milk products in the West. In South American

and Middle Eastern cultures the animal is more likely to be a sheep or a goat. By and large, their products seem to be better tolerated than those of bovine origin. There are several possible reasons for this, of which the most important is probably the A1, A2 difference (Chapter 2).

However, many people who cannot tolerate dairy products from cows find that milk from other animals causes similar difficulty.

Clinical problems associated with dairy products

Here are some of the clinical problems which can arise from a diet high in milk and its products:

- *Allergy, sensitivity and intolerance:* Allergy is a specific immune response, mediated by the IgE arm of the immune system. People who talk about 'milk allergy' may be referring to this response, but more often the correct term is 'milk sensitivity' or 'milk intolerance', often used interchangeably. Such reactions can be mediated through either immune or non-immune mechanisms. Immune reactions include IgG or IgA responses (Chapters 3 and 6). Typically, both allergy and sensitivity responses are reactions to the protein component of milk. People with these reactions may also react to other cow proteins such as beef and gelatine. IgE-mediated allergy can cause eczema, asthma and even anaphylaxis. Cot death has some biochemical features in common with anaphylaxis, and it has been proposed that cow's milk allergy could be one of the mechanisms by which cot death can occur (Chapter 9).

- *Other immunological problems:* Illnesses which may be caused by the various intolerance mechanisms, or possibly some other immune mechanism not yet identified, include inflammatory bowel diseases such as Crohn's disease and ulcerative colitis, irritable bowel syndrome, asthma, migraine, autism, learning and behavioural difficulties, psoriasis, tonsillitis, and autoimmune diseases like diabetes. All of these illnesses have multiple causes including genetic predisposition, nutritional status, and environmental exposure; milk

consumption alone is unlikely to be the culprit.
However, when such illnesses appear more frequently in
a dairy culture, the possible contribution of dairy has to
be considered.

• **Digestive problems due to the lack of the appropriate
  enzyme in the gut:** When the problem relates to the
  sugar content of milk, the person is said to have a lactose
  intolerance. This is not an allergy. Lactose-intolerant
  people, either temporarily or permanently, lack the
  enzyme lactase. They are unable to digest the sugar in
  milk, and are prone to wind and diarrhoea as a result.
  Such people can digest lactose-free milk, which has no
  benefit for those who react to the milk proteins.

• **Cholesterol content:** The cholesterol in milk products *may*
  contribute to the burden of 'bad' cholesterol in the body.

• **Casein content:** The protein called casein, especially the
  beta casein found in A1 milk, is implicated in raising
  serum cholesterol and in autoimmune disorders. Most
  of these have been discussed in Chapters 2 and 6. The
  discussion about casein-free (and gluten-free) diets
  in schizophrenia, autism and learning difficulties also
  appears in Chapter 9, and will be concluded shortly.

• **Calcium and magnesium:** Unbalanced calcium
  supplementation may be undertaken as a result of
  misguided medical advice. The dairy industry promoted
  calcium supplements and milk as the solution to the
  rising problem of osteoporosis, and yet it is only in the
  dairy cultures of the developed world that osteoporosis
  is a problem. It is true that calcium deficiency can cause
  osteoporosis and that milk overload is not the only cause
  of osteoporosis, but we should remember that the ratio
  of calcium to magnesium in cow's milk is between 15 to
  1 and 8 to 1. At a cellular level, calcium and magnesium
  compete with each other for absorption; a high-dairy
  diet is often by definition a low-magnesium diet. A calf
  nibbles on grass when it is a few weeks old, obtaining

magnesium and other essential minerals. If by the age of six weeks it is not nibbling grass, it will become sick from magnesium deficiency because it cannot get enough from milk. By about one year of age it is weaned and will not drink milk again even if it is available. In humans, by contrast, a dairy-based diet can give rise to a problem of magnesium balance. Many of the illnesses associated with magnesium deficiency are diseases of dairy cultures, rather than of affluent societies.

Which milk?

Low-fat milk

Many patients attempt to address their milk intolerance by only drinking low-fat milk. Often they are making their problem worse. When fat or cream is removed from milk, the remaining buttermilk is a generally unacceptable product. To thicken it, milk solids and other milk proteins are added, increasing the protein load and thus the intolerance burden.

If Cholesterol were a character in a medieval play, its mask would without doubt represent evil. This is a pity, and the defence of cholesterol appeared in Chapters 3, 8 and 9. The milk solids added back include casein, which can actually increase serum cholesterol. Whether this is a problem specific to A1 milk, or is true of all casein, remains unknown.

Lactose-free milk

The common problem of lactose intolerance was discussed above. It comes about because many people after the age of two permanently lose the gut enzyme known as lactase. People in dairy cultures may retain this enzyme throughout most of their lives: 80 per cent of Caucasians are in this category, although they may temporarily lose it after viral illness or other damaging event such as the consumption of gluten by people with coeliac disease. By contrast, most Asians and dark-skinned people do not retain this enzyme, and have a poor tolerance of milk. They may be able to tolerate milk from which the lactose has been removed.

Cultured milk products

Those who lack the enzyme lactase can still consume milk under certain circumstances. The lactobacilli bacteria used to produce yoghurt actually consume lactose as their own energy source, producing a by-product known as lactate. Just as a wine fermented out to 'dry' no longer contains sugar, cheese and yoghurt often contain little milk sugar; the lactose-intolerant can often enjoy a fully cultured yoghurt. For this reason we often find that milk products have persisted in cultures which are genetically predisposed to lose the lactase enzyme after infancy.

Cultured milk products are an interesting adaptation of the agricultural revolution. From the time humans first started to tend animals, the advantages of using their milk must have been obvious. The making of cultured products reduced spoilage and also renewed the supply of good gut bacteria and shared those bacteria within the tribal group. It is probable that these cultures of yoghurt were 'contaminated' in a beneficial way as the human cultivators tasted and handled the product.

Coeliac disease and the gluten-free diet

Coeliac disease was discussed in Chapters 2 and 6. It is an absolute, and (at this stage of medical knowledge) lifelong intolerance to gluten, one of the proteins found in wheat, rye, oats and barley. Of the cereals which form the basis of the food pyramid, only rice and corn among the common staples are gluten-free.

I have discussed in earlier chapters the problem of clinical coeliac disease. Relevant here is the question of the 25 per cent of the population who have the genes for coeliac disease but do not develop it. Possibly these people might feel better on a gluten-free or low-gluten diet. My experience is that many people who are not coeliac feel better when gluten-free. Very recently it has become feasible to do the blood test (HLA typing) which determines whether coeliac genes are present. It is impressive just how many of these people are carrying coeliac genes.

Then there are researchers like Alessio Fasano (Chapter 6) who seem to feel that we'd all be better off without gluten. It may be that those doctors who regard gluten-free diets as faddish may end up eating some humble (gluten-free) pie.

In Western culture it is hard to avoid gluten; but before the arrival of the white man the diet of the Australian Aboriginal, like many other aboriginal diets, would have done so.

The casein-free, gluten-free diet

Based on the considerations in Chapters 2, 6 and 9, this diet has been proposed to manage conditions such as autism, specific learning defects and schizophrenia. There is a strong belief that schizophrenia is a disorder of dopamine metabolism, hence the idea of removing dopaminergic and opiate foods.

As early as the 1960s, Dohan was proposing a link between cereals and schizophrenia.[19] The clinical evidence that such diets make a difference is considerable.

The low-salicylate, low-amine diet

Salicylates illustrate Tudge's concept that an ideal diet contains natural medicines.[20] A little salicylic acid acts as an anti-inflammatory, reduces our risk of heart attacks and bowel cancer, and all round seems like a good idea. But the chronic neglect of bowel health, combined with green harvesting of fruit, has caused many people to become sensitive to salicylates. All manner of allergies seem to follow.

We now have the ludicrous situation where half of the population is taking aspirin to make up for the lack of fresh fruit and vegetables in their diet, and the other half is avoiding some of nature's healthiest bounty because they suffer from a 'salicylate sensitivity'.

Blood group diets

The varying incidence of coeliac disease and milk intolerance according to culture gives some credibility for the concept of the blood group diet.

A number of research centres now support the idea that some people require an individual food pyramid. Blood groups give a clue to our racial origins. The Children's Hospital Oakland Research Institute in California and the Cornell Institute for Nutritional Genomics are just two of the centres looking at diets to match our genetic makeup. The science has been named nutrigenetics, and is as yet in its infancy.

The limitation of current blood group diets is that they are based on the red blood cell or ABO Rh system. If we could type the white cells, we would be able to determine the status of the HLA class II genes of the individual. The HLA groups determine our vulnerability to some illnesses where dietary intervention may be significant, such as coeliac and diabetes. HLA typing is technically straightforward, but at the moment prohibitively expensive. That is changing, and we can now look at two class II genes, HLA-DR and HLA-DQ, with relatively cheap tests. These tests detect the increased risk for coeliac (plus or minus diabetes). The alleles for HLA class I genes, expressed on all cells, also offer diagnostic potential. Class I HLA B27 alleles can determine a risk for Crohn's disease and can be easily tested. Watch this space.

In future, typing may show us not only what to avoid, but what we need to seek out. Some racial groups may have actually become dependent upon certain foods. It is hard to imagine that Inuit, after thousands of years living on fish and fish oils, would tolerate deprivation of omega-3 fatty acids. (It has been suggested that Inuit might not need to ingest Vitamin C. This has not been confirmed, and probably will not be, but it is an interesting concept.)

Elimination diets

The diets mentioned both above, and in other parts of this book, are often referred to as elimination diets. The principle is that, if sensitivity to a particular food or food chemical is provoking a certain reaction, the strict removal of the offending substance/s from the diet may help recovery. Elimination diets are most commonly used in treating eczema, irritable bowel, migraine and, of course, coeliac disease, but the management of many medical conditions can involve an elimination diet.

The food list in Appendix 2 can be useful here. Not only does it remind us that there is more than wheat and milk to eat, but it also lists a rich variety of foods that we might never have thought of eating. This list groups foods in families because members of the same food family often share similar proteins and chemicals. Sensitivity to one food in a family may warn of problems with related foods. If mangoes give you migraine, don't be surprised if cashews have the same effect. People with peanut allergy may react to curries containing fenugreek, and so on.

RESPONSES TO MASS FOOD PRODUCTION

Bad food, contaminated food, refined diets, loss of diversity, loss of unique food cultures—these things have not gone unnoticed. An attempt by the McDonald's chain to open a branch in an area of France known for its regional produce ignited outrage. The outbreak of diseases like BSE (mad-cow) and avian flu has caused people to question where their food has come from. The appearance of diseases in cultures where they were unknown has forced attention at the highest levels. In the case of Australian Aboriginals, suffering one of the highest incidences of diabetes, coronary artery disease and hypertension in the world, the message has been stark:

> Replacing fatty, sugar-laden foods with a traditional meat, fish and root diet … was not just about improving lifestyle … It is simply about ensuring the survival of Aboriginal culture and people. If we don't, children and adults will continue to die and the only need for land will be for cemeteries.[21]

The response to the globalisation of food production comes from many quarters. It is impossible to separate the food from the grower, the culture, the economy or the health of the consumer. As a sober world reflects on the damage as well as the benefits of 20th-century globalisation, many questions are being asked about the price we pay for agribusiness. I will discuss a few of the responses to this situation.

The Policy Commission on the Future of Farming and Food

In 2001, the British Labour Government set up the Policy Commission on the Future of Farming and Food to enquire how agriculture could meet the diverse demands of the economy, sustainability, the environment, human health and animal welfare. Its approach was multidisciplinary. The medical input was endorsed by several august bodies, including the Faculty of Public Health Medicine of the Royal Colleges of Physicians and the National Heart Forum. It is not possible here to do justice to its 59-page report, *Why Health is the Key to the Future of Food and Farming*. Here are some of my favourite extracts:

The key purpose of food and farming is — or should be — to advance the health and well-being of the population. Other considerations such as the economy, trade liberalisation, CAP reform, etc., should all meet this goal of improved public health; if they do not, they should be rejected ... Farming and food should give equal weight to both human and environmental health. Policy and practice should encourage diversity of foods and biodiversity in fields. The food chain should decrease its reliance on non-renewable energy over and above global, European and UK commitments. Food costs should more fully reflect their real costs of production, distribution and mal-consumption. Food chains should be as short as possible ... Financial measures currently encourage policy confusion: [between] conventional 'efficiency' ... and ecological efficiency. Food policies should ... encourage local food suppliers, providers and retailers to reduce in 'food miles' [more shortly], ensuring that all citizens are within walking or bicycling distance of food shops ... health goals need not conflict with other goals for a sustainable, competitive and diverse farming and food sector ... environmental goals and health goals are entirely complementary. In order to advance both environmental and health goals there needs to be a switch from animal based foods to plant-based foods — particularly vegetables and fruit ... There is evidence that diet is a factor in some mental ill-health conditions. [pp 3–11]

On pesticides, the report says:

In 1995 when the Working Party on Pesticide Residues found excessive residues in carrots ... the Chief Medical Officer issued advice in 1997 to peel carrots ... there is currently some negotiation ... whether the CMO's advice ... is still needed. *Whether this is so or not is almost beside the point. The fact that so-called Good Agricultural Practice allowed application of pesticides to carrots in such quantities that consumer safety was even slightly in doubt suggests that agricultural production was coming before consumer safety* [p 19 — my italics].

On antibiotics, it has this to say:

Recent best estimates indicate that more antibiotics are used in agriculture each year than in treating humans. Evidence now links widespread use of antibiotics in animal feed, common to confined animal feeding operations, with rising numbers of humans infected with bacteria that respond poorly or not at all to treatments with these same antibiotics, or closely related drugs. [p 29]

Other observations included:

- In Europe, the most heavily subsidised crop per hectare was tobacco. [p 40]
- The loss of local greengrocers had produced urban 'food deserts'. [p 20]
- The relocation of food outlets to supermarkets on the edges of large towns committed the public to using fuelled transport to purchase food. The consequences of this were: increase in greenhouse gases; reduction in physical exercise; loss of social capital as neighbours encountered one another less; and money saved on cheaper food was matched by increased transport expenditure. [p 37]
- Ready-made meals and better cleaning agents saved the average person 2 hours and 41 minutes in domestic chores per week. This was balanced by an increase of 2 hours and 48 minutes travelling to, and spent in, shopping outlets. [p 33]
- It is naive to believe that this trend will be reversed by increases in individual responsibility and self-management alone. [p 37]
- 'Universities ... agricultural and veterinary colleges rely for their research support on government departments, the research councils, the private sector.' Such bodies are 'in many cases well placed to respond to new incentives to research into producing safer foods and healthier diets, but the current pattern of incentives are pushing academic researchers in contrary directions.' [p 52]

This report prompts some what-if questions. What if governments stopped spending money on highways and diverted the funds into public transport, shopping buses for the elderly, dedicated bicycle paths? What if the lands used to build the highways that transport vegetables were given over to the growing of those vegetables instead? What if public and private moneys spent on exercise regimes for young and old were diverted to enable people to exercise as they weeded the nation's food-gardens?

What if the price of an apple grown on one continent, flown to another, and finally trucked the length of that country, were truly costed in environmental terms? (Australian orchardists have pulled out productive orchards because they can't compete with the prices of oranges grown in the United States.) This is no abstract concern. The benefits of eating good food are diminished if its transport increases pollution and global warming. Some 2003 'food miles' statistics from Britain make us think:

- *Apples:* 76 per cent of those consumed came from overseas — many from the United States, a journey of 10,133 miles. Meanwhile, 60 per cent of Britain's orchards had been destroyed in the last three decades.
- *Pears:* from Argentina, 6886 miles. Local production had fallen 22 per cent in the last decade.
- *Grapes:* from Chile, 7247 miles — with a lot of packaging to prevent damage. Where does this packaging go?
- *Lettuce:* from Spain, a mere 958 miles. The authors estimated that it cost 127 calories of energy (in aviation fuel) to import 1 calorie of lettuce-energy.
- *Strawberries:* also from Spain, but sometimes from California. The authors estimated that the energy cost of importing 1 kg of out-of-season strawberries from California was the equivalent of keeping a 100-watt light bulb on for eight days.
- *And the rest:* broccoli and spinach came from Spain; potatoes from Israel, 2187 miles; tomatoes from Saudi Arabia, 3086 miles (long-life varieties picked early — less flavour, fewer nutrients); prawns from Indonesia, 7278 miles; brussels sprouts from Australia, 10,562 miles; wine from New Zealand, 14,287 miles; carrots and peas from South Africa, 5979 miles.[22]

In conclusion we have to ask what if governments were obliged to take the social and moral costs of cheap overseas foods into account when they negotiated trade deals? None of these what-ifs are technically difficult.

The Slow Food Movement

Blessed are the cheesemakers.— Monty Python's Life of Brian

A small market town in the foothills of the Italian Alps was the birthplace of a movement known as Slow Food. The year was 1986, and the triggering event was the opening of a McDonald's restaurant in the famous Piazza di Spagna in Rome. The founder of the movement was a man called Carlo Petrini who, in an interview in *The Nation* said, 'A hundred years ago, people ate between 100 and 120 species of food. Now our diet is made up of, at most, 10 or 12 species.'[23]

No matter how this story is played out, or which statistics are given, the estimates and themes are consistent. Within any one production line, the range is dictated by the demands of commerce. The vegetables we can buy are not the healthiest, or even those that taste the best. They are the ones which crop in a convenient time band, pack easily, endure transport. The medical consequences of this have been the subject of much of this book. These health considerations, the risk of famine when monocultures fail, the loss of gastronomic delights and of traditional livelihoods—all of these factors have boosted the Slow Food Movement.

Spurred on by factors like mad-cow disease and the risk of GM monocultures, support for Slow Food has spread to many countries. Membership has increased beyond the 1.4 million members it had when Petrini first discussed the organisation with Ralph Nader.

Slow Food extends its concern beyond the range of available foods to the production methods. To meet modern hygiene standards, governments prohibit such activities as the traditional production of cheese. Yet a master cheesemaker, perhaps the sixth or seventh generation to practise the craft, may pose less threat than a factory where commercial interest is the driving force. The same is true of traditionally produced breads, wines, and many other foods.

In fact, when we consider the factors raised in Chapter 6: The Gut, it is probable that the friendly micro-organisms in our intestines actually *depend* on the products of natural fermentation processes to maintain their own health and balance. The pathogens in naturally produced cheeses, such as *Listeria monocytogenes*, may pose a health risk only when intestinal florae are out of balance. And this lack of balance comes largely as a result of the use of antibiotics, preservatives and sugar in the modern production of food, none of which is countermanded by food safety laws. The members of the Slow Food Movement understand this well.

Permaculture

The term Permaculture was coined by Australian bio-geographer Dr Bill Mollison in the 1970s as a contraction of 'permanent agriculture'. He developed guidelines for the design and maintenance of agriculturally productive ecosystems. These guidelines cover the inter-relationships of landform features (slopes, watercourses), plant species and built structures (dwellings, gardens, roads, lakes). The objective is to achieve a harmonious integration of landscape and people, providing their material and non-material needs in a sustainable way. Although the focus is on agriculture, the guidelines extend to the design of buildings and to social and organisational structures.

Permaculture draws on the patterns found in natural ecosystems, and it encourages protracted and thoughtful observation, as opposed to protracted and thoughtless action. By getting the design right, needless expenditure of energy (both human and mechanical) can be avoided. The diversity of products needed for quality of life can be produced.

Permaculture is now an international movement. As well as several books written by Mollison, there is the *International Permaculture Journal* and a Permaculture Institute involved in training (see www.permaculture.org.au and www.tagari.com). Permaculturists follow design principles that are generally supportive of human health, for example:

- Short supply chain for food from point of production to consumption, resulting in fresh produce with minimal nutrient loss.
- Diversity and density of plants and animals similar to that found in natural ecosystems, leading to resilience and stability on one hand, and continuity of production

on the other, while avoiding any need for poisons or artificial fertilisers.

A design based on Permaculture principles might use warmth generated by a compost heap or a fowl house to protect frost-tender plant species. Manure from ducks and hens fertilises the vegetables growing nearby. The ducks and hens keep insects and grubs under control. Pesticides are avoided or eliminated altogether.

Ancient crops and rare breeds

In a seaside village in Cornwall there is a sign on a tiny cottage which reads: 'Here lived Dolly Pentreath, the last person to speak the Cornish language as a mother tongue until her death in 1777 aged 102.' There is a haunting image of an ageing Dolly standing at her front gate, the sole reservoir of a precious Gaelic heritage. Such loss of language is poignant. Language, culture, food — how can we separate these? Some linguists argue that languages have spread not by conquest and exploration, but by farming and agriculture. But as languages and cultures have spread, others have been lost.

Certain plants, aided by the forces of the global economy, seemed bent on conquest, as if they were malevolent vegetable imperialists. As linguists strive to preserve tongues which are on the brink of extinction, so many rare species have found their defenders.

Inspired by movements such as Permaculture and Slow Food, many farmers are now beginning to recognise the value in preserving ancient crops and rare animal breeds. Cultivated over centuries, these species resulted in rich diversity and had many adaptive benefits. The problems of monocultures were avoided, and biodiversity was maintained. Sustainability was not mentioned because it was taken for granted.

Seed-saving organisations, with names like Seeds of Change, Heritage Crops and Eden Seeds, have appeared around the world. Some have been started by altruistic bodies to help poor nations recover the means of feeding themselves. Others are the efforts of biologists and field scientists appalled by loss of diversity. Many have been started by small-scale farmers and gardeners of the First World.

Some wonderful stories have emerged from this quest — an onion was thought to be extinct until it was found growing in a tiny country cemetery; a pear tree producing fruit weighing half a kilogram; rare varieties are found growing beside country roads, railway lines, in abandoned lots and old vineyards. Seeds and cuttings from these plants are traded and cultivated through national and international seed-saving organisations. Some are available through commercial outlets.

Not long ago, few had heard of bread made from quinoa, spelt or kamut, progenitors of modern wheat. Amaranth is an ancient grain used by the Aztecs for cereals and bread; something of a wonder plant, its leaves are rich in protein, vitamins and minerals and its seeds are a good source of amino acids. We might ask how such a useful grain was all but lost to agriculture. The answer is not attractive. When Cortes invaded Mexico, he and his Spanish army burned the amaranth plantations and forced the Indians to grow barley.

Slowly these heritage plants are being rediscovered, along with their nutritional and environmental advantages. Amaranth, cassava, yams, arrowroot and taro are gluten-free. Whole cultures lived well on diets which to Western eyes are severely limited simply because they lack gluten and dairy products.

Bush foods

In Australia a growing awareness of the value of bush foods has paralleled the interest in rare breeds. They are the foods which sustained hunter-gatherers in ancient times and were only passively cultivated by humans. These fruits, nuts, berries, herbs and vegetables are an untapped resource. They can provide food with minimal ecological impact. They promise a wide array of novel medicines. Only a fragment of the total number appears in Appendix 2. As with the ancient crops, scientists, researchers and ethno-botanists are seeking to intervene before it is too late.

In 1989 the journal *Nature* published a paper described as seminal. Entitled 'Valuation of an Amazonian Rainforest', it argued that the revenues from the sale of rainforest fruit alone would exceed the one-off sale of trees to loggers. This original research has led to the production of a simple book for locals, explaining in pictures the subsistence value of the fruits, fibres, game and medicines preserved when logging was avoided. Described as a 'blend of hard science and local knowledge', the book (also known as the 'fruit book'), has been well received by locals, politicians in Western Amazonia, and even Brazil's environment minister.[24]

The consumption of a bush food diet has so many benefits that it makes the development of agriculture seem like a backward step. Agriculture's obvious benefits are social rather than nutritional. Bush food by contrast is fresh, seasonal, varied, and possibly uniquely suitable to meet the biochemical needs of the inhabitants of the local region. Both in Australia and the rest of the world, many local foods have been ignored. Edible nettles, dandelions, sorrels and brambles have been regarded as weeds. They have been sprayed with expensive poison, while we rush to import vegetables which are neither fresh nor free of agricultural chemicals.

Wild game also has many adaptive benefits. It is rich in omega-3 fatty acids because wild animals graze on the algae and seeds which are a source of omega-3s. The eggs and meat of these animals are similarly enriched. Nowadays animals used in native diets may be endangered, so there is understandable resistance to promoting them as a food source. The sensitivities of the Western world recoil at the idea of eating our primate cousins or cute animals, yet we countenance overfishing and the use of primates in inhumane experiments. Another irony. 'Primitive' peoples, who throughout the ages respected their food supply, suffer under rules imposed by an 'advanced culture', responsible for all the commercial misuse and most of the extinctions in the first place.

Australia: a case in point

The macadamia nut is one of the few native foods which most Australians know, yet we are surrounded by bush foods of high nutritional value. For instance, Warrigal greens are leafy tender greens which grow in abundance on sand dunes, stony beaches and salt marshes. They are sought by chefs overseas, but few non-indigenous Australians would recognise them as food. Also growing on dunes and otherwise unpromising land is a plant called pigface; its fleshy succulent leaves and fruit are both edible.

Not all Australian bush foods grow on hostile terrain: many are the product of rich rainforest environments. But as Australia's fragile ecosystems are further degraded by attempts to grow inappropriate crops, the foods which do are of special interest. The native peach or quandong, *Santalum acuminatum*, which thrives in desert country, is a good source of Vitamin C, and the large seed contains an edible, oil-rich nut.

Thousands of edible tubers, fruits, nuts and seeds are native to Australia, and further variety is provided by seaweed, algaes, edible wattle gums and nectars. They are so numerous that no complete list exists. In the least food-rich environment, the Western Australian desert, the Aboriginal inhabitants still were able to avail themselves of an estimated 150 foods. Compare this with the estimate by chef Vic Cherikoff, in his landmark books on Australian native cuisine, that even the most adventurous eater in Sydney has a repertoire of 80–85 foods.[25]

Many of the animals once used by Aboriginals are now 'protected'. Often this means that commercial operations have a quota for the numbers of fish, shellfish or kangaroos that they can harvest. Other animals are completely protected. Recent gains have been made in making exemptions for traditional hunters. There is still a long way to go in this regard.

Farmers' markets and food co-operatives around the world

Concerns about mass food production have come together in the growing phenomenon of farmers' markets. The atmosphere at these events is often festive and a spirit of camaraderie flourishes as people try nettle soups and bush foods, and buy free-range eggs from farmers who can tell you the names of all the hens who laid them. Much of the produce is organically grown. Organic produce is also a fast-growing sector within the general retail market. Available, too, at these markets are seeds from the seed-saver organisations mentioned above.

LIFESTYLE AND CULTURE

Heard melodies are sweet, but those unheard
Are sweeter; therefore, ye soft pipes, play on;
Not to the sensual ear, but, more endear'd,
Pipe to the spirit ditties of no tone ...
— John Keats, 'Ode on a Grecian Urn'

In these beautiful lines Keats captures some of the complexity of human experience. Western medicine has neglected these abstract and subtle aspects of life, and their impact on health. Fortunately, lifestyle is now making its appearance on the health agenda. Everything that happens to us, from cradle to grave, has some impact on our physical and mental well-being. Some of this experience comes to us through sight, smell, and touch, and some is cued more subtly. A baby in the womb responds to its mother's anxiety, probably as a result of her neurotransmitters. Women in group housing menstruate in synchrony, completely unaware of the pheromones that drive this phenomenon.

Our senses are far more than the transmission of electrical signals from the receptive organs. We come into a room and sense an atmosphere. We talk about seeing with our inner eye, or hearing the silence between two phrases of music.

With no full understanding of the impact of sensory — or even extra-sensory — phenomena, we have made changes in the modern world which are unique in human and animal experience. The impact of these on health, 'hael' or 'wholeness' is the subject of the remainder of this book. Many of the lessons we are learning come from cultural and anthropological studies. Some come from studying animals as they function in natural groups in the wild.

Lifestyle includes areas as wide as literature, art and music, sport and recreation, and it also covers how and where we live, and with whom. Do we live in large family groups, or alone in an inner-city studio flat? Do we get up at dawn to meditate or read our email, or are we night-owls whose day starts around 11 am with a cup of strong black coffee? Do we deal with stress by listening to Mozart, fighting with our neighbour, or going for a jog? Perhaps we are a Renaissance woman or man and do all of the above. In the remaining pages I will look at a few aspects of lifestyle which may affect our health.

A walk in the forest

If you come to me on a Monday morning and say that you feel tired, unwell and unable to face work, I may ask you how you spent the weekend. If you tell me that you stayed back late at work on Friday, slept in on Saturday, had a few beers too many on Saturday night, and loafed around on Sunday after doing some essential chores, you might not be surprised if I suggested that next weekend you plan a camping trip or a bushwalk in the nearest National Park.

But if you take up my suggestion, do you have any idea how powerful the 'medicine' I have prescribed might be? One biologist might be able to help you understand. Joan Maloof says that 120 chemical compounds were found in the mountain forest air of the Sierra Nevada.[26] Among them were volatile organic compounds, including the monoterpenes used by aromatherapists as 'essential oils'. Edible monoterpenes, Maloof says, have been shown both to prevent and to cure cancer. Of the 120 plant chemicals, only 70 were identifiable: 'when we lose our forests, we don't know what we are losing ...'

Even if you don't have a cancer you need to treat, I'm pretty sure you'll feel better for that walk in the bush.

Biological clocks

The lifestyle of individuals is largely directed by the culture they live in but, as any parent of adolescent and young adult children knows, two different shifts of people can live in the same household with almost no overlap at all. This has been made possible largely by the advent of the electric light. We have not taken into account the effect that living across varied time zones can have on our biorhythms.

We know about jet lag, produced by the disturbance of the circadian rhythm—a sick feeling that is independent of the amount of sleep lost. The word circadian is derived from two Latin words: *circa*, 'about'; and *diem*, '(within) a day'. It describes the changes that occur approximately every 24 hours in the human body. Many important bodily functions are affected by circadian rhythm.

Circadian rhythm explains many things. It makes us wake up at the usual time, often within minutes of our weekday pattern, even on weekends when we don't have to. It prevents us from opening our bowels in the middle of the night, although we sometimes wake to urinate. It causes us to reach for an extra blanket just before dawn, even though the ambient temperature has not dropped. It explains why we are most at risk of heart attacks first thing in the morning and why people with a fever have a temperature 'spike' in the late afternoon.

In the mid-1990s researchers discovered four genes that regulate the circadian cycles of flies, mice and humans (a good cross-section of the Ark). These genes were found to be expressed in *every cell* of the body. Indeed, they were found to operate *outside* the body. Not only do your pineal gland and your kidney keep an eye on the time, but so do your cells when they have been taken and grown in a laboratory somewhere. What's more, your liver cells run on a different time schedule to your heart cells, your gut cells, and so on.

Although the circadian clock runs on a 24-hour schedule, it needs continual resetting. This is done in two centres in the hypothalamus, each known as a suprachiasmic nucleus (SCN). These centres affect the daily fluctuations of body temperature, blood pressure and alertness level. The SCN also tells the pineal gland when to secrete melatonin. Cells in the retina (known as ganglion cells) give the SCN information about light levels. These cells can respond to light levels over long periods, ignoring brief fluctuations such as switching on a light in the middle of the night or entering a dark space in the daytime. Several neurotransmitters are involved in the setting of the clock. Dopamine, which has many and varied roles, is thought to act as a timekeeper when released in bursts by the substantia nigra in the brain.

If every cell in the body is paced by the circadian rhythm, we can begin to understand why disruption of these body rhythms can affect our health. Most, if not all, of our hormones and organs are running to some type of clock. This explains why nurses and other shift workers are prone to thyroid and fertility problems. At the level of cell division, there is known to be a mitotic clock. Both accelerated ageing and cancer are possible consequences of a disturbed mitotic clock. The increased levels of cancer and other serious health problems in shift workers are a warning that we meddle with biological clocks at our peril.

The circadian day

Significant melatonin secretion begins around 9.00 pm and ceases around 7.30 am: this is the time-frame in which we should do our sleeping. Within that, there are 90-minute sleep cycles. Deepest sleep occurs around 2.00 am, in the fourth cycle of an 'ideal' pattern. These 90-minute cycles continue throughout the day, but are much weaker in daylight. If you are jet-lagged or have had a bad night's sleep, you will notice periodic waves of fatigue. Timed, they will be found to occur about every 90 minutes. If you resist them you can probably stay awake, but this can be a dangerous practice, especially when driving a car.

The commonest time for planes to crash is said to be 6.00 am, and 'human error' is often listed as the cause. This is when the pilot and the air traffic controller should be entering the final phase of a good night's sleep. Their alarm clocks probably woke them during the REM phase of the deepest sleep cycle. (Do this with volunteers for several days and you will induce psychotic symptoms.) If they have drunk black coffee with sugar, the caffeine gives an adrenalin kick which interferes with the ability to adjust the biological clock. The sugar causes a spike in the blood glucose, followed by a precipitous fall, and they may experience functional hypoglycaemia, symptomatically akin to inebriation. (Many of the features of drunkenness are due to a drop in blood sugar. Children found in a coma after drinking punch at the family barbecue need urgent intravenous glucose to save them from fatal hypoglycaemia.)

Other functions have predictable timing. DHEA, known as a 'longevity hormone', surges at dawn, but this surge is suppressed by the first food of the day (Chapter 8). Surely a case for a late breakfast following the overnight fast.

At 4.30 am the body temperature reaches its lowest point, and we may reach for that extra blanket. At 6 am there is a cortisol surge, often accompanied by a fall in blood sugar. The (transient) hunger associated with this starts to stir the body into action. At 6.45 am, there is the sharpest rise of blood pressure. In a healthy person, this helps prepare for the day's activities. In someone with cardiovascular disease, it may precipitate a heart attack.

At 8.30 am, just as most people are rushing off to work, there is a natural cycle for a bowel action. At 10.00 am, there is a period of high alertness — at least we get that one right.

In addition to these daily rhythms, there are seasonal rhythms.

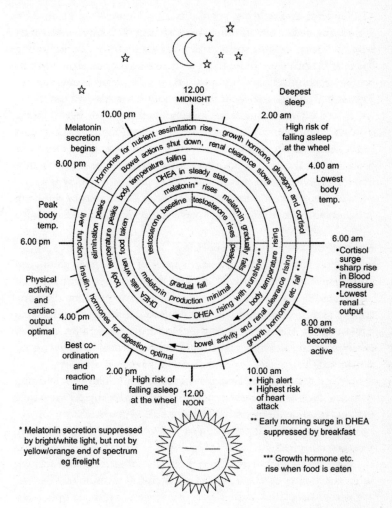

Chart 10.1: Circadian rhythms

Before the industrial revolution dictated the rhythms of life by mechanical clocks, people adjusted their circadian rhythm to suit the seasons. The advantage of having a clock which could be reset by melatonin is obvious. When days were long, they got up earlier and went to bed later. In the long nights of a northern winter, while not actually hibernating, they probably slowed down, slept more. In the long dark winters, many of our cultural pursuits arose. This became a time for repairing nets, weaving cloth, telling stories.

There is a tantalising possibility that some racial groups are genetically more tolerant of seasonal change than others. This may help to throw some light on disease patterns which vary according to racial origin. If we argue that the disruption of circadian rhythms results in significant health impacts, then disruptions brought about by seasonal change may be tolerated better by some than others.

Racial variation aside, what evidence is there of the health effects of disrupted cycles? Apart from the sleep disturbance which occurs in jet lag, there are several indicators. The phenomenon known as SAD (seasonal affective disorder) is suspected to be a disjunction between the circadian rhythm and the demands of a society which runs to the clock. Waking to an alarm clock interrupts deep sleep and causes surges of stress hormones such as adrenalin and cortisol.

Dopamine and time perception

Schizophrenia and non-seasonal depression are two psychological conditions associated with altered dopamine metabolism. In vulnerable people, disruption of biological rhythms could be the trigger that precipitates the illness. We know that there is a seasonal variation in the birth month of people who later develop schizophrenia, although the implications of this have yet to be unravelled.

Type 2 diabetes may be another case in point. Two people eating the same diet will have different outcomes depending on *when* they eat the food, as discussed in Chapter 8: Obesity. Eating out of synchrony with the rhythms of liver and gut cells is almost certainly a part of this effect.

Earlier it was noted that dopamine plays a role in the timekeeping process. Conditions characterised by altered dopamine metabolism are often associated with altered time perception. People with Parkinson's disease release less dopamine from the substantia nigra, and these patients consistently underestimate the amount of time which has passed. Marijuana and alcohol have a similar effect because they lower the availability of dopamine. Stimulants such as cocaine and amphetamines do the opposite. With increased dopamine available, time appears to speed up (hence, 'speed'). Stress, via the action of adrenalin and cortisol, also leads us to believe that an unpleasant event lasted interminably, when in reality it was all over in a short time.

Altered dopamine levels affect both the perception of time and the actual function of the biological clock. It is not difficult to see how stress and drugs, by altering dopamine metabolism, increase the risks of certain medical conditions.

Meditation, music and the arts

Volumes have been written on the health benefits of meditation, which in one form or another has been practised by many different cultures. It is now assumed that many activities—watching a flickering fire and gardening, as well as meditating—exert their beneficial effects by inducing alpha brain waves and releasing feel-good hormones such as dopamine.

The association between longevity and involvement in the arts has often been noted. The greatest longevity by occupation seems to be that of conductors of classical music. Long after many of their contemporaries are in nursing homes or deceased, these people can be found treading the boards of some of the world's most famous concert platforms. The tasks they perform require executive functions that would challenge people half their age. It is not just a metaphor that the role of the conductor is literally to harmonise, to bring all themes together.

Music therapy is an established discipline, which probably began with the observation that children with Down syndrome are unusually responsive to music. Perhaps also the striking association between the savant syndrome and artistic genius alerted people to this aspect of the arts.

Many argue that the brain is actually hard-wired by evolution to respond to pleasing musical sounds. When we hear an incomplete set of arpeggios the brain cries out for, even indeed 'hears', the resolution to the tonic or home chord. The 'incompleteness' is identifiable regardless of formal musical training. Similarly the ability to distinguish chord from discord does not need to be learned. Play a chord in a major and then a minor key and ask a five-year-old which is sad and which is happy. The response is impressively consistent.

One of the devices used by composers is the insertion of notes known as accidentals. These are notes which are in the 'wrong' key or timing. They give colour to the music and they work because they are unexpected. But why is the brain 'expecting' anything, if it has not heard the piece before? We can only assume that the brain has been drawn into the pattern, is responding to the harmony, and is startled by the unexpected.

There are, of course, cultural variations in scale, harmony and tone. However, even people exposed to a totally alien music form usually recognise it as music, and can apply words such as sad, happy, angry or contemplative to describe it. Indeed, the range of adjectives used to describe music from any genre encompass wide-ranging concepts such as 'narrative', 'ceremonial' 'grandiose'.

Some argue that because music expresses to a significant degree the type of emotions that we express in speech, it has co-evolved with language. A falling cadence expresses sadness, even depression, whether in music or in speech. Music by Elgar is said to express English sound patterns, while European composers express the European languages. The idea that language and music intertwine is demonstrated in the musicality of animal, and particularly bird, vocalisations. Even a narrow range of notes has a musical quality. Buddhist or Gregorian chants may lack 'melody' as such, but the impact can be electrifying.

The visual arts, of course, date from the earliest cave drawings and rock carvings, and include jewellery, decorations on vases and drinking vessels, spears and woven fabrics. The tattoos that are popular today presumably fulfil some primeval need. Self-decoration, indeed, seems to have significant psychological benefit. A depressed woman who cheers herself up with a new hairdo or hat shows a healthier response than one who reaches for Prozac.

We need music and artistic endeavour for the 'wholeness' which makes us human. The most convincing evidence of this is that no human cultures are devoid of the arts. As a means of recording experience, marking ceremonies, or simply relaxing, art is abundant and it predates our own era by tens of thousands of years.

Cultural practices

The insidious loss of cultural practices is only now being appreciated. Many were the result of communal living.

Sleep
Along with all the factors already considered in the causation of insomnia, we need to remember that for most of human history the tribe slept within a heartbeat of one another. Insomniacs describe

the nightmares and anxieties that recur in the sleepless hours. Children worry about monsters and burglars in the dark. Parents once of necessity slept with their children. Perhaps now the seeds of insomnia are sown in early childhood. In later years, under multiple assaults of alcohol, disturbed biorhythms and stress, insomnia is waiting to happen.

Communal living

The tribe has become redefined, and is often alien. People living in a high-rise apartment block may not know each other, not even the person who sleeps the thickness of one brick away. By contrast, on a 'lonely' farm road, in all probability, every neighbour knows all the others and watches out for them.

If telling stories and making music around the campfire has been with us for centuries, is the B-grade movie on television an adequate substitute? Does it set up the brain-wave patterns which will aid digestion, relieve stress, prepare us for sleep?

Contrast the average night in our suburban home to the holiday taken with friends in a congenial environment—the discussions over the evening meal, the night fishing expedition, shared endings to shared days. Children fall asleep around the campfire and are carried to their tents. Sounds idyllic doesn't it? We have to contrive the artifice of the holiday to re-create the pattern which was the norm for most of human history.

Some people are taking the problem of cultural isolation into their own hands. I know of two extended friendship groups, one in Canberra, Australia, and another in Davis, California, who are building their own retirement villages. This makes a lot of sense in an age where biological families are scattered over the globe and 'family' is more a friendship group than shared genes. If eventually one needs residential care, why not share it with the friends of a lifetime? It will be interesting to track the health profile of such groups. We can reasonably anticipate an improvement in both the quality and length of life.

Pica

The practice of pica, also known as 'geophagy', might cause us to marvel at the wisdom of old cultures. A child who eats dirt in our culture is regarded as disturbed, and an adult who does the same thing is assumed to be retarded or psychotic. But perhaps they are self-medicating?

Several cultures regard mud-eating as normal and even make expeditions to find just the right sort of mud to consume. Women, especially when pregnant, may become real connoisseurs. We are accustomed in our culture to the idea that a pregnant woman may crave some tasty snack food. We can only guess at the minerals she might be seeking—perhaps her needs might be better served by a good dose of mud.

In her book *Wild Health*, Cindy Engel discusses the various reasons for which animals are thought to benefit from this practice.[27] She gives the dramatic example of a mineral-rich cave in Kenya that has been visited by countless generations of elephants and other animals, despite an arduous and dangerous access. Some animals need sodium in particular. But as salt often occurs in the presence of other minerals, the drive for salt may also reflect a primitive instinct for a mineral-rich supplement.

Soil or clay can bind to the poisons which occur in many natural diets, just as we administer charcoal when people have been poisoned. This can reduce absorption, or by forming a new compound it can reduce toxicity. Clays have been shown to bind to man-made chemicals, fungi and bacteria as well as to plant toxins. Clay is antihelminthic, reducing the burden of parasitic worms by binding to eggs or larvae. By binding to water it can also reduce the catastrophic dehydration of parasitic disease. Without this 'medicine', death from diarrhoea is a real risk.

The properties of clay are such that it can also act as an antacid, aid digestion, and prevent damage to the lining of the gut. When we consider the proportion of Western medicines taken up by gut medications, clay is clearly a polypill.

No-one would suggest that we take our children down to the nearest park, contaminated with arsenic on the playground equipment and the faeces of dogs and cats, and feed them dirt. The difficulties of translating this type of knowledge into useful action are apparent.

'Taking the waters'

The benefits of bathing in water steeped in minerals have already been discussed in Chapter 4: Magnesium. Long before modern chemistry, people knew that many ailments could be helped or cured by immersion in natural spas. In 1995, a mainstream international dermatology journal reported that sunbathing in the Dead Sea for 28 days produced a significant reduction in the lesions of psoriasis, and that 58 per cent of the 1448 people in the study had complete clearing of the skin.[28]

When we were medical students, we were told that psoriasis was the commonest chronic skin condition. Students in the years ahead of us advised that in the dermatology exam, if we didn't recognise the problem in the sample of skin, 'psoriasis' was the safe answer. Together, the minerals in the Dead Sea and the effects of Vitamin D are an effective treatment for most cases of psoriasis.

Sunshine

Previous cultures respected the sun, even worshipped it. Now we are seeing a whole range of illness brought about by sun-deficiency, as we spend daylight hours indoors in our offices. Cancer, depression, osteoporosis are some. While some people avoid the sun, others are out getting burnt by it, giving themselves skin cancer.

Observations from the animal world

In her book, which has rightly received international recognition, Engel details the many ways in which animals in the wild manage to stay healthy. Her preface comes from the book of Job, 12:7: 'Ask now the beasts, and they shall teach thee; and the fowls of the air, and they shall tell thee.' The strength of this book is its refusal to romanticise or anthropomorphise the lives of animals. The things animals do are not intentional in the human sense, nor do they always work. But where they do work, it seems that the animals are obeying the instincts built into them over eons of time. The themes of this and other writings indicate we could acquire a wealth of wisdom from the study of our fellow creatures.[29]

Earlier in this chapter I discussed food and herbs as Nature's pharmacy. Animals avail themselves of this drugstore all the time. People observe it in their pets: a cat eats grass when it is 'sick', a horse turns to weeds when it is 'missing something'. Farmers know that animals that chew the fence posts and barbed wire of their enclosures probably have a dietary deficiency.

Sometimes the animals on my farm eat heliotrope and Paterson's curse. These purple weeds are toxic because of their alkaloid content. But alkaloids can have anti-helminthic properties, that is, they are active against worm infections. The weeds also contain copper, which is anti-bacterial and anti-helminthic. The current wisdom is that animals should be wormed annually, but animals got along for millennia before 20th-century medicines. Of course, they roamed widely, effectively resting the pasture, but perhaps they also 'know' that a feed of certain plants fixes the discomfort of an overdose of gut worms. Many other plants will serve. Tannins in the barks of many trees are directly anti-helminthic. Certain leaves and fruits cause purging, and this has a flushing effect on parasites. Animals use a wide range of other plants whose properties await identification with a resultant lowering of worm and parasite count. Good field studies have demonstrated that animals which have access to these plants do not have the same parasite burden as those which do not.[30]

Tribal peoples who share the same habitat as these creatures use the same plants for various medicinal purposes. These include plants which are anti-bacterial, anti-viral, anti-protozoal and anti-helminthic. Even plants which are active against schistosomiasis and malaria have been identified.

If we were to make a clearing in the forest, drape a few vines around, and fashion a counter from a fallen tree, we could open Nature's Pharmacy — Local Ailments a Specialty. We already have enough stock to make a respectable start on the 'antibiotic' shelf. How about the anti-inflammatories? The most widely used anti-inflammatory in the world is aspirin, first isolated from willow bark as we have seen. But the aspirin in willow bark is very concentrated, so if our customers are getting enough salicylates from the many fruits and vegetables in their diet, there might not be much demand.

What else might be protecting animals from arthritis and pain? Let's go back to my horses and their Paterson's curse. A recent analysis showed that its seeds contained a high level of omega-3 fatty acids similar to the omega-3 content of flax seeds.[31] Many nuts and seeds of grasses and plants are rich in these EFAs, so perhaps we won't do too much business from this shelf either. My horses also eat St John's wort. This is known to be good for depression and in laboratory analysis it has been shown to have anti-viral properties, including action against cytomegalic virus and HIV-AIDS.[32] It is has been shown to be useful in arthritis. Perhaps we had better market this one as a polypill.

The last area I will mention is cancer. Animals in the wild are not free of this health problem, but they do seem to have a lot less of it than humans. When cancer is prevalent in wild populations, it seems to have more to do with the results of human activity, such as pollution, than with 'cancer genes'. To be sure, animals do not smoke or engage in other activities associated with cancer risk, but their greatest protection probably comes from the fresh natural diet to which they have adapted over time. Rich in vitamins, minerals and essential fatty acids, and containing all the fibre they need, it provides a defence afforded by few Western diets. It is also possible that Nature's Pharmacy supplies continuous doses of anti-cancer medicines that arrest cancers before they become anything larger than a few cells. Something like 70 per cent of all anti-cancer drugs currently employed have been derived from plants, algae, crustaceans and other 'simple' life forms.

IN CONCLUSION

The foods and natural medicines discussed in the last few pages strike at the core market of the pharmaceutical bestsellers. These natural medicines surround us in abundance. They are products whose evolution has taken place alongside our own: the local product is wondrously fitted to the local problems. In the Darwinian struggle, plants and animals only co-survived when there was mutual benefit.

This book argues that we have right in front of us solutions to the pressing health problems of our age — both of the affluent world and of developing countries. It is not the lack of a magic bullet which keeps us in poor health, nor the lack of scientific breakthroughs. Current scientific understanding enables us, more than any previous generation, to learn from nature. Such thinking is alive with possibility.

EPILOGUE

In this book I have attempted to explore 'health', but I have not offered a definition.

The World Health Organisation defines health as: 'a state of complete physical, mental and social well-being, not merely the absence of disease and infirmity'. Although this definition has had many challenges since its original inception in 1948, it serves as a useful and simple model.

More poetic and more relevant to a world facing catastrophic climate change, and far more luminous, however, might be the words of the Australian poet Robert Gray, from his poem, 'To the Master, Dōgen Zenji (1200–1253 AD)':

> After years, home from China,
> and he had brought no scriptures; he showed them
> empty hands.
>
> This in Kyoto,
> at someone-else's temple. He said, All that's important
> is the ordinary things.
>
> Making a fire
> to boil the bathwater, pounding rice, pulling weeds
> and knocking dirt from their roots,
>
> or pouring tea — those blown scarves,
> a moment, more beautiful than the drapery
> in paintings by a master.
>
> 'It is this world
> of the *dharmas* (the atoms)
> that is the Diamond.'

(Reproduced with the kind permission of the author.)

Appendixes

APPENDIX 1: DIETARY REQUIREMENTS

The definitions and usage of dietary requirements of vitamins and minerals started in the United States with Recommended Dietary Allowances (RDA), defined in 1941. These were updated from time to time, until in 1997 a new term, Dietary Reference Intake (DRI), was introduced.

The DRIs are designed to overcome some of the shortcomings of the RDAs and are intended to replace them. By using quantitative statistics where available, the DRIs recognise variations in individual requirements, which the single-value RDAs could not do. DRIs consist of four reference values:

- *EAR, Estimated Average Requirement:* intake to meet the requirement of 50 per cent of people
- *RDA, Recommended Dietary Allowance:* intake to meet the requirement of 98 per cent of people
- *AI, Adequate Intake:* intake observed in healthy people (to be used when no RDA is available)
- *UL, Tolerable Upper-intake Level:* highest level of intake likely to pose no health risk to almost all people.

In Australia, Recommended Dietary Intake (RDI) is now used instead of RDA. In the UK the Reference Nutrient Intake (RNI), the amount of vitamins and minerals that should meet the needs of the majority was set by the Commitee on Medical Aspects of Food and Nutrition in the 1990s. Food labelling by contrast uses different terminology—Daily Values. These are divided into two:

- *DRV, Daily Reference Value:* applies to macronutrients, such as fats and carbohydrates; calculated to provide adequate energy content in the diet
- *RDI, Reference Daily Intake:* in general, these are the same as the RDAs.

The following table gives some values for adult males and females. Values for pregnant women, and for children, may be different: for instance, they may be lower due to lower body mass or higher due to growth requirements. Values have been drawn from a variety of sources, and do not necessarily correspond to any official or authoritative publications.

The requirements in the table relate to total dietary intake. The question of supplementation needs to be addressed in the context of what is in the diet, as well as individual variability of requirements and tolerance. Most supplements come as combinations; an all-purpose multivitamin is often adequate, with extras taken under advice from a health-care practitioner.

Confusion is often caused by varying terminology from manufacturer to manufacturer; quantities may be given by weight (milligrams, mg, or micrograms, mcg) or in International Units (IU).

Nutrient	Australian DRI data[1] — Adult males				Females	US Daily Value		UK Males	UK Females
	EAR	AI	UL	RDI	RDI	DRV	RDI	RNI	RNI
Vitamins									
Vitamin A	0.63 mg 2100 IU		3 mg	0.9 mg 3000 IU	0.7 mg 2333 IU		1.5 mg 5000 IU	0.7 mg 2333 IU	0.6 mg 1800 IU
Thiamin (B1)	1.0 mg			1.2 mg	1.1 mg		1.5 mg	1 mg	0.8 mg
Riboflavin (B2)	1.1 mg			1.3 mg	1.1 mg		1.7 mg	1.3 mg	1.1 mg
Niacin (B3)	12 mg		35 mg	16 mg	14 mg		20 mg	17 mg	13 mg
Vitamin B6	1.1 – 1.4 mg		50mg	1.3 – 1.7 mg	1.3 – 1.5 mg		2 mg	1.4 mg	1.2 mg
Biotin		30 mcg					300 mcg	100-200 mcg	100-200 mcg
Pantothenic Acid		6 mg					10 mg	5.4 mg (AI)	5.4 mg (AI)
Folic Acid	0.32 mg		1.0 mg	0.4 mg	0.4 mg		0.4 mg	0.2 mg	0.2 mg
Cobalamin (B12)	2.0 mcg			2.4 mcg	2.4 mcg			15 mcg	15 mcg
Vitamin C	30 mg		1g	45 mg 10g[2]			60 mg	40 mg	40 mg
Vitamin D		5 – 15 mcg	80 mcg	sunlight	sunlight		2 mcg 400 IU	sunlight	sunlight
Vitamin E		10 mg	300 mg				30 IU	4 mg	3 mg
Vitamin K		70 mcg						1 mcg/kg bw	1 mcg/kg bw
Choline		550 mg	3.5 g						

Minerals							
Sodium	0.46 – 0.92 g	2.3 g		2.4 g		1.6 g	1.6 g
Potassium	3.8 g			3.5 g		3.5 g	3.5 g
Calcium (Ca)	0.84 – 1.1 g	2.5 g	1 – 1.3 g	1 – 1.3 g		700 mg	700 mg
Phosphorus (P)	0.58 g	4 g	1 g	1 g	1 g	550 mg	550 mg
Iodine (I)	100 mcg	1.1 mg	150 mcg	150 mcg	150 mcg	140 mcg	140 mcg
Magnesium (Mg)	350 mg	350 mg³	420 mg	320 mg	400 mg	300 mg	270 mg
Zinc (Zn)	12 mg	40 mg	14 mg	8 mg	15 mg	5.5-9.5 mg	4-7 mg
Copper (Cu)	1.7 mg	10 mg			2 mg	1.2 mg	1.2 mg
Selenium (Se)	60 mcg	400 mcg	70 mcg	60 mcg		75 mcg	60 mcg
Manganese (Mn)	5.5 mg					5.5 mg (AI)	5.5 mg (AI)
Iron (Fe)	6 mg	45 mg	8 mg	18 mg		8.7 mg	14.8 mg
Fluorine (F)	4 mg	10 mg				0.05 mg/kg bw	0.05 mg/kg bw
Chromium (Cr)	35 mcg					25 mcg	25 mcg
Molybdenum	34 mcg	2,000 mcg	45 mcg	45 mcg	45 mcg	230 mcg (AI)	230 mcg (AI)

UK Prison Trial supplements as an example

The UK Prison Trial (Chapter 9) provides a convenient example of the sort of supplementation that can be beneficial. The daily supplement in that trial was:

- four capsules of omega-3 oil (fish oil)
- one Forceval multi-mineral/vitamin tablet containing the amounts in the following table.

I regard this as a reasonable one-size-fits-all regime for adults. I would probably add a good magnesium supplement (magnesium aspartate or magnesium orotate) in doses as recommended on the label.

Ingredient	Amount	Ingredient	Amount
Vitamin A	2,500 IU (750 mcg RE)	iron	12 mg
Vitamin D2	400 IU (10 mcg)	copper	2 mg
Vitamin C	60 mg	magnesium	30 mg
Vitamin E	10 mg	zinc	15 mg
Vitamin B1	1.2 mg	iodine	140 mcg
Vitamin B2	1.6 mg	manganese	3 mg
Vitamin B6	2 mg	potassium	4 mg
Vitamin B12	3 mcg	phosphorus	77 mg
folic acid	400 mcg	selenium	50 mcg
biotin	100 mcg	chromium	200 mcg
nicotinamide	18 mg	molybdenum	250 mcg
pantothenic acid	4 mg		
calcium	100 mg		

APPENDIX 2: FOOD GROUPS

This list is confined to plant foods. Every living creature that has ever has walked, crawled, flown, hopped or swum has at some stage been eaten by some other creature, and so a complete taxonomy of the animal world is not necessary here. It might be useful to consider, however, that many creatures that we consider as pests are consumed rather than poisoned in other cultures. These include grubs, larvae, locusts and other insects, and even deep-fried tarantulas.

Actinidiaceae: Chinese gooseberry or kiwi fruit (*Actinidia chinensis*)

Algae: agar-agar, carrageen, dulse, kelp or seaweed

Alliaceae: chives, garlic, leek, onion, shallot (all *Allium* species)

Amaranthaceae: Chinese spinach or hinn choi (*Amaranthus tricolor*), grain amaranth (*A. hypochondriacus*), green amaranth (*A. viridis*)

Araucariaceae: bunya nuts (*Araucaria bidwilli*)

Arrowroot family, *Marantaceae:* arrowroot (*Maranta arundinacea*)

Arum family, *Araceae:* ceriman (*Monstera*), dasheen (*Colocasia*), taro, malanga, yautia

Asclepiadaceae: bush banana (*Leichhardtia australis, Marsdenia vividiflora*) — leaves, flowers, tubers

Banana family, *Musaceae:* arrowroot (*Musa*), banana, plantain

Basellaceae: creeping spinach or basella (*Basella alba*), ulluco (*Ullucus tuberosa*)

Beech family, *Fagaceae:* chestnut (*Castanea sativa*), dwarf chestnut or chinquapin

Birch family, *Betulaceae:* hazelnut or filbert (Corylus avellana), oil of birch (wintergreen)

Bombacaceae: durian fruit (*Durio zibethinus*)

Borage family, *Boraginaceae* **(herbs):** borage, comfrey (leaf and root)

Buckwheat family, *Polygonaceae:* buckwheat (*Fagopyrum esculentum*), garden sorrel, rhubarb (stems only), sea grape

Buttercup family, *Ranunculaceae:* golden seal

Cactus family, *Cactaceae:* prickly pear

Canna family, *Cannaceae:* Queensland arrowroot

Caper family, *Capparidaceae:* caper

Carpetweed family, *Aizoaceae:* Warragul greens (*Tetragonia tetragniodes*), various pigface (*Carpobrutus* species)

Carrot family, *Umbelliferae* **a.k.a.** *Apiaceae:* angelica, anise, carraway, carrot, celeriac, celery, chervil, coriander, cumin, dill, fennel, gotu kola, lovage, parsley, parsnip, sweet cicely, skirret

Cashew family, *Anacardiaceae:* burdekin plum (*Pleiogynium timorense*), cashew, mango, pistachio

Citrus family, *Rutaceae:* lime, lemon, orange, grapefruit, citron (*Citrus* and *Microcitrus* species); cumquat (*Fortunella* species)

Combretaceae: kakadu plum (*Terminalia ferdinandiana*), native almond (*T. grandiflora*), nut tree (*T. arostrata*), sea almond (*T. catappa*)

Composite family, *Compositae* **a.k.a.** *Asteraceae:* alpine yam daisy, boneset, burdock root, cardoon, chamomile, chicory or endive, coltsfoot, costmary, dandelion, escarole, globe artichoke, goldenrod, Jerusalem artichoke, lettuce, pyrethrum, romaine, safflower, salsify, santolina, scolymus (Spanish oyster plant), scorzonera, shungiku (*Chrysanthemum coronarium*), southernwood, sunflower (*Helianthus annus*), tansy, tarragon, witloof chicory or French endive, wormwood (absinthe), yam daisy, yarrow

Conifer family, *Gramineae:* juniper (gin), pine nut (pi-on)

Custard-apple family, *Annona* species: custard-apple, papaw or pawpaw

Cyatheaceae: soft tree fern (*Dicksonia antarctica*)

Cycad family, *Coniferae:* cycad seed (*Cycas media*), Florida arrowroot (*Zamia*)

Davidsoniaceae: Davidson's plum (*Davidsonia pruriens*)

Ebony family, *Ebonaceae:* persimmons (Japanese and American), black plum, date plum (all *Diospyros* species)

Flax family, *Linaceae:* flaxseed

Fungi, *Agaricaceae:* yeasts, moulds, mushrooms, truffles

Ginger family, *Zingiberaceae:* cardamon, East Indian arrowroot (*Curcuma*), ginger, turmeric

Ginseng family, *Araliaceae:* American ginseng, Chinese ginseng

Goosefoot family, *Chenopodiaceae:* beetroot, chard, quinoa, silverbeet, spinach, sugar beet, tampala

Gourd family, *Cucurbitaceae:* bitter melon, choko, cucumber, gherkin, squashes (butternut etc.), pumpkins, sweet melons (cantaloupe etc.), watermelons, zucchini

Grape family, *Vitaceae:* grapes, raisins, wine, wine vinegar, brandy

Grass family, *Gramineae* a.k.a. *Poaceae:* barley (*Hordenum vulgare*), corn (*Zea mays*), millet, oats, rice, sorghum, triticale, wheat, bamboo shoots, sugarcane, lemongrass, wild rice, woollybutt grass (*Eragrostis eriopoda*)

Heath family, *Ericaceae:* bearberry, blueberry, cranberry, huckleberry, tree strawberry (*Arbutus unedo*)

Honeysuckle family, *Caprifoliaceae:* elderberry

Horsetail family, *Equisetaceae:* shavegrass (horsetail)

Iris family, *Iridaceae:* orris root, saffron (*Crocus*)

Lamiaceae: bush tea leaf (*Ocimum tenuiflorum*), hairy basil (*O. americanum*)

Laurel family, *Lauraceae:* avocado, bay leaf, cassia bark, cinnamon

Legume family, *Leguminoseae,* a.k.a. *Fabaceae:* alfalfa (sprouts), beans (numerous varieties), soy beans, peas (numerous varieties), peanuts, lentils, carob, fenugreek, jicama tubers, tamarind

Lily family, *Liliaceae:* Aloe vera, asparagus, bulbine lily or wild onion (*Bulbine bulbosa*), chocolate lily or grass lily (*Dichopogon strictus*)

Linden family, *Tiliaceae:* basswood or linden, melokhia (*Corchorus olitorius*)

Madder family, *Rubiaceae:* coffee (*Coffea arabica, C. canephora*), woodruff

Mallow family, *Malvaceae:* althea root, cottonseed oil, roselle or rosella (*Hibiscus sabdariffa*), okra (*H. esculentus*)

Malpighia family, *Malpighiaceae:* acerola (Barbados cherry)

Maple family: sap of sugar maple (*Acer saccharum*)

Mint family, *Labiatae* (herbs): various mints, basil, bergamot, catnip, chinese artichoke, clary, dittany, horehound, hyssop, lavender, lemon balm, marjoram, oregano, pennyroyal, perilla, rosemary, sage, summer savory, thyme, winter savory

Morning-glory family, *Convolvulaceae:* bush potato (*Ipomoea costata*), sweet potato (*I. batatas*), kangkong (*I. aquatica*)

Mulberry family, *Moraceae*: breadfruit (*Artocarpus incisa*), various figs (*Ficus* species), jackfruit, mulberry

Mustard family, a.k.a. Cabbage family, *Cruciferae* a.k.a. *Brassicaceae*: various rockets (*Cakile* species, *Heperis* species, *Eruca* species), broccoli, brussels sprouts, cabbage, watercress, canola, cauliflower, cress, horseradish, kale, kohlrabi, mizuna, komatsuna, radish, rutabaga, turnip

Myrtle family, *Myrtaceae*:

- nectar: various bottlebrush (*Callistemon* species)
- fruit: lilly pilly, brush cherry, durobby (*Szygium* species), myrtles (*Austromyrtus* species)
- edible sap: cider gum (*Eucalyptus gunnii*)

Nasturtium family, *Tropaeolaceae*: nasturtium

Nutmeg family, *Myristicaceae*: nutmeg

Olive family, *Oleaceae*: olive (green or ripe)

Orchid family, *Orchidaceae*: vanilla

Oxalis family, *Oxalidaceae*: carambola or star fruit (*Averrhoa carambola*), oxalis or oca (*Oxalis tuberosa*)

Palm family, *Palmaceae*: coconut (*Cocos nucifera*), date, palm cabbage, sago palm

Papaya family, *Caricaceae*: papaya

Passion Flower family, *Passifloraceae*: granadilla or passion fruit

Pedalium family, *Pedaliaceae*: sesame (*Sesamum indicum*)

Pepper family, *Piperaceae*: peppercorn (*Piper* species)

Pineapple family, *Bromeliaceae*: pineapple

***Pittosporaceae*:** appleberry (*Billardiera scandens*), purple appleberry (*B. longiflora*), sweet appleberry (*B. cymosa*)

***Podocarpaceae*:** brown pine (*Podocarpus dispersus*), illawarra plum (*P. elatus*), mountain plum pine (*P. lawrencei*),

Pomegranite family, *Punicaceae*: pomegranate (*Punica granatum*)

Poppy family, *Papaveraceae*: poppyseed

Potato family, a.k.a. Nightshade family, *Solanaceae*: tomato, bush tomato, tree tomato, eggplant, capsicum, chilli, potato, tobacco

Protea family, *Proteaceae*: geebungs (*Persoonia* species), bush nut (*Macadamia tetraphylla*), nectar from various banksias, grevilleas and hakeas

Purslane family, *Portulaceae*: pigweed or purslane (*Portulaca oleracea*)

***Rhamnaceae*:** Chinese jujube (*Zizyphus jujuba*), Indian jujube (*Z. mauritania*)

Rose family, *Rosaceae*:

- pomes: apple, azarole, crabapple, loquat, medlar, pear, quince, rosehips
- stone fruits: almond, apricot, cherry, peach (nectarine), plum (prune), sloe
- berries: blackberry, boysenberry, dewberry, loganberry, longberry, youngberry, raspberry, strawberry

***Santalaceae*:** various ballart (*Exocarpus species*), broad-leaved native cherry (*E. latifolius*), quandong (*Santalum acuminatum*)

Sapodilla family, *Sapotaceae:* chicle (chewing gum)

Sapucaya family, *Lecythidaceae:* Brazil nut (*Bertholletia excelsa*), sapucaya nut (paradise nut)

Saxifrage family, *Saxifragaceae:* currant, gooseberry

Sedge family, *Cyperaceae:* Chinese water chestnut (*Eleocharis dulcis*), chufa (groundnut), nalgoo tuber (*Cyperus bulbosus*)

Smilacaceae: sweet tea (*Smilax glyciphylla*)

Soapberry family, *Sapindaceae:* akee apple (*Blighia sapida*), litchi or lychee, longan (*Dimocarpus longan*), rambutan (*Nephelium lappaceum*)

Spurge family, *Euphorbiaceae:* candlenut (*Aleurites moluccana*), cassava or yuca (*Manihot dulcis, M. esculenta*), castor bean

Sterculia family, *Sterculiaceae:* chocolate (cacao), cocoa, cola nut, kurrajong tree seeds

Tacca family, *Taccaceae:* Fiji arrowroot (*Tacca* species)

Tea family, *Theaceae:* tea (*Camellia sinensis*)

Valerian family, *Valerianaceae:* corn salad (*Valerianella locusta*)

Verbena family, *Verbenaceae:* lemon verbena

Walnut family, *Juglandaceae:* various walnuts (*Jugland* species), hickory nuts and pecan (*Carya* species)

Waterlily family, *Nymphaeaceae:* lotus (*Nelumbo nucifera*)

Wattle family, *Mimosaceae:* seed and edible gum or sap from various wattles (*Acacia* species), mulga (*A. aneura*)

Winteraceae: dorrigo pepper (*Tasmannia stipitata*), mountain pepper (*T. lanceolata*)

Xanthorrhoeaceae: grass tree (*Xanthorrhoea australis*)

Yam family, *Dioscoreaceae:* various types of yam (*Dioscorea* species).

APPENDIX 3: GUT HEALTH

- *Exclude serious conditions:* See your doctor to make sure you do not have coeliac disease, IgA deficiency, food allergies, helicobacter overgrowth, etc. If helicobacter is found to be present in overgrowth, consider the possibility that *low* levels of stomach acid may be the cause.

- *Avoid* food that is picked before it is ripe (green harvested): It will be high in salicylates and will set you up for salicylate sensitivity.

- *Don't make holes in the gut:* Gluten and dairy sensitivity, sugar, aspirin and chlorine — all increase gut permeability and allow large allergenic molecules through undigested.

- *Chew food:* Mechanical grinding by the teeth is the first major step in digestion. Also, there are enzymes in the saliva which occur nowhere else in the gut. This stage of digestion is lost when you bolt food.

- *Sit down to eat:* By doing this you increase hydrochloric acid production, which facilitates digestion and efficient passage to the duodenum. The acid also helps to kill pathogens, control helicobacter levels and denature toxins. You may need vinegar, lemon or hydrochloric acid tablets from the chemist or health food shop to aid this process. *Antacids may make things worse,* while giving temporary relief.

- *(Pancreatic) enzymes:* Many gut conditions respond to supplementation with digestive enzymes. Pancreatic enzymes are derived from animals and are usually expensive. Vegetable enzymes, such as bromelain and papain, are cheap and often adequate.

- *Acidophilus and bifidus:* These friendly bacteria help the digestive and elimination processes, destroy toxins and keep the bowel mucosa healthy. Get advice from your pharmacist or natural health practitioner. Your gut bacteria use lentils, legumes, asparagus, onions and garlic as their own food source, so feed them some of these foods.

- *Avoid things which destroy good gut bacteria:* This list includes chlorine (therefore filter your water), sugar, antibiotics and food preservatives.

- *Consume things which heal the gut:* Honey, especially from the leptospermum plants, has been shown to be kill undesirable bacteria and encourage regrowth of good bacteria. 'Manuka' is a good variety. Sap from wattle trees was a traditional Australian Aboriginal food, and serves a similar purpose in the gut. Magnesium, molybdenum, zinc, selenium and EFAs all help heal the gut.

ABBREVIATIONS

5HT: 5-hydroxy tryptophan
ACE: angiotensin-converting enzyme
ACNEM: Australasian College of Nutritional and Environmental Medicine; it trains doctors in natural medicine and provides a referral service for the public.
See *www.acnem.org*

ADD:	attention deficit disorder
ADHD:	attention deficit hyperactivity disorder
AIDS:	acquired immune deficiency syndrome
ARMD:	age-related macular degeneration
ASD:	autistic spectrum disorders
BCME:	bis(chloromethyl) ether
BH4:	tetrahydro biopterin
BMR:	basal metabolic rate
BPH:	benign prostatic hypertrophy
BSE:	bovine spongiform encephalitis (mad cow disease)
COX:	cyclo-oxygenase (enzyme)
DGLA:	Dihomogamma linolenic acid
DHA:	Docosahexaenoic acid
DHEA:	dehydroepiandrosterone
DHT:	dihydro-testosterone
DNA:	deoxyribonucleic acid: the genetic material of nearly all life forms, with four bases, adenine, thymine, guanine, cytosine
EPA:	Eicosapentaenoic acid
FHM:	familial hemiplegic migraine
GALT:	gut-associated lymphoid tissue
GI:	glycaemic index
GORD:	gastro-oesophageal reflux disease
HDL:	high-density lipoproteins
HRT:	hormone replacement therapy
IGF-1:	insulin-like growth factor
LDL:	low-density lipoproteins
MMR:	measles, mumps, rubella
mRNA:	messenger RNA
MRSA:	multiple resistant *Staph aureus* (resistant to many antibiotics)
NHS:	National Health Service (UK)
NK cell:	natural killer cell
NNT:	number needed to treat
NSAID:	non-steroidal anti-inflammatory drug
PAF:	platelet-activating factor
PAHs:	polycyclic aromatic hydrocarbons
PCBs:	polychlorinated biphenyls
PCOS:	polycystic ovary syndrome
RCT:	random controlled trial
RDA:	recommended dietary allowance; see Appendix 1
RDI:	reference daily intake; see Appendix 1
SAH:	s-adenosyl homocysteine (abbreviated as *adohcy* in some texts)

SAMe:	s–adenosyl methionine
	(abbreviated as *adomet* in some texts)
SHBG:	sex-hormone-binding globulin
SCFA:	short-chain fatty acid
SCN:	suprachiasmic nucleus
SLE:	systemic lupus erythematosus; also known as lupus
SNRI:	serotonin and nor-adrenalin reuptake inhibitor
SSRI:	selective serotonin reuptake inhibitor
THM:	trihalomethanes
tRNA:	transfer RNA
VLDL:	very low-density lipoproteins

NOTES

CHAPTER 1: MEDICINE AND PROGRESS

1   Philip and Phyllis Morrison, '*Wonders*', *Scientific American*, February 2000.
2   Bob Holmes, 'Manna or Millstone', *New Scientist*, 18 September 2004, p. 29.
3   *American Scientist*, vol. 89 no. 6, November–December 2001, pp 558–9, reviewing a textbook by the archaeologist Lewis Binford.
4   J. G. Vaughan and C. A. Geissler, *The New Oxford Book of Food Plants*.
5   Jennifer Isaacs, *Bush Food: Aboriginal Food and Herbal Medicine*.
6   Colin Tudge, 'The Best Medicine', *New Scientist*, 17 November 2001.
7   *Habitat*, the magazine of the Australian Conservation Foundation, December 1998, p. 2.
8   'Organic Foods, Hard Evidence for their Superiority', *New Vegetarian and Natural Health*, Autumn 2000, p. 34.
9   *Sydney Morning Herald*, 26 February 2001, reprint of an article by Matthew Engels, 'That Green Vegetable', from *The Guardian*, 2001.
10 Emma Young, 'Why It's Good for You', Health and Science, Sydney Morning Herald, 14 April 2005, p. 6.
11 Dr Elaine Ingham, lecture on soil chemistry at University of Western Sydney, Richmond campus, 1 July 1999.
12 Jean D. Wilson et al., Harrison's Principles of Internal Medicine, 12th edition, McGraw Hill, 1991; Thomas Gordon Hungerford, Diseases of Livestock, 9th edition, McGraw Hill, 1990.
13 Extract from letter from Dr T.G. Hungerford, 8 June 1989.
14 Latifa Shamsuddin et al., 'Use of Magnesium Sulphate among Eclampsia Cases at Community Level Before Referral to Tertiary Hospitals', *International Journal of Gynecology and Obstetrics*, vol. 70, Supplement 2, 2000, p. 47.
15 'Feed Your Dog's Brains', *New Scientist*, 26 January 2002, p. 25.
16 Dr Ian Billinghurst, *Grow your Pups with Bones*, Ian Billinghurst, 1999.

17   Cindy Engel, 'Nutritional Wisdom', *Wild Health*, Weidenfeld and
     Nicholson, 2002, p. 27.

CHAPTER 2: THE POLITICS OF HEALTH

1   Michael S. Simmons et al., 'Unpredictability of Deception in Compliance
     With Physician-Prescribed Bronchodilator Inhaler Use in a Clinical Trial',
     Chest, vol. 118, 2000, pp. 290–5.
2   B. Moosman and C. Behl, 'Selenoprotein synthesis and side-effects of
     statins', *The Lancet*, 13 March 2004, vol. 363 (9412), pp. 892–4.
3   Danny Penman 'No Pain, No Gain?', *New Scientist*, 8 June 2002, p. 6.
4   Carmia Borek, 'Antioxidants and Cancer', *Science and Medicine*,
     November–December 1997, pp. 52–61.
5   W. V. E. Doering, 'Antioxidant Vitamins, Cancer and Cardiovascular
     Disease', *New England Journal of Medicine*, 3 October 1996, vol. 335,
     pp. 1065–9.
6   'Duped by Drugs', *New Scientist*, 8 June 2002, p. 5.
7   Paul A. Komesaroff and Ian H. Kerridge, 'Ethical Issues Concerning the
     Relationships between Medical Practitioners and the Pharmaceutical
     Industry', *Medical Journal of Australia*, 4 February 2002.
8   T. Fahey, S. Griffiths and T. J. Peters, 'Evidence-Based Purchasing:
     Understanding Results of Clinical Trials and Systematic Reviews',
     British Medical Journal, 21 October 1995, vol. 311, pp. 1056–60.
9   Ray Moynihan, 'Drug Firms Hype Disease as Sales Ploy, Industry Chief
     Claims', *British Medical Journal*, 13 April 2002, vol. 324, p. 867.
10   'No Double Standards', editorial, *New Scientist*, 27 April 2002, p. 3.
11   Samuel S. Epstein, *The Politics of Cancer Revisited*, East Ridge Press, 1998.
12   Bob Beale, Linda Morris and James Woodford, 'Sydney Choking on Its
     10-Cigarettes-a-Day Air', *Sydney Morning Herald*, 28 May 1996.
13   Samuel S. Epstein, *The Politics of Cancer Revisited*, p. 201.
14   Epstein, *The Politics of Cancer Revisited*, p. 641.
15   Alison McCook, 'Lifting the Screen', *Scientific American*, June 2002, p. 12.
16   Heather O. Dickinson and Louise Parker, 'Leukaemia and Non-
     Hodgkin's Lymphoma in Children of Male Sellafield Radiation Workers',
     International Journal of Cancer, 20 May 2002, vol. 99, no. 3, pp. 437–44.
17   Deborah Josefson, 'Mammography Is No Better than Physical Breast
     Examination, Study Shows', *British Medical Journal*, 30 September 2000,
     vol. 321, p. 788.
18   O. Olsen and p. C. Gotzche, 'Cochrane Review on Screening for Breast
     Cancer with Mammography', *The Lancet*, 20 October 2001, vol. 358
     (9290), pp. 1340–2.
19   Alexandra Barratt et al., 'Model of Outcomes of Screening
     Mammography: Information to Support Informed Choices', *British
     Medical Journal*, April 2005, vol. 330, p. 936.
20   Sharon Batt and Liza Gross, 'Cancer, Inc.', *Sierra Magazine*, September–
     October 1999, at *www.sierraclub.org/sierra/199909/cancer.asp.*
21   Trevor Powles et al., 'Interim Analysis of the Incidence of Breast
     Cancer in the Royal Marsden Hospital Tamoxifen Randomised
     Chemoprevention Trial', *The Lancet*, 11 July 1998, vol 352, pp. 98–101.

22 Batt and Gross, 'Cancer, Inc.'.

23 Theo Colborn, Dianne Dumanoski, John Peterson Myers, *Our Stolen Future*, Little, Brown and Co., 1996.

24 Bianca Nogrady, 'Risk Outweighs Benefit in HRT Heart Prevention', *Australian Doctor*, 15 August 2003, p. 3.

25 Sylvia Pagan Westphal, 'New Data Halts Largest HRT Trial', *New Scientist.com* news service, 9 July 2002.

26 Collignon, '*Virus Fears Cloud Future of Animal Organ Transplants*', *Sydney Morning Herald*, 10 January 2002.

27 Mark Metherell, '$200m Mass Vaccination to Combat Killer Disease', *Sydney Morning Herald*, 10–11 August 2002.

28 Debora Mackenzie, 'Bird Flu's Ticking Time Bomb', *New Scientist*, 27 March 2004, p. 6.

29 'The Lessons To be Learnt from Animal Vaccine Research', *Private Eye Magazine Special Report*, May 2002, p. 20.

30 'The Lessons To be Learnt from Animal Vaccine Research', *Private Eye Magazine Special Report*.

31 Dr Robert Rogers, 'Multiple Vaccines Hinder Immune Response', *Medical Observer*, 21 August 1998, based on the journal *Infection and Immunity*, 1998, vol. 66, p. 2093.

32 Debora MacKenzie, 'The Hidden Catch', *New Scientist*, 4 May 2002, p. 7.

33 'Polio Returns', *New Scientist*, 27 August 2005, p. 4.

34 Andrew Wakefield and Scott Montgomery, 'Through a Glass Darkly', *Adverse Drug Reactions Toxicology Review*, December 2000, vol. 19, no. 4, pp. 265–83.

35 Heather Mills, 'MMR: The Story So Far', *Private Eye Magazine Special Report*, May 2002.

36 P. Farrington et al., 'A New Method for Active Surveillance of Adverse Events from Diphtheria/Tetanus/Pertussis and Measles/Mumps/Rubella Vaccine', *The Lancet*, 1995, vol. 345, pp. 567–9.

37 James Braly and Ron Hoggan, *Dangerous Grains*, Avery Penguin Putnam, 2002, p. 113.

38 Greg Wadley and Angus Martin, 'The Origins of Agriculture: A Biological Perspective and a New Hypothesis', *Journal of the Australasian College of Nutritional and Environmental Medicine*, April 2000, pp. 3–12.

39 Keith Woodford, *Devil in the Milk*, Craig Potton Publishing, 2007

40 Batt and Gross, 'Cancer, Inc.'.

41 Professor Jane A. Plant, *Your Life in Your Hands*, Virgin Books Ltd, 2001.

42 Plant, *Your Life in Your Hands*.

43 K. M. Fairfield and R. H. Fletcher, 'Vitamins for Chronic Disease Prevention in Adults', *Journal of the American Medical Association*, 19 June 2002, vol. 287, no. 23, pp. 3116–26.

CHAPTER 3: HEALTH PROCESSES

1 Bill Mollison, *Permaculture: A Designers' Manual*, Tagari Publications, 1988.

2 Martha H. Stipanuk, *Biochemical and Physiological Aspects of Human Nutrition*, W. B. Saunders Co., 2000, p. 44.

3 Tom Brody, *Nutritional Biochemistry*, 2nd edition, Academic Press,

1999, p. 497 ff.

4   Stipanuk, *Human Nutrition*, p. 498.

5   Dr Henry Butt, BioScreen, Bio21 Molecular Science and Biotechnology Institute, University of Melbourne.

6   Garry Hamilton, 'Insider Trading', *New Scientist*, 26 June 1999, p. 43.

7   Hamilton, 'Insider Trading', p. 45.

8   F. Adlerberth et al., 'High Turnover Rate of *Escherichia coli* Strains in the Intestinal Flora of Infants in Pakistan', *Epidemiology and Infection*, 1998, vol. 121, pp. 587–98; Hamilton, 'Insider Trading'.

9   Stipanuk, *Human Nutrition*, p. 148

10 Stipanuk, *Human Nutrition*, p. 149.

11 Martin J. Blaser, 'An Endangered Species in the Stomach', *Scientific American*, February 2005, p. 24.

12 Brody, *Nutritional Biochemistry*, p. 189.

13 Kurt Kleiner, 'Power Lunch', *New Scientist*, 2 June 2001, p. 5.

14 Helen Phillips, 'Master Code', *New Scientist*, 15 March 2003, p. 44; Emma Young, 'Strange Inheritance', *New Scientist*, 12 July 2008.

15 Philip Cohen, 'You Are What Your Mother Ate', *New Scientist*, 9 August 2003, p. 14.

16 Cohen, 'You Are What Your Mother Ate'.

17 Paul A. Marks et al., 'Inhibitors of Histone Deacetylase Are Potentially Effective Anticancer Agents', *Clinical Cancer Research*, April 2001, vol. 7, pp. 759–60.

18 Anil Ananthaswamy, 'Enzymes Scan DNA Using Electric Pulses', *New Scientist*, 18 October 2003, p. 10.

CHAPTER 4: MACRONUTRIENTS AND MINERALS

1   Stipanuk, *Human Nutrition*, p. 44.

2   Stipanuk, *Human Nutrition*, p. 884.

3   Prof. Derek Bryce-Smith and Liz Hodgkinson, *The Zinc Solution*, Century Arrow, 1986.

4   Daniela Rhodes and Aaron Klug, 'Zinc Fingers', *Scientific American*, February 1993, pp. 32–9.

5   Brody, *Nutritional Biochemistry*, p. 245.

6   P. J. Fraker et al., 'The Dynamic Link between the Integrity of the Immune System and Zinc Status', *Journal of Nutrition*, 2000, vol. 130, pp. 1399S–1406S.

7   Archie Kalokerinos, *Every Second Child*, Thomas Nelson (Australia), 1974, p. 116.

8   J. Britton et al. 'Dietary Magnesium, Lung Function, Wheezing, and Airway Hyperreactivity in a Random Adult Population Sample', *The Lancet*, 6 August 1994, vol. 344, pp. 357–62.

9   A. Piekert, C. Wilimzig and R. Kohne-Volland, 'Prophylaxis of Migraine with Oral Magnesium: Results from a Prospective, Multi-Center, Placebo-Controlled and Double Blind Randomized Study', *Cephalalgia*, 1996, vol. 16, pp. 257–63.

10 L. C. Clark et al., 'Effects of Selenium Supplementation for Cancer Prevention in Patients with Carcinoma of the Skin: A Randomised

Controlled Trial', *Journal of the American Medical Association*, 1996, vol. 276, pp. 1957–63.

11 M. P. Rayman, 'The Importance of Selenium to Human Health', *The Lancet*, 15 July 2000, vol. 356, pp. 233–41.

12 Wilson et al., *Harrison's Principles of Internal Medicine*, 12th edition.

13 Stipanuk, *Human Nutrition*, p. 784.

14 Laura Spinney, 'Poor Diets Breed Deadly Viruses', *New Scientist*, 20 May 1995, p. 16.

15 Spinney, 'Poor Diets Breed Deadly Viruses'.

16 Stipanuk, *Human Nutrition*, p. 790.

17 Stipanuk, *Human Nutrition*, p. 796.

18 Rayman, 'The Importance of Selenium to Human Health'.

19 Clark et al., 'Effects of Selenium Supplementation for Cancer Prevention'.

20 Rayman, 'The Importance of Selenium to Human Health'.

21 A. Castano et al., 'Low Selenium Diet Increases the Dopamine Turnover in Prefrontal Cortex of the Rat', *Neurochemistry International*, 1997, vol. 30, pp. 549–55.

22 W. C. Hawkes and L. Hornbostel, 'Effects of Dietary Selenium on Mood in Healthy Men Living in a Metabolic Research Unit', *Biogical Psychiatry*, 1996, vol. 39, pp. 121–8.

23 J. W. Finley and J. G. Penland, 'Adequacy or Deprivation of Dietary Selenium in Healthy Men: Clinical and Psychological Findings', *Journal of Trace Elements in Experimental Medicine*, 1998, vol. 11, pp. 11–27.

24 Rayman, 'The Importance of Selenium to Human Health'.

25 Wilson et al., *Harrison's Principles of Internal Medicine*.

26 Norman Swan with Julian Mercer, 'The Role of Copper in the Body', *Health Report*, ABC Radio National, 19 September 2005; Stipanuk, *Human Nutrition*, p. 744.

27 Stipanuk, *Human Nutrition*, p. 831.

28 Igor Tabrizian, *Nutritional Medicine: Fact and Fiction*, NRS Publishing, 2003, p. 70.

29 www.mbschachter.com/Iodine.htm; www.helpmythyroid.com.

30 Search for 'iodine' at www.townsendletter.com. Articles from August 2005 are relevant.

31 Deborah Smith, 'Children at risk from lack of iodine', *Sydney Morning Herald*, 20 February 2006 (quoting from a study by Mu Li reported in *Medical Journal of Australia*).

CHAPTER 5: VITAMINS AND ESSENTIAL FATTY ACIDS

1 Stipanuk, *Human Nutrition*.

2 W. W. Fawzi et al., 'Vitamin A Supplementation and Child Mortality. A Meta-Analysis', *Journal of the American Medical Association*, 17 February 1993, vol. 269.

3 A. H. Shankar et al., 'Effect of Vitamin A Supplementation on Morbidity due to *Plasmodium falciparum* in Young Children in Papua New Guinea: A Randomised Trial', *The Lancet*, 17 July 1999, vol. 354, pp. 203–9

4 Stipanuk, *Human Nutrition*, p. 603.

5 John Boik, *Natural Compounds in Cancer Therapy*, Oregon Medical Press

LLC, 2001, p. 320; Luigi M. De Luca et al., 'Retinoids in Differentiation and Neoplasia', *Scientific American Science and Medicine*, July–August 1995, pp. 28–36.

6   Yoshitaka Tsubono, Shoichiro Tsugane and K. Fred Gey, 'Plasma Antioxidant Vitamins and Carotenoids in Five Japanese Populations With Varied Mortality from Gastric Cancer', *Nutrition and Cancer*, 1999, vol. 34, no. 1, pp. 56–61

7   Stipanuk, *Human Nutrition*, p. 468.

8   Stipanuk, *Human Nutrition*, p. 498.

9   Norman Swan with Joel Mason, 'Does Folate or Folic Acid Prevent Cancer?' *Health Report*, ABC Radio National, 4 March 2002.

10 Hazel Muir, 'Acid Test', *New Scientist*, 28 July 2001, p. 7.

11 Stipanuk, *Human Nutrition*, p. 501.

12 Brody, *Nutritional Biochemistry*, p. 550.

13 Stipanuk, *Human Nutrition*, p. 529.

14 Melvyn R. Werbach, *Textbook of Nutritional Medicine*, Third Line Press, 1999, p. 246.

15 Werbach, *Textbook of Nutritional Medicine*.

16 Stipanuk, *Human Nutrition* p. 565

17 Ian Brighthope, 'Vitamin C Is Safe and Effective: A Response to the Pennsylvania Study', *Journal of the Australasian College of Nutritional and Environmental Medicine*, April 2001, p. 2.

18 Archie Kalokerinos, *Every Second Child*.

19 Archie Kalokerinos, Glen Dettman and Ian Dettman, *Vitamin C: Nature's Miraculous Healing Missile*, Frederick Todd, 1993.

20 Stipanuk, *Human Nutrition*, p. 635.

21 Norman Swan with William Grant, Michael Holick and Nina Jablonski, 'The Body's Response to Sunlight', *Health Report*, ABC Radio National, 4 March 2002; Chang Van Den Bemd, 'Vitamin D and Vitamin D analogs in cancer treatment', *Current Drug Targets*, February 2002, vol. 3, no. 1.

22 Later published as Michael Holick, 'Vitamin D: Importance in the Prevention of Cancers, Type 1 Diabetes, Heart Disease, and Osteoporosis', *American Journal of Clinical Nutrition*, March 2004, vol 79, no. 3, pp. 362–71.

23 Stipanuk, *Human Nutrition*, p. 585.

24 'Vitamin E Vicissitudes', *Journal of Complementary Medicine*, January–February 2005, p. 12.

25 Udo Erasmus, *Fats that Heal, Fats that Kill*, Alive Books, 1986.

26 Debra Jopson, 'Fish Cuts Asthma Rate in Children', *Sydney Morning Herald*, 6 February 1996, reporting *Medical Journal of Australia*, 5 February 1996.

27 Tanveer Ahmed, 'The Good Oil Comes from Fish', *New Scientist*, 28 June 2005.

28 Robyn Williams with John McGowan, 'The Disappearing Plankton', *The Science Show*, ABC Radio National, 24 April 2004.

CHAPTER 6: A SYSTEMATIC APPROACH TO DISEASE

1   Anil Ananthaswamy, 'Best to Be Last', *New Scientist*, 17 November 2001, p. 5; Garry Hamilton, 'Let Them Eat Dirt', *New Scientist*, 18 July 1998, p. 30.

2   Amanda Dunn, 'New Research Uncovers Link between Exercise and Cholesterol Levels', *Sydney Morning Herald*, 25 March 2003.

3   William J. Rea, *Chemical Sensitivity*, vol. 1, Lewis Publishers, 1992, p. 7.
4   William J. Rea, *Chemical Sensitivity*, vol. 3, Lewis Publishers, 1995, p. 1272.
5   John K. Pollack, *The Toxicity of Chemical Mixtures*, Centre for Human Aspects of Science and Technology (CHAST), 1993 p. 32.
6   Kurt Kleiner, 'Lead May Be Damaging the Intelligence of Millions of Children Worldwide', *New Scientist*, 26 April 2003, p. 21.
7   Samuel S. Epstein, *The Politics of Cancer Revisited*, p. 641; Theo Colborn, Dianne Dumanoski and John Peterson Myers, *Our Stolen Future*, p. 184.
8   Jay Withgott, 'Popular Herbicide May Gender-bend Wild Frogs', *New Scientist*, 2 November 2002 p. 13.
9   Eugenie Samuel, 'Is There a Safe Limit for Weedkillers?', *New Scientist*, 21 September 2002 p. 10.
10 Epstein, *The Politics of Cancer Revisited*, p. 81.
11 'A Spoonful of Sugar: Medicine's Management in NHS Hospitals', UK Audit Commission, 18 December 2001.
12 Prof. Ray Kearney, 'Health Impacts of Vehicle Exhaust Emissions', lecture at Australasian College of Nutritional and Environmental Medicine, Sydney, 4 December 2003.
13 Stipanuk, *Human Nutrition*, p. 912.
14 Rea, *Chemical Sensitivity*, vol. 1, p. 38.
15 Epstein, *Politics of Cancer Revisited*, p. 53.
16 Epstein, *Politics of Cancer Revisited*, p. 115.
17 Robert Buist, *Food Chemical Sensitivity*, Collins/Angus and Robertson 1990, p. 37.
18 Buist, *Food Chemical Sensitivity*, pp. 52–4
19 Buist, *Food Chemical Sensitivity*.
20 Epstein, *Politics of Cancer Revisited*, p. 125.
21 G. R. Howe et al., 'Artificial Sweeteners and Human Bladder Cancer', *The Lancet*, 17 September 1977, 2, pp. 578–81.
22 Epstein, *Politics of Cancer Revisited*, p. 575.
23 Buist, *Food Chemical Sensitivity*, p. 47.
24 Epstein, *Politics of Cancer Revisited*, p. 135.
25 Sylvia Pagan Westphal, 'Lost Innocence', *New Scientist*, 6 April 2002, p. 6.
26 Epstein, *Politics of Cancer Revisited*, pp. 481, 572; Rea, *Chemical Sensitivity*, vol. 3, pp. 1580, 1625.
27 Epstein, *Politics of Cancer Revisited*, p. 201.
28 Rea, *Chemical Sensitivity*, vol. 3, p. 1779.
29 Fred Pearce, 'Arctic Faces Toxic Time Bomb', *New Scientist*, 1 February 2003, p. 9.
30 Colborn, Dumanoski and Myers, *Our Stolen Future*, p. 113.
31 Colborn, Dumanoski and Myers, *Our Stolen Future*, pp. 151, 162.
32 Pearce, 'Arctic Faces Toxic Time Bomb'.
33 'Hormones on the Menu', *New Scientist*, 30 March 2002, p. 23.
34 Julie Wakefield, 'Boys Won't Be Boys', *New Scientist*, 29 June 2002, p. 42.
35 'Drastic Plastic Ban', *New Scientist*, 23 April 2005, p. 6.
36 Wakefield, 'Boys Won't Be Boys'.
37 Daniel Lewis, 'Green-fingered Get Helping Hand to Grasp Chemical Laws', *Sydney Morning Herald*, 31 July 2002, p. 7.

38 'Banned Toxins Found in Cord Blood', *Australian Doctor*, 29 July 2005.
39 Epstein, *Politics of Cancer Revisited*, p. 81.
40 Kearney, 'Health Impacts of Vehicle Exhaust Emissions'.
41 Hamilton, 'Let Them Eat Dirt', p. 28.
42 Jasmine Chua, 'Asthma Due to Too Much Cleanliness', *Australian Doctor*, 12 July 1996, reporting *Medical Journal of Australia*, Jennifer Peat, Ann Woolcock.
43 Paolo M. Matricardi et al., 'Exposure to Foodborne and Orofecal Microbes Versus Airborne Viruses in Relation to Atopy and Allergic Asthma: Epidemiological Study', *British Medical Journal*, 12 February 2000, vol. 320, pp. 412–17.
44 M. Eric Gershwin, J. Bruce German and Carl L. Keen, *Nutrition and Immunology*, Humana Press, 2000, p. 319.
45 Norman Swan with Alessio Fasano, 'Coeliac Disease', *The Health Report*, ABC Radio National, 15 August 2005; see also C. E. Taplin et al., 'The Rising Incidence of Childhood Type 1 Diabetes in New South Wales, 1990– 2002', *Medical Journal of Australia*, 2005, vol. 183, pp. 243–6.
46 Norman Swan with Hugh Sampson, 'Food Allergy in Children', *The Health Report*, ABC Radio National, 15 April 2002.
47 Lissa Christopher, 'Boweled Over', Health and Science, *Sydney Morning Herald*, 23 September 2004, p. 2.
48 John Gever, 'Excess Study Deaths Prompt Concerns About Enteral Probiotics', MedPage Today, 14 February 2008, www.medpagetoday.com (reporting on a study by Hein G. Gooszen of the University Medical Centre, Utrecht).
49 M. Hadjivassiliou et al., 'The Role of Gluten Sensitivity in Neurological Illness', CME Journal Gastroenterology, Hepatology and Nutrition, 1999, vol. 2, pp. 3–5.
50 Andy Coghlan, 'Wonderful Worms', *New Scientist*, 7 August 1999, p. 4.
51 M. Kalliomaki et al., 'Probiotics in Primary Prevention of Atopic Disease: A Randomised Placebo-Controlled Trial', *The Lancet*, 2001, vol. 357, pp. 1076–9.
52 Stephen Davies and Alan Stewart, *Nutritional Medicine*, Pan Books, 1987, pp. 318–22.
53 Cindy Engel, *Wild Health*, Weidenfeld and Nicholson, 2002.
54 Nell Boyce, 'The Demon Drink', *New Scientist*, 18 July 1998, p. 18.
55 Gail Vines, 'A Gut Feeling', *New Scientist*, 8 August 1998, p. 26.
56 Norman Swan with Eric Reynolds, William Bowen, Jeff Hillman and Bruce Rutherford, 'Dental and Oral Health', *The Health Report*, ABC Radio National, 18 March 2002.
57 'Is it Worth Worrying About?', *New Scientist*, 15 June 2002, p. 17.
58 'Here We Go Again', *New Scientist*, 6 July 2002, p. 3.
59 John Vidal, 'GM Genes Found in Human Gut', *Guardian*, 17 July 2002.
60 Alsion Motluk, 'From Minor to Major', *New Scientist*, 4 May 2002, p. 9.
61 Gail Vines, 'Swallow This', *New Scientist*, 15 June 2002, p. 26.
62 Peter Hadfield, 'No Burps, Please', *New Scientist*, 15 June 2002, p. 21.
63 Jo Whelan, 'Double Diabetes', *New Scientist*, 27 October 2007, p. 48.
64 Garry Hamilton, 'Filthy Friends', *New Scientist*, 16 April 2005, p. 34.

65 Kate Benson, 'Daycare Helps Ward off Cancer', *Sydney Morning Herald*,
    30 April 2008 (reporting on the second Causes and Prevention of
    Childhood Leukaemia conference, London, UK, 29 April 2008; see also,
    J. Marshall, 'Filthy Health', *New Scientist*, 12 January 2008, p. 34.
66 J. Correale and M. Farez, 'Association between parasite infection and
    immune responses in multiple sclerosis', *Ann Neurol*, February 2007, vol.
    61, no. 2, pp. 97–108.
67 Dr James Daveson at the Princess Alexandra Hospital in Brisbane (2008),
    reported in *The Australian Coeliac*, pp. 11–13, June 2008
68 See also: Leigh Dayton, 'Gut Bug Link in Childhood Asthma: Study',
    The Australian, 9 July 2008

CHAPTER 7: SOME FIXED-NAME DISEASES

1 S. Ayres and R. Mihan, 'Acne Vulgaris and Lipid Peroxidation: New Concepts
   in Pathogenesis and Treatment', *International Journal of Dermatology*,
   17 May 1978, vol. 7, pp. 305–7.
2 James Randerson, 'Asthma Linked to Use of Antibiotics', *New Scientist*,
   5 June 2004, p. 13.
3 John S Dowden, 'Coax, COX and Cola', *Medical Journal of Australia*,
   24 October 2003, vol. 179, no. 8, pp. 397–8.
4 Werbach, *Textbook of Nutritional Medicine*, p. 671.
5 Werbach, *Textbook of Nutritional Medicine*, p. 679.
6 Gershwin, German and Keen, *Nutrition and Immunology*, p. 159.
7 Werbach, *Textbook of Nutritional Medicine*.
8 Werbach, *Textbook of Nutritional Medicine*, p. 577; Michael J. Murray and
   Joseph Pizzorno, *Encyclopaedia of Natural Medicine*, Little, Brown and Co.,
   1998, p. 697.
9 Murray and Pizzorno, *Encyclopaedia of Natural Medicine*, p. 697.
10 Alison Motluk, 'Antibiotics for Babies Linked to Asthma', *New Scientist*,
   4 October 2003, p. 16.
11 Qihan Dong and Jas Singh, 'Antioxidant cocktail shows good results in
   fight against prostate cancer', 7 December 2007,
   www.cancerresearch.med.usyd.edu.au/news.index.php.
12 Epstein, *Politics of Cancer Revisited*, p. 298.
13 Joanna Moorhead, 'The Cream Comes off Our Milky Ways',
   Sydney Morning Herald, 30 December 2004, p. 14.
14 L. C. Clark et al., 'Plasma Selenium Concentration Predicts the
   Prevalence of Colorectal Adenomatous Polyps', *Cancer Epidemiology
   Biomarkers and Prevention*, 1993, vol. 2, no. 1, pp. 41–6.
15 Zhen Zhang et al., 'Three Biomarkers Identified from Serum Proteomic
   Analysis for the Detection of Early Stage Ovarian Cancer',
   Cancer Research, 15 August 2004, vol. 64, pp. 5882–90.
16 Moorhead, 'The Cream Comes off Our Milky Ways'.
17 'Resistance Fighters', *New Scientist*, 1 May 1999, p. 23.
18 Ray Moynihan and Alan Cassels, *Selling Sickness*, Allen and Unwin, 2005.
19 Jordan Baker, 'Treat the Leakage', Health and Science, *Sydney Morning
   Herald*, 15 September 2005, p. 4.
20 *www.who.int/reproductive-health/family_planning/cocs_hrt.html*

21 'Bad Breath Bugs', *New Scientist*, 1 March 2003, p. 24.
22 Epstein, *Politics of Cancer Revisited*, p. 390.
23 Norman Swan with Eric Reynolds, William Bowen, Jeff Hillman and Bruce Rutherford, 'Dental and Oral Health', *The Health Report*, ABC Radio National, 18 March 2002.
24 Swan with Reynolds, Bowen, Hillman and Rutherford, 'Dental and Oral Health'.
25 Andy Coghlan, 'Does It Matter if Genes Can Jump from GM Food to Bugs in Human Gut?', *New Scientist*, 27 July 2002, p. 6.
26 Stipanuk, *Human Nutrition*, p. 875.
27 Stipanuk, *Human Nutrition*, pp. 875–6.
28 N. Shouji et al., 'Anticaries Effect of a Component from Shiitake', *Caries Research*, January–February 2000, vol. 34, pp. 94–8.
29 Helen Pearson, 'Could a Choc a Day Keep the Dentist Away?', *New Scientist*, 26 August 2000, p. 16.
30 Weston A. Price, *Nutrition and Physical Degeneration*, 1945, Keats Publishing Inc., 1989.
31 Douglas Fox, 'Blinded by Bread', *New Scientist*, 6 April 2002, p. 9.
32 Rachel Nowak, 'Eyes Wide Open', *New Scientist*, 1 February 2003, p. 40.
33 Fox, 'Blinded by Bread'.
34 Michael Le Page, 'Can You Train Your Eyes to See Better Underwater?', *New Scientist*, 17 May 2003, p. 14.
35 Fox, 'Blinded by Bread'.
36 Anna Evangeli, 'Zinc Plus Antioxidants Saves Sight', *Medical Observer*, 19 October 2001.
37 W. Smith, Pp. Mitchell and S. R. Leeder, 'Dietary Fat and Fish Intake and Age-Related Maculopathy', *Archives of Ophthalmology*, March 2000, vol. 118, pp. 401–4.
38 Nowak, 'Eyes Wide Open', p. 43; Matt Ridley, 'Genes Are So Liberating', *New Scientist*, 17 May 2003, p. 39.

CHAPTER 8: TWO LEADING CAUSES OF DEATH

1 Stipanuk, *Human Nutrition*, p. 11.
2 S. H. Saydah et al., 'Abnormal Glucose Tolerance and the Risk of Cancer Death in the United States', *American Journal of Epidemiology*, 15 June 2003, vol. 157, no. 12, pp. 1092–100.
3 John Hockenberry and guests Peter Bennett et al., 'Rewriting Heredity: environment and the genome', 2008, www.dnafiles.org; Linda Geddes, 'Watch out for the wrong kind of sugar', *New Scientist*, 28 June 2008, p. 9; Maribel Rios and Norman Swan, 'Appetite Control', *The Health Report*, ABC Radio National, 24 March 2008; Jo Whelan, 'Double Diabetes', *New Scientist*, 27 October 2007, p. 48; Various papers published by Joe Proietto and Katherine Samaras; Emma Young, 'Strange Inheritance', *New Scientist*, 12 July 2008.
4 Neal Baynard, 'Compulsive Eating', *New Scientist*, 13 September 2003, p. 28.
5 John Cornwall, 'Madness on Trial', *New Scientist*, 15 March 2003, p. 27.
6 Steve Bloom, 'The Fat Controller', *New Scientist*, 9 August 2003, p. 40.
7 Derek Bryce-Smith and Liz Hodgkinson, *The Zinc Solution*, p. 71.

8 Stipanuk, *Human Nutrition*, pp. 466, 828ff., 938; Murray and Pizzorno, *Encyclopaedia of Natural Medicine*, p. 60.

9 Stipanuk, *Human Nutrition*, chapter 32.

10 Murray and Pizzorno, 'Diabetes Mellitus', *Encyclopaedia of Natural Medicine*.

11 M. S. Wu et al., 'A Case-Control Study of Association of *Helicobacter pylori* Infection with Morbid Obesity in Taiwan', *Archives of Internal Medicine*, 2005, vol. 165, pp. 1552–5.

12 Geoff Watts, 'Dig in, Dine on, Pig out', *New Scientist*, 23 March 2002, p. 28.

13 Brad Lemley, 'What Does Science Say You Should Eat?', *Discover*, February 2004, pp. 43–9.

14 Jennie Brand-Miller et al., *The New Glucose Revolution*, Marlowe and Co., 2003.

15 See note 3, above.

16 Manny Oakes and Peter Clifton, *The CSIRO Total Wellbeing Diet*, Penguin, 2005.

17 Matthew Ricketson, 'CSIRO's best selling diet "ignores cancer concerns"', *The Age*, 1 April 2008

18 Ray Kearney, 'Ageing Diet, Melatonin, DHEA', lecture given at Australasian College of Nutritional and Environmental Medicine, Sydney, 1999.

19 'Why a Fruit Breakfast?', *Natural Health*, April–May 1994, pp. 2, 3, quoting *The Lancet*, October 1987.

20 E. Gueux et al., 'Effect of Magnesium Deficiency on Triacylglycerol-Rich Lipoprotein and Tissue Susceptibility to Peroxidation in Relation to Vitamin E Content', *British Journal of Nutrition*, 1995, vol. 74, pp. 849–56.

21 Scott H. Goodnight, 'The Fish Oil Puzzle', *Scientific American Science and Medicine*, September–October 1996, pp. 42–51.

22 Peter Libby, 'Atherosclerosis: The New View', *Scientific American*, May 2002 p. 47–55.

23 Stipanuk, *Human Nutrition*, chapter 41.

24 Erasmus, *Fats that Heal, Fats that Kill*, p. 57.

25 J. G. Eric et al., 'Mortality over Two Centuries in Large Pedigree with Familial Hypercholesterolaemia: Family Tree Mortality Study' *British Medical Journal*, 28 April 2001, vol. 322, pp. 1019–23.

26 K. S. McCully, 'Hyperhomocysteinemia and arteriosclerosis: historical perspectives', *Clin Chem Lab Med*, 2005; 43(10) pp. 980–6.

27 Stipanuk, *Human Nutrition*, p. 496.

28 Melvyn R. Werbach, 'Nutritional Influences on Illness: Nutrients for Lowering Cholesterol', *Journal of the Australasian College of Nutritional and Environmental Medicine*, June 1998, p. 25.

29 Julie Robotham, 'A New Prescription', *Sydney Morning Herald*, 19 December 2002; P. Whelton et al., 'Major Outcomes in High-Risk Hypertensive Patients Randomised to Angiotensin-Converting Enzyme Inhibitor or Calcium Channel Blocker vs Diuretic: The Antihypertensive and Lipid-Lowering Treatment to Prevent Heart Attack Trial (ALLHAT), *Journal of the American Medical Association*, 18 December 2002, vol. 288, no. 23, pp. 2981–97.

30 *www4.dr-rath-foundation.org/pdf_files/heart_book.pdf, p. 61.*

CHAPTER 9: MENTAL HEALTH AND NEUROLOGICAL DISORDERS

1 Dominic Murphy, 'Breaking out of the Straitjacket', *New Scientist*, 17 May 2003, p. 46.

2 Michael D. Lemonick et al., 'The Mood Molecule', *Time*, 29 September 1997, pp. 53–9.

3 *National Health Priority Areas Report on Mental Health: A Report Focussing on Depression 1998 — Summary*, Australian Institute of Health and Welfare, 4 August 1999.

4 Norman Swan with Richard Taylor, 'Increased Suicide Rates under Conservative Governments', *The Health Report*, ABC Radio National, 30 September 2002.

5 C. Bernard Gesch et al., 'Influence of Supplementary Vitamins, Minerals and Essential Fatty Acids on the Antisocial Behaviour of Young Adult Prisoners', *British Journal of Psychiatry*, 2002, vol. 181, pp. 22–8.

6 Mark Peplow, 'Full of Goodness', *New Scientist*, 16 November 2002, p. 39.

7 Phyllida Brown, 'A Mind under Siege', *New Scientist*, 16 June 2001, pp. 35–7.

8 Robert M. Carney and Allan S. Jaffe, 'Treatment of Depression Following Acute Myocardial Infarction', *Journal of the American Medical Association*, August 2002, vol. 288, pp. 750–1; editorial, pp. 701–9.

9 *New Scientist*, 24 August 2002, pp. 35–6.

10 Rayman, 'The Importance of Selenium to Human Health', p. 235.

11 Leo Sher, 'Effects of Selenium Status on Mood and Behaviour: Role of Thyroid Hormones', *Australian and New Zealand Journal of Psychiatry*, August 2002, vol. 36, no. 4, pp. 559.

12 'Prozac for Kids', *New Scientist*, 11 January 2003, p. 7.

13 Richard Lathe and Michael Le Page, 'Toxic Metal Clue to Autism', *New Scientist*, 21 June 2003, pp. 4–5.

14 www.medical-adviser.org/autism.php.

15 Patricia M. Rodier, 'The Early Origins of Autism', *Scientific American*, February 2000, p. 40.

16 Lathe and Le Page, 'Toxic Metal Clue to Autism'.

17 A. M. Knivsberg, K. L. Reichelt and M. Nodland, 'Reports on Dietary Intervention in Autistic Disorders', *Nutritional Neuroscience*, 2000, vol. 4, pp. 25–37.

18 Lathe and Le Page, 'Toxic Metal Clue to Autism'.

19 Philip Cohen, 'You Are What Your Mother Ate', p. 14

20 Helen Philips, 'The Key to Autism', *New Scientist*, 4 May 2002, p. 14; Simon Murch et al., 'Small Intestine Enteropathy with Epithelial IgG and Complement Deposition in Children with Regressive Autism', *Molecular Psychiatry*, 2002, vol. 7, pp. 375–82.

21 Darold A. Treffert and Gregory L. Wallace, 'Islands of Genius', *Scientific American*, June 2002, pp. 60–9.

22 Frances Adank, 'The Sleeping Killer', *The Bulletin*, 2 June 1992, pp. 46–8.

23 Tony James, 'Zinc, Selenium May Cut Infection in Aged', *Australian Doctor*, 30 April 1999.

24 Werbach, *Textbook of Nutritional Medicine*, p. 290.

NOTES 511

25 Werbach, *Textbook of Nutritional Medicine*.
26 Howard Weiner, 'When Nerves Break Down', *New Scientist*, 5 June 2004, pp. 44–7.
27 Murray and Pizzorno, *Encyclopaedia of Natural Medicine*, p 673.
28 Werbach, *Textbook of Nutritional Medicine*, p. 535.
29 Rea, *Chemical Sensitivity*, vol. 3, p. 1769.
30 Helen Philips, 'Pesticide Link to Parkinson's Grows Stronger', *New Scientist*, 6 November 2004, p. 18.
31 Neil Boyce, 'Slow Poisons', *New Scientist*, 11 November 2000, p. 16.
32 A. Menegon et al., 'Parkinson's Disease, Pesticides, and Glutathione Transferase Polymorphisms', *The Lancet*, 24 October 1998, vol. 352, pp. 1344–6.
33 J. M. Gorell, 'Multiple Risk Factors for Parkinson's Disease', *Journal of Neurological Science*, 15 February 2004, vol. 217, no. 2, pp. 169–74.
34 A. Seidler et al., 'Possible Environmental, Occupational, and Other Etiologic Factors for Parkinson's Disease: A Case-Control Study in Germany', *Neurology*, May 1996, vol. 46, pp. 1275–84.
35 Rea, *Chemical Sensitivity*, vol. 3, p. 1763.
36 Moussa Youdim and Peter Riederer, 'Understanding Parkinson's Disease', *Scientific American*, January 1997, pp. 52–9.
37 Neil Mahant, Victor Fung and John Morris, 'Assessing and Managing Parkinson's Disease', *Medicine Today*, January 2003, pp. 16–23.
38 M. F. Beal, 'Mitochondrial Dysfunction and Oxidative Damage in Alzheimer's and Parkinson's Diseases and Coenzyme Q10 as a Potential Treatment', *Journal of Bioenergetics and Biomembranes*, August 2004, vol. 36, no. 4, pp. 381–6.
39 Helen Phillips, 'All in the Mind', *New Scientist*, 21 June 2003, p. 36.
40 Christine Gorman and Alice Park, 'The New Science of Headaches', *Time*, 7 October 2002.
41 G. M. Terwindt et al., 'Familial Hemiplegic Migraine: A Clinical Comparison of Families Linked and Unlinked to Chromosome 19', *Cephalalgia*, 1996, vol. 16, pp. 153–5.
42 Phillips, 'All in the Mind'.
43 A. Piekert, C. Wilimzig and R. Kohne-Volland, 'Prophylaxis of Migraine with Oral Magnesium; Results from a Prospective, Multi-Center, Placebo-controlled and Double Blind Randomized Study', *Cephalalgia*, 1996, vol. 16, pp. 257–63.
44 Kathy Kramer, 'High-dose Riboflavin Can Reduce Migraine', *Medical Observer*, 13 August 2004.
45 Werbach, *Textbook of Nutritional Medicine*, p. 405.
46 Werbach, *Textbook of Nutritional Medicine*, p. 407.

CHAPTER 10: SOME CONCLUSIONS

1 'Animal Organs a Risk to Humans', *Sydney Morning Herald*, 13 January 2004, p. 3.
2 Laurie Garrett, *The Coming Plague*, Virago Press, 1994, p. 6.
3 David L. J. Freed, 'Do Dietary Lectins Cause Disease?',

British Medical Journal, 17 April 1999, vol. 318, pp. 1023–4.

4   Engel, *Wild Health*.

5   A. B. Becker et al., 'The Bronchodilator Effects and Pharmacokinetics of Caffeine in Asthma', *New England Journal of Medicine*, 22 March 1984, vol. 310, pp. 743–6.

6   Rob Edwards, 'The Natural Choice', *New Scientist*, 16 March 2002.

7   C. J. Blacklock et al., 'Acid May Be the Answer to Why Vegetarians Have Lower Rates of Cardiovascular Disease', *International Journal of Epidemiology*, 2001, vol. 30, p. 1219.

8   Parris M. Kidd, 'The Use of Mushroom Glucans and Proteoglycans in Cancer Treatment', *Alternative Medicine Review*, 2000, vol. 5, pp. 4–28.

9   Boik, *Natural Compounds in Cancer Therapy*, p. 284.

10 M. Jang et al., 'Cancer Chemopreventive Activity of Resveratrol, a Natural Product Derived from Grapes', *Science*, 10 January 1997, vol. 275, pp. 218–20.

11 Jeanelle Boyer and Rui Hai Liu, 'Apple Phytochemicals and Their Health Benefits', *Nutrition Journal*, 2004, vol. 3, p. 5.

12 Terry Lane with James Joseph, 'Blueberry Brainfood', *The National Interest*, ABC Radio National, 11 July 2004.

13 'Chocolate's Smell Takes the Cake', *Australian Doctor*, 31 January 1997.

14 Doug Payne, 'Chocolate Smell Boosts Immunity', *Australian Doctor*, 22 January 1999.

15 K. L. Koo et al., 'Gingerols and Related Analogues Inhibit Arachidonic Acid-induced Human Platelet Serotonin Release and Aggregation', *Thrombosis Research*, 1 September 2001, volume 103, no. 5, pp. 387–97.

16 Andrea Lord, 'Sweet Healing', *New Scientist*, 7 October 2000, p. 32.

17 M. L. Garg et al., 'Health Benefits of Macadamia Nuts in Borderline Hyperlipidaemic Male Volunteers', *Asia Pacific Journal of Clinical Nutrition*, 2001, p. S12.

18 Philip Cohen, 'Olive Oil May Reduce Breast Cancer Risk', *New Scientist*, 15 January 2005, p. 7.

19 Dr Richard Mackarness, *Not All in the Mind*, Pan Books, 1990 (also Harper Collins, 1994).

20 Colin Tudge, 'The Best Medicine', *New Scientist*, 17 November 2001, pp. 40–3.

21 Shane Houston, director, Office of Aboriginal Health, Western Australian Health Dept., 'Go Back to Bush Food, Blacks Told', *Sydney Morning Herald*, 28 April 1998.

22 Robyn Lewis, Felicity Lawrence and Andy Jones, 'Miles and Miles and Miles', Food, *Guardian*, 18 May 2003, pp. 18,19.

23 Alexander Stille, 'Slow Food', *The Nation*, 20 August 2001.

24 Charlie Pye-Smith, 'Fruits of the Forest', *New Scientist*, 19 July 2003 pp. 36–9.

25 Vic Cherikoff, *The Bushfood Handbook*, Bush Tucker Supply Australia, 1993; Vic Cherikoff, *Uniquely Australian*, Bush Tucker Supply Australia, 1992.

26 Joan Maloof, 'Take a Deep Breath', *New Scientist*, 6 August 2005, pp. 44–5.

27 Engel, *Wild Health*.

28 D. J. Abels, T. Rose and J. E. Bearman, 'Treatment of Psoriasis at a Dead

Sea Dermatology Clinic', *International Journal of Dermatology*, February
1995, vol. 34, no. 2, pp. 134–7.
29 Engel, *Wild Health*.
30 Engel, *Wild Health*, p. 132.
31 Deborah Smith, 'Curse Discovery Gets Good Oil Ready for Salvation
Jane', *Sydney Morning Herald*, 6 November 2003.
32 Melvyn R. Werbach and Michael T. Murray, *Botanical Influences on Illness*,
Third Line Press, 1994, p. 31.

APPENDIX 1

1 Nutrient Reference Values for Australia and New Zealand from the
National Health and Medical Research Council website,
September 2005, *www.nhmrc.gov.au/publications/subjects/nutrition.htm*. UK
Reference Nutrient Intake from the Food Standards Agency website
December 2008, *http://www.eatwell.gov.uk/healthydiet/nutritionessentials/
vitaminsandminerals/*
2 Archie Kalokerinos, Glen Dettman, and Ian Dettman,
Vitamin C: nature's miraculous healing missile, Frederick Todd, 1993, p. 363.
3 UL is for Mg given as a supplement, endpoint at onset of diarrhoea.

GLOSSARY

acetyl: A functional group with two carbons, one oxygen and three hydrogen
in a fixed arrangement.
acute: Of disease, one which rapidly develops to a crisis.
aetiology: The medical term for the cause of a disease.
allele: The term used for an 'allowed' variant of a gene. Some genes can exist
in one form only. Mutations causing other forms are incompatible with
life. Other genes can exist in many forms, allowing for variation within
the species. The genes for hair and skin colour are a good example of
genes which tolerate variety, and for which there are many alleles.
arrhythmia: Abnormal rhythm of the heartbeat.
biochemistry: Chemistry of biological organisms.
biodynamic farming: A form of organic farming described by Rudolph
Steiner, generally considered to be more strict (natural) than other variants.
carbohydrates: Organic compounds made of carbon, hydrogen and oxygen,
which can be broken down (burnt) to carbon dioxide and water with the
release of energy.
carcinogenic: Capable of causing cancer.
catabolic: The breakdown of bodily tissues to provide energy, as in starvation.
chronic: Of disease, one which is long continued. This doesn't refer to severity.
codon: In DNA and mRNA, a sequence of three bases that specifies a
particular amino acid to be placed in a protein. A few codons signal the

start and stop of transcriptions.

co-morbidity: Of medical conditions when they occur together.

concordance rate: Rate at which one feature or disease can be found in a compared individual or population.

congenital: Present at birth. This doesn't refer to whether the feature was inherited or not.

double blind: A term used to describe a research technique in which the true identity of treatment is concealed from both the patient and the provider.

ectopic: Tissue occurring beyond its normal confines. In pregnancy, the fertilisation of the ovum and growth of the foetus outside the uterus.

embryogenesis: The processes leading to the formation of the embryo.

endogenous: Internally generated or assembled.

enzymes: Proteins coded for by genes that catalyse (speed up) biological reactions. Usually their names end in -*ase*.

epigenetic: Inheritance that appears to operate outside genetic coding.

eugenics: Study of the means by which human populations might be improved by the application of genetics.

functional group: A chemistry term for an atom or group of atoms acting as a unit to carry out a specific function. For example, a carbon atom with three hydrogens attached is called a 'methyl group'. When the molecule to which this methyl group is attached donates the methyl group to another molecule to carry out methylation reactions, the methyl group is referred to as 'the functional group'.

genetic code: Like most codes, an 'alphabet' or set of symbols is used to denote the real message. In the genetic code, the same four amino acids are arranged in various combinations to denote the recipe the cell must use to make a particular protein. The manufacture of proteins is the goal of the genetic code. These recipes will be specific to the species bearing that code. Another layer of specificity comes in as each member of that species has a slightly different code to each other member.

genome: The collection in its entirety of genes for that species.

genotype: The particular alleles (gene variants) that an individual has for the characteristic in question.

half-life: The time taken for a reaction to be completed on half of the material.

hepatocyte: Liver cell.

heterozygous: When an individual has one copy of a particular gene allele, they are said to be heterozygous for the characteristic caused by that gene. For example, if they have one copy of the gene for haemochromatosis, they are 'carriers' for haemochromatosis, or heterozygotes. (They will not get the disease, because in this case, a double dose is required. If a gene variant is seriously deleterious, one copy may be enough to cause disease. Such a gene is regarded as dominant, and the heterozygous state is sufficient to cause trouble.) The term not only applies to disease states; it can also apply to normal gene variants such as hair colour.

homeostasis: Maintenance of the desirable status quo in a specified biological system.

homozygous: If an individual has a double dose of a particular gene variant, they are said to be homozygous for the gene. If the characteristic is unfavourable, the homozygous state can cause significant illness. Again, the term is not confined to disease-causing genes.

immunogenic: Refers to the ability of a substance to provoke an immune response from any cell or organ of the immune system.

in vivo: Taking place in a living organism.

in vitro: Taking place in an artificial environment (e.g. a test tube).

incidence: The frequency with which new cases of a given disease present during a specified period for a given population.

inherited: Passed from parents to offspring.

leucopenia: Low white-cell count.

lipids: A family of biological compounds with a non-polar structure and poor solubility in water: includes fats, waxes and steroids. 'Non-polar' is a chemical term that refers to molecules with a symmetrical charge distribution. The expression 'hydrophobic' is also used, which means 'repelling water'.

lipoprotein (a): Is formed when low-density lipoprotein (LDL) combines with a second protein, apo(a), and then links to another lipoprotein called apo B. Confusingly named, the significance of lipoprotein (a) is its apparent association with cardiovascular disease. Although there are genetic aspects involved, the Western diet seems to be the main determinant for lipoprotein (a) to become a troublemaker.

macrophages: These cells are one of the more primitive parts of the immune system. They can be found in the blood or lymph, are large single white cells, and are good at ingesting things, especially harmful bacteria, which pose a danger to the organism.

methyl: A functional group of three hydrogens attached to one carbon (CH_3).

mitochondria: These are small structures found within the cytoplasm of the cell. They are often referred to as the 'powerhouse of the cell' because they contain the enzymes for burning—by oxidation—nutrients for the production of energy.

An interesting feature of mitochondria is the fact that they have their own DNA; they do not use the DNA which is located in the nucleus of the cell. This knowledge is now being utilised to trace various aspects of our ancestry.

mutagen: A substance that is capable of causing mutations.

mutation: Any permanent change in the genetic code of the DNA.

myocardial infarction: 'Heart attack'—death of cardiac muscle due to lack of oxygen.

nulliparous: A female who has never given birth.

organelle: A generic term used to describe specialised tiny membrane-wrapped structures within the cytoplasm of the cell. A mitochondrion and an endoplasmic reticulum are examples of organelles.

organic farming: Farming without use of poisons or chemical fertilisers, while maintaining soil health by natural means; exact definitions and standards vary.

organic chemistry: Chemistry of compounds containing carbon.

phenotype: The appearance and other measurable characteristics of an organism.

pica: 'Unnatural' craving for unusual food; eating dirt or mud.

polymorphism: The presence in a population of two or more alleles of a particular gene.

presbyopia: Long-sightedness and impairment of vision caused by reduced ability to adjust the focus of the eye, typically due to advancing age.

prion: An infectious agent that contains protein but no nucleic acid.

prophylactic: Tending to prevent or protect against an unwanted event.

protein: Protein is one of the four major classes of organic molecules of which all biological systems are composed. Its nitrogen component is one of its defining characteristics, but it is the amino acids (the building blocks of protein) that determine our dietary need for protein.

On average, we need a little less than one gram of quality protein per kilogram of body weight, per day—to meet our body's demand for the amino acids required for growth and repair .

rhabdomyolysis: Catabolic breakdown of muscle.

saturation of fats: Saturated fats are those with no double bonds (that is, they are 'saturated' with hydrogen atoms). Unsaturated fats are those with at least one double bond. Polyunsaturated fats are those with at least two double bonds.

steroid: The definition of a steroid is quite broad because it includes all substances that are based on the classic four-ringed sterol structure as depicted in Chart 3.5.

The most important application of the term in animal biology relates to the hormones and to Vitamin D, which are derived from the sterol molecule, cholesterol. Plant sterols are usually poorly absorbed from the intestines of humans, but their contribution to human biology is not negligible.

Some drugs, such as digoxin from plants, have a steroid nucleus.

Synthetic steroids are widely used as drugs, both legal and illegal.

teratogenic: Producing abnormal embryos.

transcription: The synthesis of an RNA molecule complementary to a DNA strand. The information encoded in the DNA is transcribed into the RNA.

FURTHER READING

Billinghurst, Ian, *Grow Your Pups with Bones*, Ian Billinghurst, 1998

Boik, John, *Natural Compounds in Cancer Therapy*, Oregon Medical Press, 2001

Brody, Tom, *Nutritional Biochemistry*, 2nd edn, Academic Press, 1999

Bryce-Smith, Derek, and Hodgkinson, Liz, *The Zinc Solution*, Century Arrow, 1986

Buist, Robert, *Food Chemical Sensitivity*, Angus & Robertson, 1990

Campbell, Colin T., and Campbell II, Thomas M., *The China Study*, Wakefield Press, 2007

Carson, Rachel, *Silent Spring*, Penguin Books, 1965

Colburn, Theo, Myers, John Peterson, and Dumanoski, Dianne, *Our Stolen Future*, Little, Brown, 1996

Epstein, Samuel S, *The Politics of Cancer Revisited*, East Ridge Press, 1998

Goldstein, Martin, *The Nature of Animal Healing*, Alfred A Knopf, 1999

Greenfield, Susan, *The Human Brain*, Phoenix, 1997

Holford, Patrick, and Braly, James, *The H Factor*, Piatkus, 2003

Illich, Ivan, *Limits to Medicine*, Marion Boyars, 2001

Isaacs, Jennifer, *Bush Food: Aboriginal Food and Herbal Medicine*, Weldon International, 1987

Kalokerinos, Archie, *Every Second Child*, Thomas Nelson (Australia), 1974

Moynihan, Ray, and Cassels, Alan, *Selling Sickness: How Drug Companies Are Turning Us All into Patients*, Allen & Unwin, 2005

Murray, Michael, and Pizzorno, Joseph, *Encyclopaedia of Natural Medicine*, rev. 2nd edn, Little, Brown, 1998

Plant, Jane A, *Your Life in Your Hands*, Virgin Books, 2001

Ravnskov, Uffe, *The Cholesterol Myths*, New Trends Publishing Inc, 2000

Sutton, David, and Spratt, Philip, *Climate Code Red*, Scribe, 2008

Tudge, Colin, *So Shall We Reap*, Allen Lane, 2003

Vaughan, J G, and Geissler, C A, *The New Oxford Book of Food Plants*, Oxford University Press, 1997

Widmaier, Eric P, *The Stuff of Life: Profiles of The Molecules That Make Us Tick*, Times Books, 2002

INDEX